"Doctors Wanted: No Women Need Apply"

"Doctors Wanted: No Women Need Apply"

Sexual Barriers in the Medical Profession, 1835–1975

Mary Roth Walsh

New Haven and London   Yale University Press

Originally published with assistance from the foundation established in memory of Philip Hamilton McMillan of the class of 1894, Yale College.

Some portions of this book appeared in a slightly different form in *JAMWA* 31, no. 6 (June 1976), pp. 247–50.

Designed by John O. C. McCrillis
and set in Baskerville type.
Printed in the United States of America by
The Vail-Ballou Press, Inc., Binghamton, New York.

Library of Congress Cataloging in Publication Data

Walsh, Mary Roth.
  "Doctors wanted, no women need apply".
  Includes index.
   1. Women physicians—United States—History.
2. Sex discrimination against women—United States—
History. 3. Women physicians—Massachusetts—Boston—
History. I. Title [DNLM: 1. Physician, Women—
United States. 2. Health manpower—History—United
States. W21 W226d]
R692.W34   331.4'81'610973   76–44416
ISBN 0–300–02024–4 (cloth)
ISBN 0–300–02414–2 (paper)

13   12   11   10   9   8   7   6   5

Contents

Tables and Illustrations   vii

Preface   ix

Acknowledgments   xxi

Abbreviations   xxiii

1 Making the Barriers Visible   1

2 A Mistaken Ally   35

3 Feminist Showplace   76

4 Male Backlash   106

5 A Break in the Barriers   147

6 Moving Backward   178

7 Lonely Battles   207

8 What Went Wrong?   236

9 Will History Repeat Itself?   268

Research and Manuscript Collections Consulted   285

Index   289

Tables and Illustrations

TABLES

1   Designations for Boston Women Physicians, 1846–60   48
2   Decline of the Woman's Medical Colleges   180
3   Percentage of Women Medical Students Enrolled
    during Academic Year 1893–94 in U.S. Cities   183
4   Percentage of Women Physicians in U.S. Cities   185
5   Boston and the U.S.: Historical Patterns
    of Women Physicians   186
6   The Coeducational Retrenchment: 1894–1908   193
7   U.S. Medical Student Breakdown by Class, 1945–46   230
8   Enrollment Figures for Women Medical Students,
    1894–1909   240
9   Women Medical Students and Graduates, 1941–56   245
10 Women Students in U.S. Medical Schools, 1961–76   269

ILLUSTRATIONS

1   Illustration used by Samuel Gregory in lecturing   40
2   Illustration used by Samuel Gregory in lecturing   41
3   Charles Ellery Stedman notebook drawing,
    December 17, 1874   136
4   Charles Ellery Stedman notebook drawing,
    June 24, 1875   137
5   Charles Ellery Stedman notebook drawing,
    March 15, 1878   138

Preface

In the fall of 1974, a doctor in a Boston suburb introduced herself to a patient, a boy of four. The surprised child stepped back and asserted with authority: "You can't be a doctor, you're a girl." The fact that by four years of age the boy had already absorbed the idea that only men are doctors attests to the strength of sex-role stereotyping in American medicine. Only 8 percent of American physicians are women, a statistic that places the United States near the bottom in a listing of industrialized nations. Countries such as the United Kingdom and the Soviet Union have percentages ranging from 25 to 74 percent.[1]

The sharp increase in the admission of women to American medical schools in the past few years, however, appears to signify the beginning of the end of women's minority position in medicine. Many observers confidently predict that women will account for up to 50 percent of the nation's physicians by the end of the century.[2] But all of those predictions overlook

1. Marjorie Galenson, *Women and Work: An International Comparison* (Ithaca, 1973); John B. Parrish, "Women in Medicine: What Can International Comparisons Tell Us?" *WP* 26, no. 7 (July 1971), pp. 352–61; John Z. Bowers, "Wife, Mother and Physician," *JAMWA* 22 (1967), p. 761. *Hearings before the Special Subcommittee on Education of the Committee on Education and Labor, House of Representatives,* 91st Congress, 2nd Session on Section 805 of H.R. 16098, part 1 (Washington, 1970), pp. 537–39. See also, "Women Win a Place in Medicine Abroad Faster than in U.S." and "For Women, M.D. Degree Is Just Hurdle 1," in *Medical Tribune,* August 14, 1974, pp. 1 and 14; "Medical Schools Continue Demeaning Bias, Women Say," in *Medical Tribune,* August 7, 1974, p. 1; *Women in Health Careers: Chart Book for International Conference on Women in Health, June 16–18, 1975* (Washington, 1975).

2. Lawrence K. Altman, "By '85, Medical School Deans Expect 30% Women for Students and Staff," *New York Times,* April 8, 1975; Joseph A. Keyes, Marjorie P. Wilson, and Jane Becker, "The Forecast of Medical

the rise and fall in the numbers of female medical students in the late nineteenth century. They reinforce the impression that ours is the first generation to witness a breakthrough for American medical women.

This belief is so pervasive that when I began research on women physicians, I was warned repeatedly that I would find little information and that perhaps it would be more fruitful to look at that branch of medicine where sources were much more plentiful and women had a monopoly—nursing. Similarly, when I was gathering historical material in Harvard's Countway Medical Library, a medical student asked me what I expected to find in an 1886 physician's directory I was examining. When I explained that I was studying women physicians, he responded confidently: "You won't find any women doctors back then."

Even social scientists who specialize in the study of the medical profession seem oblivious to the fact that women physicians are a part of that profession and have a past of their own. In Eliot Freidson's *Profession of Medicine,* voted the prestigious Sorokin award in 1972 by the American Sociological Association, women in medicine are discussed only under the category of nursing and paramedical work. Similarly, in *Boys in White,* a participant observation study of a medical school class over several years, the four to five women in each class are entirely ignored. Although the authors note that "there is no theme . . . more interesting than the changes in the respective roles of man and woman looking after those who are sick," they warn their readers that the book is a study of how *boys become medical men.* It is almost as if the social scientists had decided to complete the work of the medical establishment and excise women physicians from the record.[3]

Education: Forecast of the Council of Deans," *J. Med. Ed.* 50 (1975), p. 321; Ronald Kotula ("Your Next Doctor May Be a Woman," *Boston Evening Globe,* November 19, 1975, pp. 1 and 18) predicts 50 percent female physicians by the end of the century.

3. Eliot Freidson, *Profession of Medicine* (New York, 1970) p. 55; Howard S. Becker, *Boys in White* (Chicago, 1961), p. 3. Judith Lorber,

It is, of course, hardly fair to condemn these writers for their ahistorical analysis when the entire question of the entry of women into the male-dominated professions has been virtually ignored by scholars.[4] Those historians who have studied American medicine, including the authors of three recent well-received books, have overlooked the role of women physicians entirely.[5] That the neglect of women doctors constitutes a serious gap in our understanding of history is now particularly being recognized by quantitative historians. Having approached the study of women's roles with a new set of questions and a rich store of demographic data, they have found them-

---

"Women and Medical Sociology: Invisible Professionals and Ubiquitous Patients," in Marcia Millman and Rosabeth Moss Kanter (eds.), *Another Voice: Feminist Perspectives on Social Life and Social Science* (New York, 1975), pp. 75–105, cites the Becker example which I quote and provides an excellent review of the sociological literature on women in medicine. Cynthia Epstein's seminal work, *Woman's Place: Options and Limits in Professional Careers* (Berkeley, 1970), remains the key sociological study on professional women. I have relied extensively on her ideas for this investigation.

4. For example, the most recent Berkshire Conference on the History of Women had 157 scholarly papers, none of which focused on women's access to the medical or legal profession—see program of Third Berkshire Conference on the History of Women, Bryn Mawr College, June 9–11, 1976. The only scholarly articles on women's access to the medical profession are: John B. Blake, "Women and Medicine in Ante-Bellum America," *Bulletin of the History of Medicine* 39 (March–April 1965), pp. 99–123; Richard H. Shryock, "Women in American Medicine," *JAMWA* 5 (1950), pp. 371–79. Other aspects of women's history are interpreted in: Lois Banner, *Women in Modern America: A Brief History* (New York, 1974); William H. Chafe, *The American Woman: Her Changing Social, Economic and Political Roles, 1920–1970* (New York, 1972); Peter Gabriel Filene, *Him, Her, Self: Sex Roles in Modern America* (New York, 1975); Mary Ryan, *Womanhood in America: From Colonial Times to the Present* (New York, 1975).

5. Martin Kaufman, *Homeopathy in America: The Rise and Fall of a Medical Heresy* (Baltimore, 1971); William G. Rothstein, *American Physicians in the Nineteenth Century: From Sects to Science* (Baltimore, 1972); Rosemary Stevens, *American Medicine and the Public Interest* (New Haven, 1971). Stevens, however, does point out on p. xiii that the study of women physicians deserves further attention.

selves seriously blocked in their attempts to offer interpretations
of the career patterns of women. As Richard Jensen, one of the
most ambitious of these new historians, has recently commented: "What we need is a systematic analysis of sex differen-
tiation and discrimination in high status occupations." [6]

In an attempt to rectify that situation, I demonstrate how
sex discrimination has prevented significant numbers of women
from entering medicine and simultaneously has seriously ob-
structed the advancement of the few women who were admitted to the profession. This discrimination became visible
when the first woman openly confronted male practitioners
and asked them to share their medical knowledge. The result
can only be described as a male backlash. I have found that the
antifeminist arguments of male physicians, so important to
the male counterattack in the nineteenth century, stemmed
from their own self-interest in maintaining control over the
profession. This survey also focuses on the ways in which
women were able to make as much progress as they did in this
hostile environment. The evidence presented here not only
explains why there are so few women doctors today but also
suggests how the lessons of the past can be used in developing
a strategy for sustaining the progress of women in medicine in
the years to come. Although there is no ineluctable connection
between the past, present, and future, the past enables us to see
the present more clearly, and our view of the future is made all
the more exact. Thus, rather than studying career patterns of
women physicians, I attempt to explain *why there are so few
careers to study.*

It might be argued that the answer lies within the general
context of sex-role stereotyping in American society. Indeed,
women are usually found in low-paying, low-status positions in
the work force. But the position of professional women in

6. Richard Jensen, "Family, Career, and Reform: Women Leaders of
the Progressive Era," in Michael Gordon (ed.), *The American Family in
Social-Historical Perspective* (New York, 1973), p. 274. See also his essay,
written with Barbara Campbell, "How to Handle a Liberated Woman,"
Historical Methods Newsletter 5, no. 3 (June 1972), pp. 109–13.

medicine is in many ways made even more discouraging by a look at the general structure of the American health care delivery system. Women are, after all, the major consumers, accounting for an estimated two-thirds of the patient visits and for 87 percent of the health workers in this country, many of whom have high technical skills compared to the majority of women in the American work force.[7] Despite this, most women have never been able to break through the barriers that prevent them from practicing medicine.

In this study I have focused on those women who identified with the standardized therapies, the so-called regulars of the nineteenth- and early twentieth-century profession. Although irregular women healers were an important part of nineteenth-century medicine, it is difficult to know how freely they chose such medical specialties since their other options were so circumscribed. Moreover, once having embarked on an irregular medical career, they were in no position to demand entrance into the regular medical schools, hospitals, and professional societies, the institutions that, for better or worse, made up the American medical establishment then as now. By concentrating on the struggles of women seeking access to regular institutions, it will be seen that the forces that have contributed to a male monopoly of medicine in the twentieth century are thrown into sharper focus.

The prominence of regular women physicians here should not, however, be interpreted as a judgment in favor of the nineteenth-century regular doctors and a condemnation of the homeopaths, hydropaths, eclectics, and other sectarian practitioners. Historians have too often dismissed the irregulars as simply quacks and dogmatists. But in an age when there were few medically valid theories available, no one had a monopoly on medical truth; it is estimated that before 1915 the average patient had little more than a fifty-fifty chance of

7. Mary Howell, "Summary Remarks," International Conference on Women in Health: Sex Roles in the Health Sector, June 18, 1975; Vincente Navarro, "Women in Health Care," *NEJM* 292, no. 8 (February 20, 1975), p. 401.

benefiting from an encounter with the average doctor.[8] Nevertheless, any explanation of why women have not been in a position to help determine the course of American medicine must focus on their efforts to gain admission to the established institutions.

Much of the nineteenth-century material presented here centers on Boston, not because it was a microcosm of the American medical world or because I wish to make it a cameo study of nineteenth-century medicine, but because the struggle of women to enter medicine in this particular city presaged that of their sisters on the national scene. Boston served as the stage for most of the crucial battles that have marked women's efforts to enter medicine. In 1835 Harriot Hunt of Boston became the first woman to practice medicine successfully. She gained her training—as did most of her male counterparts— by serving an apprenticeship. It was the same Dr. Hunt who unsuccessfully applied to Harvard Medical School in 1847 and again in 1850; thus launching a campaign that was not won until Harvard opened its doors to women medical students in 1945. More important, it was with Hunt that the battle to enter medicine was first joined. Her individual struggle was transformed into a group effort when the New England Female Medical College was founded by Samuel Gregory in 1848, the first medical college for women in the world.

Gregory's paternal attitude and the women students' struggle for greater autonomy led Dr. Marie Zakrzewska, a former faculty member of the college, to found her own hospital and clinic. This was the New England Hospital for Women and Children, a unique institution that was owned and operated by women. Not only did it provide women with the internship training denied them by other hospitals, but it also functioned as a showplace to demonstrate that women could be successful physicians. Using New England Hospital as a base, women physicians fought a sustained battle to gain access to the twin sources of medical power in nineteenth-century Boston: Harvard Medical School and the Massachusetts Medical Society.

8. Cited by Stevens, p. 135.

In both cases, the hospital women were building on the individual efforts of earlier physicians: Hunt, in the case of Harvard Medical School, and Dr. Nancy Talbot Clark of Boston, who in 1852 became the first woman in the United States to seek certification from a state medical society.

It is no surprise, in light of the fact that Boston was a hotbed of feminist medical activity, that the city became the center of the first and most sustained male physicians' counterattack. The assault was launched in the 1860s by Dr. Horatio Storer, a Boston gynecologist, who charged that women were unfit to practice medicine because of their "menstrual difficulties." This argument was picked up, expanded, and popularized by a Harvard University Overseer, Dr. Edward H. Clarke, whose book, *Sex in Education; or, a Fair Chance for the Girls,* became the bible of the foes of coeducation.

As the nineteenth century drew to a close, the efforts of Boston women to enter the medical profession became more and more closely intertwined with the campaigns of their sisters in other cities. During the period 1900 to 1920 the medical curriculum consolidated into a standardized and relatively homogenous pattern of education. At the same time a national professional structure, the American Medical Association (AMA), gained influence over both the medical colleges and the practice of medicine itself, but long before this transformation was completed, a number of women began to see that the answer to their problems in medicine required a national solution. Consequently, in the last section of this book, I gradually focus on the national scene, a necessity which reflects the steady institutionalization of American medicine.

When I first conceived of this study, I thought that I would be dealing with only a small number of women physicians in the nineteenth century. I also expected to find that the nineteenth century's institutional barriers would give way to the twentieth century's social and psychological obstacles, especially those inherent in the difficulties of combining marriage and motherhood with a career. I further assumed that these factors were the only ones responsible for the failure of women to make any significant progress in the medical profession—evidenced by the relatively static percentages of women medical students: 4.0 in 1905 and 4.9 in 1955.[9]

My first hypothesis quickly fell before the statistical material that I was able to amass. Far from being a period when women physicians were an anomaly, the late nineteenth century witnessed a remarkable increase in their numbers. In Boston, the peak was reached in 1900 when women physicians accounted for 18.2 percent of the city's doctors. In those years, the two major coeducational medical institutions, Boston University and Tufts College, were graduating the largest proportion of women in their history. In sharp contrast to today, the number of women medical students and practicing physicians was far greater in the United States than in any country in Europe. For example, at the beginning of the twentieth century there were 95 female physicians in France (chiefly in Paris), 258 in England, and more than 7,000 in the United States, at least a third of whom had medical degrees. And far from the image which historians have given us of the nineteenth-century professional woman who neither married nor had children, sizable numbers of women physicians were both wives and mothers.

What accounts for women's progress in Boston medicine between 1850 and 1900? I argue that feminism was a crucial variable. A female physician was severely stigmatized because of her sex. The woman's rights movement called for female physicians as a matter of principle, stimulated fund-raising and scholarships, and promoted feminist institutions such as the New England Hospital for Women and Children. Equally important, feminism furnished women with the moral and psychological support that enabled them to function in a culture generally hostile to feminine achievement. It is no coincidence that the recent increase in the number of women medical students parallels the rebirth of feminism. This is not to sug-

9. Carol Lopate, *Women in Medicine* (Baltimore, 1968), p. 145; Lee Powers, Harry Wiesenfelder, and Rexford C. Parmelee, "Practice Patterns of Women and Men Physicians," *J. Med. Ed.* 44 (1969), pp. 481–91; "The Case Against the Female M.D.," *Medical Economics* (December 1961).

gest that the word *feminism* was widely used in the nineteenth
century or even that it means the same thing to everyone
today. I use the term to apply broadly to the efforts of both
women and men who have consciously worked to expand
opportunities for women in any historical period.

The investigation of why women were unable to capitalize
on the nineteenth-century feminist victories led me to a new
understanding of the importance of institutions for women's
history. Leigh Marlowe has cogently argued that: "Sexism
cannot be explained on an individual basis. Its roots are cul-
tural, though it works out on a personal and interpersonal
level. Consequently, sexism has to be treated institutionally." [10]
I learned that instead of fading away, the institutional barriers
of sexism remained remarkably resilient in the twentieth century, so much so that they remained the central force in turning back the tide of women who, despite the obstacles, still
aspired to careers in medicine. As a result, there were fewer
women physicians in Boston in 1950 than there had been in
1890.

The few historians who have dealt even tangentially with
the subject of women in medicine have divided along two
lines: those who see professionalization, chiefly in the form of
extended educational requirements and licensing laws, as
responsible for the women's failure and those who argue that
women simply lost interest in becoming physicians. One problem with the former argument is that it ignores the fact that
there were few women physicians in the early nineteenth century, when neither medical school requirements nor licensing
laws played a significant role in medicine. Moreover, it does
not explain why female physicians experienced their greatest
gains in the late nineteenth century, a period of rapid professionalization, when educational requirements and licensing
laws were fast becoming the norm. Those who argue that
women voluntarily rejected medical careers hold women re-

10. "Commentary," *International Journal of Group Tensions* 4, no. 1
(March 1974), Special Issue: Who Discriminates Against Women? pp. 136–
37.

sponsible for their own lack of progress. This study challenges such a thesis. The central proposition that this book advances is that the medical establishment made a conscious effort to minimize the number of women physicians. It succeeded because despite gains in the nineteenth century women physicians were never able to exert any real power in medical institutions. As C. Wright Mills has pointed out: "No one can be truly powerful unless he [or she] has access to the command of major institutions, for it is over these institutional means of power that the truly powerful are, in the first instance, powerful." [11]

Failure to gain any degree of major institutional control meant that women physicians could do little more than protest the establishment of a quota system for medical admissions in the twentieth century, while those women who were able to squeeze through the barriers to medical school fell victim to the "old boy" network of professional patronage that shunted women into the less prestigious internship and hospital appointments. With the female portion of most medical school classes limited to 5 or 6 percent, the medical establishment could effectively accomplish its exclusionary policy while at the same time claiming that the few token women in each class proved that any qualified woman could be admitted.

The recent increase in the number of first-year female medical students, up almost 700 percent since 1959, suggests that the sexual exclusion that has characterized the twentieth century may be fast coming to an end. Consequently, one might argue that this book has little significance for today. However, the rise and fall of a previous "golden age" for women in medicine stands as a warning that hard-won victories for professional women are easily wiped away.

This book explores why women have not been given an equal chance in medicine. Almost forty years ago, Virginia Woolf received a request from a society promoting the employment of professional women. She sent the society one guinea on the condition that the society "help all properly qualified people, of whatever sex, class, or colour, gain entrance to the

11. C. Wright Mills, *The Power Elite* (New York, 1959), p. 9.

profession." Woolf's response points to the incredible complexity of women's upward mobility, encompassing as it does the manifold problems of class, ethnic, and racial barriers. I leave it to other scholars and reformers to expand our understanding of these issues and to accept her challenge to take the guinea and use it "not to burn the house down, but to make its windows blaze." [12]

12. Virginia Woolf, *Three Guineas* (New York, 1938), pp. 80 and 83.

Acknowledgments

I have accumulated many debts during the several years that this book has been in preparation. I am especially grateful to Matina Horner who first aroused my interest in women physicians in a conversation we had in 1971. Her continuing interest in my work, her advice and support, and, most important, her friendship have been of inestimable benefit.

Research funds were provided by a Boston University Summer Research Fellowship (1972) and a Ford Foundation Fellowship in Women's Studies (1973–74). David Hall's initial support of my work is deeply appreciated. Richard Bushman's encouragement and criticism played a valuable role during the first draft of this manuscript. Sam Bass Warner was a constant source of help throughout the preparation of this book. I sought and received his advice at a number of crucial stages in my research. His confidence in me and his belief in the importance of my work did much to turn a manuscript into a book. A special note of thanks is due Nathan Glazer whose interest in my work spurred me on through a critical point in the prepublication process.

Four women physicians and scientists, Ruth Kundsin, Jane Anderson, Mary Ampola, and Iolanda Low, have provided me with friendship and valuable insights into the role of women in the medical and scientific professions. A number of scholars have made useful suggestions or have shared their research with me at various stages of this work; they are G. J. Barker-Benfield, Henry K. Beecher, John Blake, James Cassedy, Lauri Crumpacker, Ann Douglas, John Duffy, Rosabeth Moss Kanter, Martin Kaufman, Joseph Kett, Sol Levine, Carol Lopate, Judith Lorber, Jean Baker Miller, James Reed, Barbara Rosencrantz, Nancy Sahli, and Ronald Takaki.

Richard Wolfe of the Harvard Countway Medical Library

was all that a researcher could ask for in a librarian. He possesses an unusual sensitivity to a scholar's needs and often provided me with material that I did not know existed. Willa Folch-Pi located Dr. Charles Stedman's drawings which appear in this book. I also thank the librarians and archivists at the Schlesinger Library of Radcliffe College and the Sophia Smith Collection at Smith College. For meticulous editing, I thank Charles Grench of the Yale University Press. Corinne Dunn typed the manuscript with care and intelligence.

Like many others, I owe much to the rebirth of the woman's movement. Although much remains to be accomplished, the movement has created an atmosphere in which achievement is possible for a larger number of women.

Finally, every author needs a facilitating personal environment. My husband, Frank Walsh, has helped me to believe in and develop my ideas and has offered valuable insights based on his own knowledge of nineteenth- and twentieth-century American history. With his enthusiasm for my work, my energy and productivity have been doubled. Moreover, the period of this research has been one of much joy and happiness.

Abbreviations

AMA	American Medical Association
AMWA	American Medical Women's Association
BCH-A	Boston City Hospital Archives
BMSJ	*Boston Medical and Surgical Journal*
BU-A	Boston University Archives
BUMS-A	Boston University Medical School Archives
CUA	Cornell University Archives
HCA	Harvard College Archives
HCL-A	Harvard Countway Library Archives
HMS-A	Harvard Medical School Archives
HWL-A	Harvard Widener Library Archives
JAMA	*Journal of the American Medical Association*
JAMWA	*Journal of the American Medical Women's Association*
J. Urol.	*Journal of Urology*
JGSB	*Journal of the Gynecological Society of Boston*
J. Med. Ed.	*Journal of Medical Education*
MWJ	*Medical Woman's Journal*
MHS	Massachusetts Historical Society
MSA	Massachusetts State Archives
NEFMC	New England Female Medical College
NEH	New England Hospital
NEJM	*New England Journal of Medicine*
NWUMS-A	Northwestern University Medical School Archives
RCE	*Records of the Commissioner of Education*
SA	Schlesinger Archives, Radcliffe College
SSC-SC	Sophia Smith Collection, Smith College
WJ	*Woman's Journal*
WMC-Pa	Woman's Medical College of Pennsylvania Archives (The Medical College of Pennsylvania)
WMJ	*Women's Medical Journal*
WP	*Woman Physician*

1

Making the Barriers Visible

In October 1835 Harriot K. Hunt and her sister Sarah, having completed their medical apprenticeship, began their practice as "female physicians" in Boston. Although Sarah Hunt practiced only a few years, Harriot, whose career spanned four decades, went on to symbolize the professional aspirations of the nineteenth-century woman's rights movement: the first woman to practice medicine successfully in this country.[1]

The fact that Elizabeth Blackwell is usually credited with being America's first woman doctor reflects a historical double standard. Blackwell's status results from having been the first woman to have received a medical degree, a standard which, if applied to her male colleagues, would have sharply reduced the number of male doctors in the country. Historians have scrutinized the credentials of female physicians more carefully than those of male physicians, many of whom practiced with no medical degree whatsoever. One writer even dismisses Blackwell because of her English birthplace and credits Dr. Lydia Folger Fowler with being "the first American woman doctor" because she was born in the United States. Hunt was by some standards an irregular practitioner, but unlike many irregulars she recognized the benefits to be derived from a

1. Elizabeth Cady Stanton, Susan B. Anthony, and Matilda Joslyn Gage, *History of Woman Suffrage* (New York, 1881; reprinted, 1969), vol. 1, *1848–1861*, p. 224. Harriot Kezia Hunt, *Glances and Glimpses; or Fifty Years Social, Including Twenty Years Professional Life* (Boston, 1856; reprinted, 1970), p. 123.

regular medical education. Her effort to obtain that education
was the opening round of the female battle to enter medicine
as full-fledged professionals.

As usual, the role of the pioneer was not an easy one. In her
autobiography, published in 1856, Hunt would remember her
first twenty years in medicine as a series of rebuffs. One medical journal greeted the announcement of the Hunt sisters'
practice with the query as to whether they "knew the difference between the sternum and the spinal column." Boston
medicine was a male club and Hunt described herself as "entirely shut out from the medical world" and denied access to
medical expertise: "a traitor, outlaw, felon—beyond their
laws." Quarantine appeared to be the most popular remedy for
the disease of feminism: "If I had had cholera, hydrophobia,
smallpox, or any malignant disease, I could not have been
more avoided than I was." [2]

Why did Harriot Hunt face so many obstacles? Was she
simply experiencing the difficulties that accompany the breaking of any barrier, be it social, religious, ethnic, or sexual?
One might even ask whether Hunt had exaggerated her difficulties, for had not women played an important role in
colonial medicine? Women had at one time dominated midwifery; in many families they provided the only available
medical care.[3] For that matter, why had not Hunt pursued
midwifery in order to satisfy her career aspirations rather than
attempting to fill the unpopular role of female physician?

The answer to these questions are important not only for
an understanding of Hunt's predicament, but also for an
insight into the larger issue: the barriers to women's achievement in medicine. The history of women in medicine during
the colonial and antebellum periods has received limited
attention, and what little has been written is impressionistic
in nature. The standard interpretation states that women
enjoyed great opportunities in medicine during the seven-

2. Hunt, pp. 127, 142, 122, 297, 154.
3. Julia Cherry Spruill, *Women's Life and Work in the Southern
Colonies* (Durham, 1938; reissued, 1969), p. 20.

teenth and eighteenth centuries—opportunities that disappeared during the first half of the following century.[4] These writers maintain that in an age of untrained or casually trained doctors, a rough equality had existed between male and female physicians.[5] Midwifery, the unquestioned province of women, is offered as further proof of their significant contribution to colonial medicine. All of this was wiped out, so the argument goes, by the rise of medical colleges, medical societies, and licensing laws. As one writer put it: "Once the public had come to accept licensing and college training as guarantees of up-to-date practice, the outsider, no matter how well qualified by years of experience, stood no chance in the competition. Women were the casualties of medical professionalization." [6]

4. See, for example, Mary Putnam Jacobi, "Women in Medicine," in Annie Nathan Meyer (ed.), *Woman's Work in America* (New York, 1891); Kate Hurd-Mead, *Medical Women of America* (New York, 1933); and Esther Pohl Lovejoy, *Women Doctors of the World* (New York, 1957). Other writers, including professional historians, who have repeated this argument include: Spruill; Gerda Lerner, "The Lady and the Mill Girl: Changes in the Status of Women in the Age of Jackson," *Midcontinent American Studies Journal* 10 (Spring 1969), pp. 5–15; Elisabeth A. Dexter, *Colonial Women of Affairs: Women in Business and Professions in America before 1776*, 2d. rev. ed. (Boston: 1931); Elisabeth A. Dexter, *Career Women of America: 1776–1840* (Francestown, N.H., 1950); Ann Douglas Wood, "The War Within a War: Women Nurses in the Union Army," *Civil War History* 18, no. 3 (September 1972), p. 197; Ann Douglas Wood, "The Fashionable Diseases: Women's Complaints and Their Treatment in Nineteenth-Century America," *Journal of Interdisciplinary History* 4, no. 1 (Summer 1973), p. 46; Jane Donegan, "Midwifery in America, 1760–1860: A Study in Medicine and Morality," Ph.D. dissertation, University of Syracuse, 1972; Ann Gordon, Mari Jo Buhle, and Nancy E. Schrom, "Women in American Society: An Historical Contribution," *Radical America* 5, no. 4 (July–August 1971), pp. 23, 58; Page Smith, *Daughters of the Promised Land: Women in American History* (Boston, 1970), pp. 55–76; Barbara Ehrenreich and Deidre English, *Witches, Midwives, and Nurses: A History of Women Healers* (Oyster Bay, N.Y., 1972 and later editions), pp. 20–28, and also a condensed version in *Monthly Review* 25 (October 1973), pp. 25–40.

5. Spruill, p. 267; Dexter (1950), p. 39; Lerner, p. 7.

6. Lerner, p. 8.

What was the condition of women in colonial medicine? Although a definitive answer must await in-depth demographic research, a survey of the existing literature (including that which argues for the significance of female practitioners) indicates that with the exception of midwifery, woman's role in colonial medicine was limited.[7] True, in an age when commercial patented medicines had yet to become widely used, a number of women did devise home remedies. Some even treated their friends or sold their mixtures in the neighborhood.[8] But the few women who have been identified as doctors seem largely to have worked in rural areas or on the frontier where physicians were absent.[9] Thus, a "doctress" who practiced in both Troy, Vermont, and Bethel, Maine, was de-

7. In addition to the Donegan dissertation cited above, there are also a number of bibliographies that bring together the existing literature on women in American medicine including: John B. Blake and Charles Roos (eds.), *Medical Reference Works 1679–1966: A Selected Bibliography* (Chicago, 1967); Genevieve Miller (ed.), *Bibliography of the History of Medicine in the United States and Canada 1930–1960* (Baltimore, 1964); National Library of Medicine, *Bibliography of the History of Medicine,* no. 1 (1964) to no. 5 (1972); Gerald N. Grob (comp.), *American Social History Before 1860* (New York, 1970), pp. 88–96, 48; Francisco Guerra, *American Medical Bibliography* (New York, 1962). Literature that deals with Boston includes: John B. Blake, *Public Health in the Town of Boston 1630–1822* (Cambridge, Mass., 1959); Edward Jacob Forster, *A Sketch of the Medical Profession from the Professional and Industrial History of Suffolk County, Massachusetts* (Boston, 1894); Walter L. Burrage, *A History of the Massachusetts Medical Society* (Boston, 1923); Samuel Abbott Green, *History of Medicine in Massachusetts: A Centennial Address Delivered Before the Massachusetts Medical Society at Cambridge, June 7, 1881* (Boston, 1881); Josiah Bartlett, *A Dissertation on the Progress of Medical Science in the Commonwealth of Massachusetts* (Boston, 1810); Henry Rouse Viets, *A Brief History of Medicine in Massachusetts* (Boston, 1930).

8. John B. Blake, "Women and Medicine in Ante-Bellum America," *Bulletin of the History of Medicine* 39 (March–April 1965), p. 107; James Harvey Young, *The Toadstool Millionaires: A Social History of Patent Medicines in America Before Federal Regulation* (Princeton, 1961).

9. Spruill, pp. 267–69; Dexter (1931), pp. 58–59.

scribed as feeling deeply chagrined when the first male physician settled in Bethel in 1800.[10]

It is certain that in Boston female physicians were not abundant during the colonial period. The sole study of medical practitioners in the town and surrounding environs of the seventeenth century reveals that only two of the seventy-six physicians were female. Both of these are usually described as midwives in other accounts, and both were later denounced as witches: Jane Hawkins, who was prohibited from further medical practice and expelled from Boston in 1641, and Margaret Jones, who was executed in 1648. From that point on, no female physicians are listed in histories of Boston until Harriot Hunt in 1835.[11]

It was not as physicians but as midwives that women are alleged to have experienced their greatest success during the colonial years. The recent renewal of interest in midwifery has led to a positive reevaluation of the role of midwifery in medicine. The traditional interpretation, which viewed the dissolution of the midwives as a significant step in the advancement of science, has come under considerable criticism. The fact that today a number of women are seeking out the services of midwives for their individual care and emotional support suggests that something of value was lost in the transition to a more "scientific" approach to childbirth.[12]

However, one must remember that no matter how valuable its services, midwifery gradually came to be considered a subordinate branch of medicine. Whereas physicians were ex-

10. Barnes Riznik, "Medicine in New England 1790–1840" (unpublished manuscript), 1965, pp. 2–3, Old Sturbridge Village, Mass.

11. Forster, pp. 232–85.

12. The traditional interpretation is found in Irving S. Cutter and Henry Viets, *A Short History of Midwifery* (Philadelphia, 1964), p. 44. In this version also, women are completedly obliterated from the historical chronicle. For a summary of the new views on this topic see Ann H. Sablosky, "The Power of the Forceps: A Comparative Analysis of the Midwife—Historically and Today," *Women and Health* 1 (January–February 1976), pp. 10–13.

pected to have had some training (usually in the form of an apprenticeship), it was assumed that a woman who had borne children and who had witnessed other women in childbirth could deliver a baby. In fact, a physician who did an extensive survey of the way in which women found themselves practicing midwifery, concluded that a majority of the women were first *catched* as they expressed it, with a woman in labor. Having managed to receive the child successfully, they were considered competent and thus, almost by accident, they became "immediately established in the profession." [13]

But advances in medicine in the eighteenth century, which amounted to an obstetrical revolution, challenged and eventually overturned female domination of midwifery. Women found it increasingly difficult to compete against physicians who possessed scientific knowledge of anatomy and parturition and who through their forceps and other instruments could shorten ordinary labor as well as relieve patients in difficult births.

In the long run, the only hope of midwives was to gain access to the information necessary to upgrade their skills, yet the few women who received training through some form of an apprenticeship remained the exception. The only formal course of study open to women during the entire colonial period was conducted by Dr. William Shippen of Philadelphia. Shippen, who had studied under the leading British obstetrician, Colin Mackensie, offered the course in 1765 to both men and women with the latter "taught privately and assisted at any of their private labors when necessary." Unfortunately, Shippen discontinued his special courses after the Revolution and henceforth lectured only to male students at the Philadelphia medical school.[14]

At first, male midwives with their iron instruments were denounced as unsafe to mother and child. Others decried the invasion of the female bedchamber as an affront to womanly

---

13. Donegan, pp. 12, 42–43; Valentine Seaman, *The Midwives' Monitor, and Mothers Mirror* . . . (New York, 1800), p. viii.

14. Donegan, p. 46.

modesty. At one point, Dr. William Smellie, an eighteenth-century British pioneer in obstetrics, went so far as to suggest that male midwives wear a feminine costume, a loose sort of nightgown, to ease the fears of their patients.[15] During the last half of the eighteenth century, male midwives gained increasing importance in urban centers such as Boston. Cries of immodesty were no match for the charges of incompetency hurled at the midwives by physicians. Dr. Shippen echoed the sentiments of his colleagues when he described the "number of women . . . in difficult labors, most of which was made so by the unskillful old women about them, the poor women having suffered extremely, and their innocent little ones being entirely destroyed, whose lives might have been easily saved by proper management." Later in the century, Boston patients found it "fashionable" to pay a doctor one guinea for a delivery because this meant that one's family had arrived on the social scene. Thus, Mary Bass, in 1772, felt compelled to move her midwife practice to Salem because "men midwives are fairly numerous in Boston." [16]

Although midwives would continue to service most of the poor and working classes throughout the nineteenth century, they had clearly lost what status they had enjoyed at the beginning of the colonial period.[17] Midwives were now marked

15. Ibid., p. 47.
16. Ibid., p. 45; *Pennsylvania Gazette,* January 31, 1765; Álice Morse Earle (ed.), *Diary of Anna Green Winslow, a Boston School Girl of 1771* (Detroit, 1970 reprint), p. 17 and n. 24; *Essex Gazette* (Salem), July 14, 1772.
17. Spruill, pp. 272–73. Sources on Boston which cite various types of evidence that midwives practiced largely among the poor and working classes include the Boston Medical Association fee tables for obstetrical cases and the following: Frances E. Kobrin, "The American Midwife Controversy: A Crisis of Professionalization," *Bulletin of the History of Medicine* 40 (July–August 1966), pp. 350–63; Thomas Darlington, "The Present Status of the Midwife," *American Journal of Obstetrics and Gynecology* 63 (1911), p. 870; J. L. Huntington, "The Midwife in Massachusetts: Her Anomalous Position," *BMSJ* 168 (1913), p. 419; Dexter (1950), p. 41; [Walter Channing], *Remarks on the Employment of Females as Practitioners in Midwifery, by a Physician* (Boston, 1820), p. 7; Hurd-Mead, p. 17; Ednah D. Cheney, "The Women of Boston," *Memorial*

as amateurs, unorganized, with no scientific equipment or knowledge. As late as 1835 midwives were charging only a dollar to deliver a baby. Male midwives, with access to formal training and often organized in medical societies, were clearly the professionals, which enabled them to charge from twelve to twenty dollars that year for the same service.[18]

Dr. Walter Channing, professor of obstetrics at Harvard Medical School, summed up the case against female midwifery in 1820. The thrust of his argument was that no one could be considered fully competent to practice obstetrics unless that person had been thoroughly trained in medicine. Channing then went on to close the door to any woman who might aspire to undertake that necessary training:

> It is obvious that we cannot instruct women as we do men in the science of medicine; we cannot carry them into the dissecting room and the hospital; many of our more delicate feelings, much of our refined sensibility must be subdued, before we can submit to the sort of discipline required in the study of medicine; in females they must be destroyed.[19]

History of Boston, vol. 4 (Boston, 1880), p. 347; letter signed by "C" in the Boston Daily Courier, April 18, 1856.

18. Samuel Thomson, New Guide to Health: or, Botanic Family Physician, Containing a Complete System of Practice, on a Plan Entirely New; with a Description of the Vegetables Made Use of, and Directions for Preparing and Administering Them, to Cure Disease, to Which is Prefixed, a Narrative of the Life and Medical Discoveries of the Author, Third Edition (Boston, 1832), pp. 131–34; George Rosen, Fees and Fee Bills (Baltimore, 1946), pp. 7–10; Henry B. Shafer, The American Medical Profession, 1783–1850 (New York, 1936), pp. 154–60, contains a detailed discussion of medical fees. William G. Rothstein, American Physicians in the Nineteenth Century: From Sects to Science (Baltimore, 1972), notes on p. 139: "[Physicians] had apparently driven out of practice many midwives and other part-time practitioners who were not able to compete with the more prestigious M.D.'s. This enabled physicians to raise their prices well beyond what the part-time practitioners charged." The idea that midwives were "part-time" is not supported by any evidence either in the primary or secondary sources since an in-depth demographic study of midwives in America has not yet been done.

19. [Channing], p. 7.

Channing's argument hinges on his assumption that the female personality is entirely distinct from that of the male; his rhetoric reflects what other writers of the nineteenth century referred to as "the cult of true womanhood." For example, in the same essay Channing denied that women were the intellectual inferiors of men. Rather, he noted, "moral qualities . . . render them in their appropriate sphere, the pride, the ornament, and the blessing of mankind." [20] Physicians were, of course, no different from their counterparts in other professions in employing the argument that women must remain masters of their appropriate and separate sphere—the home.

However, unlike other professionals, physicians seized upon the separate spheres argument to prevent an existing subgroup—the midwives—from making inroads into the profession. As Channing put it: "It was one of the first and happiest fruits of improved medical education in America, that . . . [women] were excluded from practice; and it was only by the united and persevering exertions of some of the most distinguished individuals our profession has been able to boast, that this was effected." [21]

20. Ibid., p. 3. In 1820, when this pamphlet was published, Channing's views appeared in the context of a general denial by society that women could practice medicine as men did. Channing claimed female midwives were not even needed. Since an attempt by two Boston physicians had been made only two years earlier to educate midwives and the opposition of male practitioners had brought the effort to a halt, it is likely that Channing's writing was actually an ideological attack on the advances of females into medicine. For a brief allusion to the midwifery episode, see Edward Warren, *The Life of John Collins Warren* (Boston, 1860), vol. 1, pp. 219–20, and vol. 2, pp. 275–76; Elizabeth Bass, "More than One Hundred Years Ago," *JAMWA* 7 (1952), p. 381. For analysis of the whole question of midwifery in America in the context of intellectual-cultural history, see J. G. Barker-Benfield, *The Horrors of the Half Known Life* (New York, 1976), especially part 2 where he discusses the absence of midwives in America and the campaign rhetoric against midwives. For an essay outlining the ideological attack of American physicians against women's demands for more personal and social power see Carroll Smith-Rosenberg and Charles Rosenberg, "The Female Animal: Medical and Biological Views of Woman and Her Role in Nineteenth-Century America," *Journal of American History* 60, no. 2 (September 1973), pp. 332–56.
21. [Channing], p. 21.

What of the argument that female physicians were sacrificed on the altar of professionalization? [22] A survey of the early development of medical professionalization in America raises serious doubts as to the adequacy of this thesis. It is true that all of the medical societies formed in colonial Massachusetts, beginning with the short-lived society established in Boston in 1735, were composed only of men. But the "gentlemen" who took part in these early medical societies were not forced to formally exclude women, for there were no women physicians to apply. Although some have claimed that the effort of the societies to license practitioners was the culminating blow to midwives, there is little evidence to indicate that midwives had anything approaching professional status before these events took place.

Women in colonial society derived their social position from their kinship attachments to men: a father or a husband. Current research gives no support to the notion that midwives acted as if their social status was equal to that of a physician. Certainly society did not treat them as such. Thus, the women, whose social role forced them to put domestic considerations first, stayed at home while the men—in this case physicians— gathered together in their medical societies "to support the characters of its members and discountenance quacks and pretenders in physick." [23]

22. The term "professionalization" has been used here in the sense defined by both Rothstein, p. 8, and Eliot Freidson, *Profession of Medicine* (New York, 1970), pp. 71–84.

23. This assumption is based, of course, on the writings of the historians who have provided accounts of these early years of the medical profession. See, for example, Burrage, p. 6; Green, passim. It is now generally recognized that male social scientists (and some female ones as well) have been blinded by the male-dominated culture and have not "seen" females even where they appeared. Lerner notes that the colonial woman's "occupations were, by and large, merely auxiliary, designed to contribute to family income, enhance their husbands' business or continue it in the case of widowhood. . . . The underlying assumption of colonial society was that women ought to occupy an inferior and subordinate position" (p. 7). Lerner then goes on to conclude that "the occasional 'doctoress' was fully accepted and frequently well rewarded" (p. 8). In Boston the fact that

Those writers who have viewed licensing as the male physicians' ultimate weapon evidence little understanding of the practice. First, licensing was not legislated in Massachusetts until 1781, when doctresses were no longer part of the Boston medical scene. In that year the Massachusetts legislature granted licensing power to the newly formed Massachusetts Medical Society, but the function of licensing before the Civil War has not been clearly understood. In Massachusetts as in many other states, licenses were not required in order to practice. The licensed practitioner received few legal advantages. In 1818 he was granted sole power to sue for fees, but this privilege was terminated in 1835 when all physicians gained this right. Then, in 1859, Massachusetts repealed all licensing legislation, creating a fluid situation that lasted until 1895.[24]

"doctresses" were not called upon in their capacity as health experts in time of medical testimonies would seem to refute the assertion that they had full acceptance—see Green, passim. Sociologists and social historians are just beginning to examine the whole question of social stratification for women—see Joan Acker, "Women and Social Stratification: A Case of Intellectual Sexism," *American Journal of Sociology* 78, no. 4 (January 1973), pp. 936–45. Historical studies on social stratification have usually ignored women; for example, see James A. Henretta, "Economic Development and Social Structure in Colonial Boston," *William and Mary Quarterly* 22 (January 1965), pp. 75–92. An attempt which includes women but finds them at the bottom of the social ladder, especially if they were widowed, is Allan Kulikoff, "The Progress of Inequality in Revolutionary Boston," *William and Mary Quarterly* 28 (July 1971), pp. 375–412.

24. I have relied extensively on the best of the histories of medical licensing: Joseph F. Kett, *The Formation of the American Medical Profession: The Role of Institutions, 1780–1860* (New Haven, 1968). See also Richard H. Shryock, *Medical Licensing in America, 1650–1965* (Baltimore, 1967), for the later period; Rothstein has a chart of the licensing legislation on pp. 332–39; Reginald H. Fitz, "The Rise and Fall of the Licensed Physician in Massachusetts, 1781–1860," *Transactions of the Association of American Physicians* 9 (1894); Reginald Fitz, "The Legislative Control of Medical Practice," *Medical Communications of the Massachusetts Medical Society* (1894), p. 30. *Laws and Resolves of Massachusetts. Acts of 1894,* chap. 458, pp. 371–73 (approved June 7, 1894, to take effect January 1, 1895). I could find no example of a scholar writing on women's history who viewed the licensing as only honorific. Most works having references

The purpose of virtually all medical licensing during the first half of the nineteenth century was honorific—to provide physicians with a means of enhancing their position in the community.[25] During this period, physicians were educated as apprentices or received their training in medical colleges of varying quality. When the graduated apprentice or medical students sought to open their own practice, evidence of professional training was either a letter of commendation from the tutor or the medical degree, which was meaningful only if the client knew the tutor or recognized the college. A license, on the other hand, represented the collective judgement of a board of recognized physicians, and therefore gave the new doctor a certified stamp of approval.[26]

Although the societies could not limit the number of practitioners, they did develop codes which would elevate the status of their members in the community while at the same time reserving for them a substantial part of the medical market. Thus, although the codes of the various societies varied a good deal, all sought to regulate consultations. The most important parts of the code provisions were those which limited consultations to members of the same society and specified who was and was not an acceptable consultant.[27] Clearly, licensing laws were important, but they could not in themselves bar women from practicing.

The early history of formal medical education also raises doubts as to the adequacy of the argument that professionalization blocked any opportunity for women in medicine. Since the majority of early physicians had obtained their training

---

to women doctors of the early nineteenth century denigrate their achievements as "unlicensed" or "illegal," for example, Mary Elizabeth Massey, *Bonnet Brigades: American Women and the Civil War* (New York, 1966), p. 9. The distortions of historians have in turn been perpetuated by contemporary sociologists. See Lillian Kaufman Cartwright, "Conscious Factors Entering into Decisions of Women to Study Medicine," *Journal of Social Issues* 28, no. 2 (1972), p. 201.

25. Rothstein, p. 79.
26. Ibid., p. 79.
27. Ibid., p. 83.

through an apprenticeship and in turn trained others, it is easy to understand why they viewed the new medical colleges with trepidation. The difficulties surrounding the establishment of Harvard Medical College reflected this conflict. In 1788, six years after the school opened, a single medical faculty member sent his only two students to be examined by the licensing committee of the Massachusetts Medical Society. The committee, fearing that the licensing of students would encourage Harvard to expand its medical program and grant degrees, rejected them, even though a physician who had observed the interview claimed that the two students were better qualified than any of the previous candidates accepted by the board.

The strategy backfired as Harvard immediately began a course of lectures, intending to award degrees to the students at the next commencement. The society urged the Harvard administration to halt the courses, but to no avail. At the end of the academic term, a public examination was held to demonstrate the competence of the students, and the society members realized that they would soon be confronted with a usurpation of their power as a certifying body. Consequently, during the week preceding commencement ceremonies, the society quietly held a reexamination of the two men, at which time "a few questions were asked, and they were passed." The issue had been resolved in favor of the school, whose degrees were thereafter considered equivalent to the society's licenses, which were then automatically given to all students of Harvard Medical College upon graduation.[28]

The development of medical schools and their success in

28. Viets, *A Brief History of Medicine in Massachusetts*, pp. 108–09. Bartlett, *A Dissertation on the Progress of Medical Sciences in the Commonwealth of Massachusetts* (Boston, 1810), p. 25; Ephraim Eliot, "Account of the Physicians of Boston," *Proceedings of the Massachusetts Historical Society* (November 1863), pp. 183–84; Peter D. Gibbons, "The Berkshire Medical Institution," *Bulletin of the History of Medicine* 38 (1964), p. 54. The Berkshire Medical Institution (founded 1823) did not obtain Harvard's privilege of automatic membership in the Massachusetts Medical Society until legislation was passed in 1837.

obtaining licenses for their graduates led to a rapid supplanting of the old apprenticeship system. In 1770 there were only two medical schools in the colonies, in 1800 there were four in the United States, and by 1850 there were forty-two. The number of graduates multiplied even more rapidly. During the period of 1840–49 alone, there were 11,828 medical degrees awarded in the United States.[29]

In summary, there are a number of problems connected with the argument that professionalization led to the expulsion of women from medicine. One must ask why the professionalizing process served to bar only females and not the male physicians in Massachusetts. One careful survey of New England physicians between 1790 and 1840 has located 896 practitioners, all of whom were male and many of whom had not gone to medical school or been accepted by a medical society.[30] In an intensive examination of Worcester County, Massachusetts, for the same period, it was found that only 27 percent of the physicians had graduated from medical colleges and less than half (42 percent) belonged to a medical society.[31]

At this point, it is important to raise the question: did professionalization offer women their first real opportunity in medicine? Were not those women who might have been interested in medicine in the preprofessional period subject to numerous unwritten laws and assumptions which served to hold them in close check? Professionalization, with its carefully delineated medical prerequisites, spelled out in detail the requirements for being a doctor. If one must acquire a medical degree, interested women could apply to medical colleges and if rebuffed could then go on to establish their own. If one must gain entrance into a medical society or obtain a license,

29. John S. Billings, "Literature and Institutions," in Edward H. Clarke et al., *A Century of American Medicine* (Philadelphia, 1876), p. 359.

30. Riznik, "Medicine in New England 1790–1840" (unpublished). For comparative statistics on New York, see Edward Atwater, "The Medical Profession in a New Society—Rochester, New York, 1811–1860," *Bulletin of the History of Medicine* 47 (May–June 1974), pp. 221–35.

31. Riznik, "Medicine in New England 1790–1840" (unpublished), p. 117. See also Barnes Riznik, *Medicine in New England 1790–1840* (Meriden, Conn., 1965), p. 23.

women could rise to meet the requirements and, if rejected, could go on to raise the cry of injustice to gain support. In short, it is possible to argue that it is easier to overcome a series of known obstacles than tilt at a series of shadowy spectres.

This is not to contend that medical schools, societies, and licensing laws were unimportant. Medical schools and societies, especially, presented major hurdles, some of which have remained intact to this very day. Nevertheless, women practitioners needed the advantages of professionalization more than men. Female physicians, already suspect because of their sex, required corroboration of their expertise to meet a disbelieving public. Although the line between irregular and regular medicine for most of the nineteenth century was a spurious one with neither side holding a monopoly on scientific truth, in retrospect, the future clearly lay with the regulars. And, as the regulars gradually came to dominate the mainstream of medicine, those women who hoped to successfully navigate these medical waters had to secure the quality education offered by leading medical colleges such as Harvard. Similarly, later in the nineteenth century women physicians would exert every effort to gain entrance to the Massachusetts Medical Society. In the absence of licensing laws, society membership was the women's only other means of separating themselves from the "charlatans and quacks."

The problem, of course, with professionalization is that it did not develop in an ideological vacuum. Rather, its evolution was shaped by the sexual biases within American society. The colonies were established on a strong patriarchal foundation, and female opportunities outside the home and family have been circumscribed ever since. A number of historians have tended to exaggerate the relative freedom granted to colonial women; one has even talked of a "feminist bias," which he views as stemming from the shortage of women during frontier conditions.[32] No doubt their short supply increased

32. See, for example, Dexter (1931) and (1950), and, most recently, Roger Thompson, *Women in Stuart England and America: A Comparative Study* (Boston, 1974). The "feminist bias" statement is from Carl N. Degler,

their value, but one must distinguish between value and equality. To take what perhaps is an extreme example, in seventeenth-century Virginia wives were exchanged for 150 pounds of good tobacco,[33] making women a valuable commodity, but a commodity nevertheless, and quite clearly, subject to the husbands who purchased them.

American women may have worked side by side with their husbands, but there was no doubt who was master. Women were designated as inferior persons in law, in education, in theology, in church affairs, and in political and property rights. Recent research has even challenged the long-held view that colonial widows, through their wealth and control over family businesses were able to gain a good deal of independence. A study of sixty-five marriages that took place between 1701 and 1710 in Winthrop, Massachusetts, demonstrates that widowhood was a social problem and that the widows, more often than not, remained "relatively poor, dependent, and lacking in other options." Just how restricted their options were is indicated in another study which found that women's literacy declined relative to that of men during the colonial period. From Anne Hutchinson on the eve of the colonial period to Abigail Adams at its end, a woman's role was carefully circumscribed. Thus Anne Hutchinson was told by the Calvinist Church fathers in Massachusetts Bay: "[Y]ou have stept out of your place, *you have rather bine a Husband than a Wife and a preacher than a Hearer; and a Magistrate than a Subject.*" [34] Clearly, men were to lead and women to follow.

"Revolution Without Ideology: The Changing Place of Women in America," in Robert Jay Lifton (ed.), *The Woman in America* (Boston, 1965), p. 193. Degler does not repeat this thesis in his more recent essay, "Is There a History of Women?" (Oxford, 1975).

33. Spruill, p. 9.

34. Alexander Keyssar, "Widowhood in Eighteenth-Century Massachusetts: A Problem in the History of the Family," *Perspectives in American History* 8 (1974), pp. 83–119; Kenneth A. Lockridge, *Literacy in Colonial New England: An Enquiry into the Social Context of Literacy in the Early Modern West* (New York, 1974); James Kendall Hosmer (ed.), *Winthrop's Journal: "History of New England," 1630–1649, Original Narratives of*

One and a half centuries later, patriarchy was still an issue as in one of Abigail Adams's letters to her husband during the Revolution reminding him: "Remember the Ladies, and be more generous and favourable to them than your ancestors." She even threatened that "we are determined to foment a Rebelion, and will not hold ourselves bound by any Laws in which we have no voice, or Representation." John Adams's answer was in harmony with what would become the classic male response to such feminist protest: that men held only nominal power. "We are obliged to go fair, and softly, and, in Practice you know We are the subjects. We have only the Name of Masters." Adams's claim that men were only nominally masters in the Revolutionary era has come under close scrutiny by recent scholars in women's history. The objective evidence that exists—court records, demographic information, literacy rates, records of occupational freedom for women, legal statutes—all support the argument that the status of women actually deteriorated during this period.[35]

Nor did the colonial-frontier situation that Frederick Jackson Turner saw as a force for freedom do much for American women. As one writer observed, the frontier is "all right for

Early American History (New York, 1908), vol. 1, p. 234; "The Examination of Mrs. Anne Hutchinson at the Court of Newtown," in David D. Hall (ed.), _The Antinomian Controversy, 1636–1638: A Documentary History_ (Middletown, Conn., 1968), p. 263. For an excellent historical overview of Hutchinson, see Lyle Koehler, "The Case of the American Jezebels: Anne Hutchinson and Female Agitation during the Years of Antinomian Turmoil, 1636–1640," _William and Mary Quarterly_ 31 (January 1974), pp. 55–78. For a psychohistorical analysis of Governor Winthrop, see Ben Barker-Benfield, "Anne Hutchinson and the Puritan Attitude Toward Women," _Feminist Studies_ 1, no. 2 (Fall 1972), pp. 65–95.

35. L. W. Butterfield (ed.), _Adams Family Correspondence_, vol. 1 (Cambridge, Mass., 1963), pp. 369–70, 381–83. For a thorough synthesis of the secondary literature on women in the Revolutionary period see Joan Hoff Wilson, "The Illusion of Change: Women and the Revolution," in Alfred F. Young (ed.), _The American Revolution_ (Dekalb, Ill., 1976). Wilson is currently doing a systematic study of the legal status of women beginning with the Revolutionary era (personal communication, March 1976).

men and dogs, but it's hell on women and horses." [36] In fact, opportunity for American women began pretty much where the frontier left off. It was the twin forces of industrialization and urbanization that stimulated at least some women to aspire to equality of opportunity. Although industrialization condemned many women to factory work, while creating a domestic prison for their middle-class sisters, it did liberate some women.

This formation of a leisured female middle class touched off a variety of responses. Many fell victim to "the cult of true womanhood," which paralleled the rise of a new class. In a rapidly changing society, one thing would remain constant— "a true woman was a true woman." The qualities of true womanhood by which a woman judged herself and was judged by others were the four cardinal virtues: piety, purity, submissiveness, and domesticity. Submission consisted of behavior which was "timid, doubtful, and clingingly dependent; a perpetual childhood." [37] As long as women occupied themselves with domestic affairs, submission was relatively easy.

True womanhood held out obvious rewards for those who subscribed to it. Men would hold sway in the world of politics and business, while women, from the vantage point of their position on the pedestal, would rule the domestic scene. But true womanhood could be interpreted (and some women did so) in a different light. If women possessed so many virtues, why could they not use them to reform the larger society? Certainly, the volume of the editorials, articles, poetry, and books glorifying domesticity attests to the fear of the writers that some women were straying into the public arena.

36. David Potter, "American Women and the American Character," in Michael McGiffert (ed.), *The Character of Americans: A Book of Readings,* revised edition (Homewood, Ill., 1970), p. 321. The seminal impact of Potter's ideas has recently been reexamined by Betty Chmaij and Patricia Kane in *Image, Myth and Beyond: American Women and American Studies,* vol. 2 (Pittsburgh, 1972), pp. 56–65, 203–18.

37. Barbara Welter, "The Cult of True Womanhood: 1820–1860," in Jane Friedman and William G. Shade (eds.), *Our American Sisters* (Boston, 1973), p. 104.

These women channeled their anger and sense of superior righteousness into the reform movements of the first half of the nineteenth century. Thus, one of the main themes of the New York Female Reform Society was an attack on the sexual double standard. Its weekly, *The Advocate of Moral Reform,* asked: "Why should a female be trodden under foot . . . while common consent allows the male to habituate himself to this vice, and treats him as not guilty." It seems that much of the reform society's crusade against the males' lack of sexual accountability "served as a screen for a more general—and less socially acceptable—resentment of masculine social preeminence." Thus an editorial in the *Advocate* in 1838 declared: "A portion of the inhabitants of this favored land are groaning under a despotism, which seems to be modeled precisely after that of the Autocrat of Russia." [38]

Other women turned their energies to the abolitionist movement, and by 1837 made up more than half of the membership of the various antislavery societies.[39] Abolitionism, with its petitions, meetings, and debates, gave a number of women their first taste of politics. For some women, like Lucretia Mott and Elizabeth Cady Stanton, the abolitionist crusade was marred by its sexual discrimination. Consequently, in 1848 in Seneca Falls, New York, Mott, Stanton, and others raised the banner of the woman's rights movement.

Many of the declarations adopted at Seneca Falls (such as those dealing with female subordination and the double standard) bore a marked similarity to the complaints raised by the

38. Carroll Smith-Rosenberg, "Beauty, the Beast and the Militant Woman: A Case Study in Sex Roles and Social Stress in Jacksonian America," *American Quarterly* 23 (October 1971), p. 572. See also Carroll Smith-Rosenberg, "The Hysterical Woman: Sex Roles and Role Conflict in 19th Century America," *Social Research* 39, no. 4 (Winter 1972), pp. 652–78. In this latter essay the author argues that women found in hysteria a socially acceptable outlet for their role frustrations and that a large number of women who could not vent their anger used hysteria or exaggerated femininity.

39. Smith, p. 111. See also Aileen S. Kraditor, *Means and Ends in American Abolitionism* (New York, 1969), especially chapter 3.

New York Female Moral Reform Society. But whereas the
Reform Society limited itself to the moral and social sphere,
the Seneca Falls participants went on to charge men with
monopolizng "nearly all the profitable employments. . . .
He closes against her all the avenues to wealth and distinction. . . . As a teacher of theology, medicine, or law, she is
not known." [40]

Although Harriot Hunt had not been an active participant
in any of the woman's organizations during this period, her
decision to enter medicine must be viewed as part of a larger
movement to break existing sex barriers. In March 1834, before the founding of the New York Female Reform Society,
she had embarked on a medical apprenticeship, and in 1847
her decision to apply to Harvard Medical College preceded
the Seneca Falls convention by one year. Hunt's role as the
first successful female physician in the United States offers us
valuable insights into the obstacles to female medical achievement which existed in the antebellum period.

There was little in Hunt's earlier years to distinguish her
from other middle-class Boston girls. Her father was a ship
joiner and a qualified navigator whose investments in ship-
ping provided a comfortable childhood for both Harriot, born
in 1805, and her sister Sarah, born three years later. In 1810
Harriot Hunt entered a private school which she attended for
the next eleven years. Although Hunt later recalled that "even
at that early period, I always felt I was to do something different," she spent the six years after leaving school at home, a
not unusual decision in an era when the best preparation for
a young woman's future was the perfection of her domestic
skills.[41]

Her father's declining health, however, coupled with busi-

40. Stanton et al., p. 71.
41. Hunt, p. 21. See also Harvey J. Graff, "Patterns of Dependency and
Child Development in the Mid-Nineteenth Century City: A Sample from
Boston, 1860," *History of Education Quarterly* (Summer 1973), pp. 129–43.
Graff's account, although referring to the years after Hunt attended school,
provides an overview of girlhood patterns. For a useful summary of the
Boston opposition to public school education for women, see Mary F. East-

ness reverses led Hunt to open a school in her house in 1827 to support her family. Her father's death later that year transformed Hunt into the sole support of her family, and her initial enthusiasm for the work quickly gave way to dejection.[42] Schoolteaching was not a particularly profitable career, a situation which Hunt considered even more intolerable because female teachers received lower wages than their male counterparts.[43]

Hunt came to loathe a system in which "miserable remuneration" undermined a woman's self-respect. Furthermore, a woman's low wages and status put her at the mercy of any suitor,

> and the poor teacher . . . her services underrated and underpaid,—her self respect gone—her toil thankless— her life disgusting—herself an underling—pinched, degraded, condemned, accused, weary, and miserable,— escapes from her daily heart-break into private civility and public respect, by marrying an imbecile.[44]

Hunt's frustration with teaching was no doubt heightened by the realization that she had no choice in terms of career

---

man, "The Education of Women in the Eastern States," in Annie Nathan Meyer (ed.), *Woman's Work in America* (New York, 1891), pp. 20–23.

42. Hunt, pp. 54–55.

43. Ibid. Published salary schedules in the *Boston Directory, 1849* indicate that the top salary for women was $900 yearly while men earned up to $2,400. Men were always in the highest paid positions while women were always in the lowest paid positions. Men had titles such as "masters"; women were either "assistants' or "ushers." Even in the girls' schools a man was always listed as "master." Thus women were barred from leadership even among women, and young girls had role models who were always subordinates to men. James Wallace, "The Feminization of Teaching: A Case Study: Massachusetts, 1840–1860," seminar paper for Harvard Graduate School of Education, October, 1972, questions the assumption that the economic factor was the most important one in the shift in the nineteenth-century Massachusetts teaching force to 81.5 percent female by 1861. His convenient tables and statistics on salary schedules show that women earned, on the average, one-third of the male salary.

44. Hunt, pp. 103–104.

alternatives. Not surprisingly, she experienced moments of deep depression which forced her to take periodic rests in the country.[45] But it was the prolonged illness of her sister Sarah (who had followed her into teaching) which finally triggered Harriot's decision to enter medicine. She later recalled how shocked she had been at the realization that male physicians were helpless in the face of feminine diseases. Doctors interspersed recommendations of rest for her sister with applications of leeches, blisters, mercurials, and prussic acid. All of this, despite the fact that the only specific diagnosis that emerged after forty-one weeks of illness and 106 house calls, was that Sarah was suffering from a "disease of the heart." [46]

In desperation, the Hunt sisters turned to a husband and wife medical team, Dr. and Mrs. Richard D. Mott, who had arrived in Boston in 1833. The Motts, who administered "Systematic Vegetable Medicines" and "Patent Champoo and Medicated Baths," were regarded as quacks by the regular physicians. Actually, the Motts' line of vegetable compounds was part of a much larger medical movement, Thomsonianism, estimated to have reached, in one form or another, from one-third to one-half of the population of this period. A comparison of the basic texts for both the Thomsonian system of treatment and Mrs. Mott's *Ladies Medical Oracle* reveals a similar set of remedies and a denunciation of the "instruments of death," dangerous and unknown chemicals advocated by the "regular" medical professionals. Given the quality of medical knowledge of the day, there was much to be said in favor of the irregulars' charges. Doctors may, in fact, have killed almost as many as they cured. One certainly could do worse than allowing nature's own cures to produce relief. In Sarah's case, where the "regulars" had failed, Mrs. Mott's gentle treatment proved successful. Moreover, Mrs. Mott proved to be a sympathetic practitioner, willing to openly discuss the case

45. Ibid., p. 7.
46. Ibid., pp. 81–83; other interpretations of Hunt include: Wood, pp. 44–47; and Regina Markell Morantz, "The Perils of Feminist History," *Journal of Interdisciplinary History* 4, no. 4 (Spring 1974), pp. 649–60.

with Harriot, in sharp contrast to the previous physicians who had visited often and explained little.[47]

Sarah's recovery under the Motts' care became a turning point for her sister: "Here was my first thought of woman as a physician." Harriot eagerly accepted an offer by the Motts to study medicine with them. Her decision to apprentice to them was influenced not only by their success with Sarah, but also by their "prosperity"—an important consideration for someone who had to support a family. Finally, it is important to remember that Hunt had no choice. Even if she had found a physician willing to grant her an apprenticeship, an unlikely event, Hunt would have to face the inevitable scandal touched off by a woman working alone with a man under intimate conditions. Since Mrs. Mott practiced with her husband (and thus served as a chaperon), Hunt had an opportunity that was unavailable elsewhere in the city.[48]

Once again, Sarah followed her sister, and both along with their mother moved into the Motts' home in 1834. Much of their apprenticeship seems to have involved corresponding

47. Hunt, pp. 110–11, 87. What Hunt could not know, because she was not a member of the Massachusetts Medical Society (and being a female meant she was not eligible for membership), was that male physicians were merely following patient protocol specified in *Rules and Regulations of the Boston Medical Association* (Boston, 1830). See also Elizabeth Mott, *Ladies Medical Oracle . . .* (Boston, 1834), pp. 1–11, 199–207 for the quotation cited here. Joseph Kett deals with the medical background of this era in Kett, pp. 100–31. See also Thomson; Rothstein, pp. 130–31. Barbara Rosencrantz's lecture on Botanism at Harvard University, March 5, 1974, has also given me valuable perspective on the topic.

48. Hunt, pp. 111, 125. Scholars in women's history who describe more opportunities for seventeenth- and eighteenth-century female physicians do not explain how these women got their training, if they got any at all. The difficulties of women in obtaining preceptorships are well documented in the manuscripts for the New England Female Medical College (BU-A). The beginnings of medical colleges formalized the procedure for obtaining preceptors (which were still required in an era when internships were nonexistent) and increased opportunities for women physicians. Often the medical college faculty sponsored students in the months the college was not in session.

with the Motts' patients. The extent of advice they offered can be gleaned from the contents of Mrs. Mott's medical handbook, published in Boston in 1834. The Mott system relied for the most part on domestic remedies: "herbs, roots, flowers, vegetables, and essential oils, gums, balsams, and simples." The Hunts' apprenticeship, however, was terminated abruptly when Dr. Mott died in 1835 and Mrs. Mott returned to England.[49]

That year, with only haphazard training and no medical degrees, the Hunts began their medical practice in Boston. This pattern was not at all uncommon among male physicians. No doubt the Hunts were further encouraged by the Thomsonians who advocated that women be treated by physicians of their own sex because "we cannot deny that women possess superior capacities for the science of medicine." Still, Hunt was fully aware of the advantages which some of the city's male physicians possessed: especially one who had " 'regularly' studied—had passed through an approved college . . . ; and with . . . an M.D. placed at the end of his name . . . had capital to start upon. He had older heads to sustain him—a code of laws to obey—a mistake would not be fatal to him, though it might be to the patient." As much as she envied medical graduates, there is no indication that Hunt thought of applying to a college during this period. As she later remarked, women simply did not dare apply.[50]

It is almost impossible today to appreciate the courage it took for two women to establish a medical practice in that period. The tenuous nature of their situation quickly forced them to abandon all housecalls. At first, they had made an occasional visit to a bedridden patient, "but we found too often that there was so much opposition to the attendance of a woman as physician among the friends of the invalids, that the good of our visits was neutralized." [51]

49. Ibid., p. 124; Mott, p. 1.
50. Hunt, p. 381.
51. Ibid., pp. 135–36.

Mrs. Mott had advised the Hunts—as if they had a choice—
to limit their practice to women and children. Their approach
to medicine was unorthodox, partly the result of haphazard
training, and based on the conviction that male physicians
were incapable of treating female ailments which the Hunts
believed were psychosocial in origin. Male physicians were
limited not only by their inability to understand the female
psyche, but by their identification with a male society, which
was often the root cause of a woman's illness. Hunt was convinced that most "physical maladies" stemmed from "the heart
histories of women which were revealed to us [only] as
women." She argued: "From male physicians the causes of the
diseases of women, as well as the extent of those diseases, are
often concealed!" She looked forward to the day when "woman
will be allowed to come into [hospitals] as physicians, and
. . . open books that are sealed." [52]

Much of Hunt's autobiography concerns itself with her con-
tempt for "regular medicine" which she dismissed as "worse
than useless." An eclectic who experimented with a variety of
sectarian treatments, Hunt proudly described herself as "the
disciple of no medical sect." But it would be a mistake to view
Hunt, as others have done, as "flaunting her anti-professional-
ism" or as an opponent of science.[53]

The course of Hunt's career was in large part dictated by
her isolation from the medical community. Forced to become
their own teachers during the first months of their practice,
the two sisters "studied with unwearying zeal . . . reciting
our lessons to each other—investigating every case that had
been presented to us through the day—often thankful that we
had declined cases . . . till we were prepared to meet them."
The only public course of instruction open to them was atten-

52. Ibid., pp. 156, 251, 139, 158. At a convention Hunt gave a speech on
the medical education of women and outlined the reasons necessitating
female physicians; see *Proceedings of the First National Woman's Rights
Convention Held at Worcester, October 23rd and 24th, 1850* (Boston, 1851),
pp. 45-49.
53. Hunt, p. 171; Wood, p. 46.

dance at the lectures delivered by touring sectarian advocates.[54]

Hunt is best understood not as one who rejected science,
but rather as one whom science had rejected. Nothing illustrates this better than her decision at age forty-two to enter
Harvard Medical College. Her mother's death in the spring of
1847 appears to have forced Hunt to reassess her situation.
Sarah, who had left medicine in 1840 to marry and was now
the mother of six, invited her sister to live with her. Harriot
refused: "I concluded to continue in Green Street, and throw
all my energies into my profession." At this point, a number
of friends suggested that she apply to Harvard Medical College—"you have been in practice so many years in Boston that
such a request could not be refused." Furthermore, public
opinion in Boston was becoming more conscious of the importance of the need for a medical degree. An avid reader of
the *Boston Evening Transcript,* she could not help but be
aware of editorials such as the one which appeared on May 11,
1847, warning: "Physicians: Quacks are at a premium!" It

---

54. Hunt, pp. 128, 361, 129, 140. Earlier scholarship that mentions
Hunt's gravitation toward sectarian medicine fails to view this in the context of sexism and medical isolation. See, for example, Thomas Francis
Harrington, *Harvard Medical School: A History, Narrative, and Documentary 1782–1905* (New York, 1905), pp. 1218–19. Harrington makes no mention of Hunt's forty-year practice, and he tries to pigeonhole her before
quickly dismissing her importance: "She was a Swedenborgian in faith, and
an advocate of woman's rights." Aside from being incorrect in stating that
she had been "brought into the family of Valentine Mott," Harrington
makes a number of factual errors, most notably that Hunt was at Gregory's
School in 1862 which she was not. Recent scholarship on women in sectarian medical history represents much more accurate as well as fair-
minded attempts. See, for example, Madeline B. Stern. *Heads and
Headliners: The Phrenological Fowlers* (Norman, Okla., 1971); John B.
Blake, "Mary Gove Nichols, Prophetess of Health," *Proceedings of the
American Philosophical Society* 106, no. 3 (June 1962); Blake, "Women and
Medicine in Ante-Bellum America," pp. 99–123. It is important to under-
stand why women were attracted to sectarian medicine as well as the
forces blocking them from advancing in orthodox medicine.

advised the public that the only guarantees that a physician could offer as evidence of professional competence were "testimonials of his education." [55]

Hunt claims to have confided her intention to apply to Harvard to a faculty member who, in turn, passed the message on. Unknown to Hunt, and for reasons which are not clear, Dr. Walter Channing, at a meeting of the medical faculty, asked: "If a woman might be admitted to medical lectures, and to an examination for a Degree?" The question was forwarded to President Everett and the Harvard Corporation, who at a special meeting on August 14, concluded that it was inadvisable to alter "the existing regulations of the medical school, which imply that the students are exclusively of the male sex." There is no indication that this decision was communicated to Hunt.[56]

Spurred on by Elizabeth Blackwell's entrance into Geneva Medical College in November 1847 Hunt applied to Harvard one month later for permission to attend the school's public medical lectures, citing the Blackwell precedent in her letter. She made no mention of any intention to pursue the medical degree. Hunt was not as optimistic as friends who had assured her that Harvard would welcome her: "Your age, your birthright as a Bostonian, must have weight with them." Nevertheless, she regarded it as her "duty to try to become stronger and stronger and stronger . . . [although] it really seemed to me farcical to ask whether a woman, who had been practicing medicine many years—a mind thirsting for knowl-

55. Hunt, pp. 214, 215.

56. Minutes of the Meetings of the President and Fellows of Harvard College, August 14, 1847, HWL-A; Hunt, pp. 214, 215, 218. The college records are extremely brief and the correspondence lacks detail so we are forced to rely on Hunt's own commentary pieced together from fragments in her autobiography. Although no individual is named in the July–August 1847 discussions regarding a female applicant, it is likely that this person was Hunt. She writes: "Having a conversation with one of the professors I told him my intention. I think he informed the clique, and that law [August 14, 1847] was passed to meet my application . . ." (p. 218).

edge, . . . *might be allowed* to share the privilege of drinking
at the fountains of science, a privilege which would not im-
poverish them, but make me rich indeed." [57]

Hunt included in her letter of application the condescending editorial printed in the *Boston Medical and Surgical
Journal,* which noted that Geneva had survived the arrival of
Miss Blackwell: "She is a pretty little specimen of the feminine gender. . . . She comes to class with great composure,
takes off her bonnet and puts it under the seat (exposing a fine
phrenology), takes notes constantly. . . . The effect on the
class has been good, and great decorum is preserved while she
is present." Describing herself as at "that mature age when the
duties of life are more clearly seen than at any other period,"
Hunt declared that she hoped to obtain from Harvard a
"scientific light." She concluded her letter by assuring Harvard
that she had *not* applied out of "love of novelty, [or] bravery
in an untried position, [or] want of patronage" but out of "a
simple and single desire for such medical knowledge, as may
be transmitted through those professors, who from year to
year, stand as beacon lights to those who would be aided in a
more full knowledge of the healing art." [58]

Once again, the medical faculty passed the issue on to the
corporation for action. Hunt's aplication was accompanied
by a letter from Oliver Wendell Holmes, Dean of the Medical
College, suggesting that if the corporation decided to act
favorably, no better candidate could be found than Hunt.
"The applicant is of mature age and might be fully trusted,
so far as appearances go. She is full of zeal for science and may
become hereafter the worthy rival of 'Madame le Docteur
Boivin' of the Parisian faculty." [59] The corporation's reply was
to the point: "It was voted, that it is inexpedient to reconsider

57. Hunt, pp. 215–16.
58. Ibid., pp. 217–18. *BMSJ* 37 (1847), p. 405.
59. Oliver Wendell Holmes to President Everett, Harvard College
Papers [Communications addressed to the President and Fellows of Harvard College], 2d. ser. 15, December 11, 1847, HWL-A.

the vote of the corporation, of the 14th of August, relative to a similar request." [60]

Harvard's decision served to radicalize Hunt. Depicting the decision as "semi-barbaric," she attacked a refusal based simply on inexpediency: "Expedient for us to enter hospitals as patients, but inexpedient for woman, however well qualified, to be there as a physician. . . . That word *inexpedient* I had always abhorred—it is so shuffling, so shifting, so mean, so evasive, . . . an apology for falsehood, a compromise of principle. . . . It had always been a *little* word in my lexicon, and it became still *littler,* when used by a medical conclave. Any kind of reason might have been accepted, but this *inexpedient* aroused my risibles, my sarcasm, my indignation." [61]

Heretofore Hunt had been a private person who had shunned the reform movements which were demanding a reordering of the social system. Although a friend of the Grimke sisters, she had to this date never attended an antislavery meeting.[62] She saw the beginnings of the woman's rights movement less than a year after Harvard's rejection as fortuitous— "a ray of light penetrated the gloom." [63] In 1850 she crossed what she termed her "equatorial line" and attended her first

60. Hunt, p. 218; Minutes of the Meetings of the President and Fellows of Harvard College, December 27, 1847.

61. Hunt, p. 219.

62. Ibid., p. 250. On the basis of the dates of correspondence between the Grimke sisters and Hunt that has been preserved, it is likely that these friendships developed in the late 1840s and grew out of Hunt's fame as a female physician. Angelina Grimke Weld had developed a prolapsed uterus, according to correspondence between Sarah Grimke and Harriot Hunt. See references to this in Gerda Lerner, *The Grimke Sisters from South Carolina. Pioneers for Woman's Rights and Abolition* (New York, 1967), p. 290. The William L. Clements Library Archives at the University of Michigan has twenty-four letters directed to Harriot Hunt but only *one* letter from Hunt. Hunt's correspondence is scattered and has been preserved mainly by those to whom she wrote. The second volume of her autobiography was never published although she anticipated in her will that it would be. See "Records of the New England Woman's Club," SA.

63. Hunt, p. 249.

woman's rights convention in Worcester, Massachusetts, and spoke on the need for trained female physicians.[64] It was then that she began the practice of regularly paying her property taxes under protest, complaining of taxation without representation. Where once she had taken pride in her birthright as a native Bostonian, she now cried: "Faneuil Hall was not *our* Cradle of Liberty. We had no hand in the rocking. If we *had* had, perhaps the child would have turned out better. But *men* rocked *that* cradle!" [65]

On November 12, 1850, buoyed up by the expanding feminist crusade, and encouraged by the recent graduation of Elizabeth Blackwell, Hunt again applied to Harvard for permission to attend the medical lectures. Dismissing her previous rejection as unjust, Hunt pointed to the "progress of the age" as reason for reconsideration. She reminded the school that it was no longer a question of female physicians, but rather whether or not female physicians would receive adequate training.[66]

For a moment it looked as if the progress of the age had struck Harvard. On November 23, the medical faculty voted five to two to allow Hunt to attend lectures "provided that her admission be not deemed inconsistent with the statutes." Dean Holmes's letter to the corporation echoed Hunt in pointing out that public opinion had shifted in favor of female practitioners. Holmes reminded the governing board that a female medical college had recently been established in Boston.[67]

Two weeks later, Harvard informed Hunt that there were no objections to her attendance at medical lectures. The decision, of course, related only to attendance at lectures, and Harvard was not forced to confront the more difficult question

64. Ibid., p. 250, n. 52.
65. Ibid., p. 44.
66. Ibid., pp. 265–67.
67. Oliver Wendell Holmes to President Sparks, Harvard College Papers [Communications addressed to the President and Fellows of Harvard College], 2d ser. 17, November 25, 1850.

of awarding a degree to a woman. Both the medical faculty and the corporation had made it clear that she would not be allowed to take the examination for the degree.[68] Hunt's age may also have initially acted in her favor. At forty-five, she would not have created the "sexual tensions" that might have been triggered by the presence of a younger woman. In her 1850 letter she even alluded to this matter: "In opening your doors to woman, it is mind that will enter the lecture room, it is intelligence that will ask for food; sex will never be felt where science leads for the atmosphere of thought will be around every lecture." Photographs of Hunt present her as a dignified matron, and Oliver Wendell Holmes himself reassured the board members that "as far as appearances go, she can be trusted." The existence of a medical school for women in Boston since 1848 must also be considered as influential in spurring Harvard to act in her favor. In that year, Samuel Gregory had opened the Boston Female Medical College. The school was a proprietary institution, and Gregory himself had no medical training whatsoever. Hunt clearly sought to use the absence of any adequate source of medical training for women in Boston as an additional point in her favor. She warned the officials that there was a danger in the city of "unprepared, uneducated women . . . going forth to prescribe, urged by this necessity." [69]

In their November meeting the medical faculty had also decided to admit three black men—Martin Delany, Daniel Laing, and Isaac Snowden—who were to emigrate to Liberia once they had completed their studies.[70] Before Hunt could attend her first lecture, the medical students met to protest her admission and that of the black men. Resolutions were

68. Hunt, p. 268; Jared Sparks to Oliver Wendell Holmes, Harvard College Papers [Communications addressed to the President and Fellows of Harvard College], 2d ser. 17, December 2, 1850.

69. Hunt, pp. 265–67; see also n. 68.

70. Hunt, pp. 270–71. The admission of the black men was to a degree program unlike the case of Hunt which was merely to attend lectures. See Harvard Medical Faculty Minutes, November 4 and 23, 1850, HCL-A.

drawn up which charged that the "socially repulsive" blacks
would undermine the value of their diploma. Similarly, Hunt
would be kept out "to preserve the dignity of the school, and
our own self-respect." No woman of "true delicacy," they
claimed, would be willing to attend medical lectures with men.
And they, in turn, would be unwilling to mix with any
woman who "unsexed" herself, thereby sacrificing her own
modesty." [71] Unfortunately, there is no recorded explanation
of the steps involved in Harvard's decision to reconsider its
position. All we know is that the school retreated in the face
of the protests and that the "leading members of the faculty"
met privately with Hunt and persuaded her not to attend the
lectures.[72]

Hunt never again attempted to penetrate Harvard's ivy
walls. The only degree she ever received was an honorary one,
awarded by the Female Medical College of Pennsylvania in
1853. Undaunted by Harvard's second rejection, she spent an-

71. The student resolutions were published in the *Boston Evening Transcript*, January 3, 1851; Hunt's letter was published January 7, 1851.
E.D.L.'s letter regarding the same incident was published January 1, 1851.
(Note that Hunt gives the date of July 5, 1851, for all of these communications and this is obviously a typographical error—see pp. 268–70 of Hunt.)
The language of the student resolutions bears close resemblance to the
text of John Ware's introductory lecture to the Harvard Medical School
class on November 6, 1850. See pp. 519–20 of the full text reprinted in the
BMSJ 43 (1851), pp. 496–504; 509–22). The title of the lecture was "Success
in the Medical Profession." Unfortunately Ware and the other members of
the faculty have left behind no papers which would explain their simul-
taneous opposition of female physicians and vote for the admission of
Hunt.

72. Letter signed "E.D.L.," cited in n. 71, above. Harvard Medical
Faculty Minutes, December 13, 1850, HCL-A. The blacks also withdrew
but there is a continuing debate on the case of Martin Delany and whether
or not he received a degree from the Harvard Medical School, see Theo-
dore Draper, "Martin Delany: The Father of American Black Nationalism,"
New York Review of Books, March 12, 1970; "An Exchange on Black
History," ibid., May 21, 1970; "Writing Black History," ibid., July 2, 1970.
Cited by Ronald Takaki, "Aesculapius Was a White Man: Antebellum
White Racism and Male Chauvinism at Harvard Medical School," paper
read at the meeting of American Historical Association, December, 1971.

other quarter-century in active medical practice, determined "to awaken public thought to the positive need of women entering the profession." [73]

Some historians have viewed professional women as individuals who must pay the price of personal unhappiness. One writer, for example, concluded that Elizabeth and Emily Blackwell personified the unhappiness and dissatisfaction of Victorian professional women: "the delight of these women lay in the search for freedom in a new field, not in the enjoyment of that freedom gained." [74] But the life of Harriot Hunt along with the lives of other female physicians demonstrate that a number of professional women, despite the obstacles in their way, were able to gain both happiness and satisfaction in their careers.

Nowhere is this better illustrated than in Hunt's silver wedding anniversary which celebrated her first twenty-five years of medical practice. She had often remarked that since her love had been channeled into her profession, she intended to celebrate her silver wedding, which she did in the summer of 1860. One of the 1,500 guests, Ednah Cheney, later described the ceremony: "Her many friends gathered about her, her home was overwhelmed with a profusion of flowers, and her own and her sister's heads were wreathed with double wreaths; a pure gold ring was given her to consecrate the marriage to her profession." Events like these made one proper Bostonian

73. Hunt, pp. 272, 155. In 1856 Harriot Hunt was listed as a "friend" of the New York Infirmary "Appeal in Behalf of the Medical Education of Women" and, along with Mrs. James Freeman Clark, collected funds in Boston for the project. See Elizabeth Blackwell, *An Appeal in Behalf of the Medical Education of Women* (New York, 1856), p. 13.

74. Andrew Sinclair, *The Emancipation of the American Woman* (New York, 1965), p. 147. A number of writers in women's history simply avoid the controversial issue of feminine achievement, but many others, like Sinclair, argue that this achievement is linked to neurosis: James R. McGovern, "Anna Howard Shaw: New Approaches to Feminism," *Journal of Social History* 3, no. 2 (Winter 1969–70), pp. 135–53; Smith, p. 300; Ferdinand Lundberg and Marynia F. Farnham, *Modern Woman:The Lost Sex* (New York, 1947), *passim;* Oliver Jensen, *The Revolt of American Women* (New York, 1952), p. 92.

comment, "[Harriot Hunt] makes every aesthetic hair rise up on my head," but Hunt's celebration, in fact, became a model for later feminists.[75]

Visitors such as Elizabeth Blackwell in 1865 were always impressed by Hunt's cheerfulness: "I called on Harriot K. Hunt, as jolly as ever, who poured out a tide of her own peculiar life, and read me her fifteenth annual protest on paying her taxes." [76] And three years before her death, she told a young woman physician: "I have been so happy in my work; every moment is occupied; how I long to whisper it in the ear of every listless woman, 'do something if you would be happy.'" [77] But beneath her sunny disposition, there always lingered the bitter recollection that she had been blocked in her attempt to gain the knowledge which would have expanded her career. "Shall I ever forgive the Harvard Medical College," she asked, "for depriving me of a thorough knowledge of . . . science . . . a knowledge only to be gained by witnessing dissections in connection with close study and able lectures?" [78]

75. Ednah Dow Cheney, *Reminiscences* (Boston, 1905), p. 52; Elizabeth Cady Stanton comments on Hunt's silver wedding celebration: "quite properly the initiative has been taken in late years, of doing honor to the great events in the lives of single women" (*Eighty Years and More: Reminiscences 1815–1897* [New York, 1971; originally printed in 1898], p. 172). Susan B. Anthony held a similar reception but without the wedding attire, p. 173. See also Stanton et al., *History of Woman Suffrage,* vol. 1, p. 260.

76. Elizabeth Blackwell to Kitty Barry Blackwell, Boston, November 18, 1865, Blackwell Family Papers, Box 79, Library of Congress. I am indebted to Nancy Sahli for bringing this quote to my attention.

77. Mary Safford Blake, *WJ,* November 23, 1872, p. 376.

78. Hunt, p. 122.

2

A Mistaken Ally

In the fall of 1847 while Harriot Hunt was preparing to apply to Harvard for the first time, Samuel Gregory, a self-styled lecturer in physiology, was busy soliciting funds for the medical education of women. Encouraged both by the positive public response and the negative response of Harvard to Hunt, Gregory opened the Boston Female Medical College on November 1, 1848. It was the first medical college for women in the world.[1]

The appearance of the college seemed to signal a new chapter in the history of women in American medicine. But, although it did demonstrate that women could be educated as doctors (albeit on a segregated basis), Gregory's college never realized its potential. Rather than marking a major breakthrough, the twenty-six year history of the school illustrates how subtle and complex were the barriers to women's achievement in medicine. For although the school provided students with what was at best a mediocre education by the standards of the day, they did receive more formal training than many of their male colleagues. Still, the lesson of the Female Medical College was that a mediocre education was not enough for a woman, though it might be for a man. Some women would have to gain access to the best medical education available if women physicians were to be taken seriously.

1. Newspaper advertisements and response to Gregory's activities date from September 7, 1847, when he began annotating a scrapbook kept until the end of 1865, at which point legislative investigations of the college were initiated. The scrapbook is in the Rare Book Room of the Harvard Medical School's Countway Library.

Ironically, while Gregory gave women their first opportunity to pursue any medical education at all, he was also
responsible in good part for the failure of the experiment.
Even though Gregory was far in advance of the public opinion
of his age regarding professional education for women, he held
an ambivalent view of the role of women. His was a progressive rhetoric accompanied by paternalistic and prejudiced
actions. A careful distinction must be made, therefore, between his ideas, which seemed to defy all that was deemed
holy by the Boston medical establishment, and his school,
which consciously set minimum standards for students who
were expected to have limited objectives—second-class professionals who would know their place in the medical world.

Nothing better underscores the isolated position of women
in mid-nineteenth-century medicine than the fact that the
founder of the first woman's medical college had no medical
training and only an honorary medical degree. Gregory was
born in Guilford, Vermont, in 1813, and like many upwardly
mobile New Englanders, was forced to teach a number of years
before he could afford to go to college. He later traced his
interest in medicine to a series of lectures on physiology and
anatomy offered by the medical department in the summer of
his senior year at Yale. Graduating in 1840 at the age of
twenty-seven, Gregory returned to Yale five years later to
receive a master's degree. Meanwhile he supported himself by
touring New England, first as a teacher of English grammar,
then, as a "Lecturer on Physiology." [2] In 1841 he published a

2. The most complete biographical study of Gregory appears in Allen
Johnson (ed.), *Dictionary of American Biography*, vol. 2 (New York, 1931),
pp. 604–05. This account is based on obituaries, Gregory's own writing,
and a few references by Marie Zakrzewska, a physician who taught at his
college from 1859 to 1862. Frederick C. Waite, *History of the New England
Female Medical College* (Boston, 1950), discusses Gregory's life on pp. 11–
16 using the same sources. Waite's account is essentially a history of the
college based on Gregory's own writings. It is incomplete insofar as it does
not refer to the critical evaluations written about Gregory and the
college. Most surprisingly it has an antifeminist bias as Waite totally
ignores the lady managers' minutes as a source of information about the

pamphlet, *Facts and Important Information for Young Men on the Self-Indulgence of Sexual Appetite*, which sold 42,000 copies in seven years and went through eight editions.[3]

The idea of a medical college for women grew out of Gregory's pamphleteering and lectures on physiology. Gregory claims to have first raised the issue in a pamphlet entitled *Licentiousness, Its Causes and Effects*, published in February 1846. He pointed out: "There is demanded now, as formerly a supply of female accoucheurs; also a class of female physicians, qualified at least to attend to the peculiar complaints of their own sex." [4] The thrust of Gregory's argument was that male midwifery was tainted with immorality.

Although male midwives had made considerable progress in the nineteenth century, the opposition had yielded ground grudgingly. Criticism of male midwifery was not a purely American phenomenon. In 1793 in London, S. W. Fores, who

---

college's treatment of women. Waite even goes so far as to omit all mention of the lady managers in his appendix of names, although he provides full lists of all the male trustees and directors. After generally disregarding the feminist point of view in his narrative, he concludes that the women did not try to fight male prejudice and that female faculty were to blame for their brief tenure at the college—see pp. 85, 63. In treating the idea of a female college just like any other college, Waite fails to confront the sexist issues that were fundamental in the history of the college.

3. Lecturing and writing on sexual hygiene was a popular way of making a living in the mid-nineteenth century. Stephen Nissenbaum has located 196 such books written and published from 1830 to 1880 and he includes only one pamphlet by Gregory on this list. The best known and most financially successful lecturer of this period was Sylvester Graham (1794–1851), a New Englander whose *Lecture to Young Men on Chastity* went through ten editions between 1834 and 1848 and was translated into several languages. By 1840 Graham was able to retire as a result of his earnings. See Stephen Nissenbaum, "Careful Love: Sylvester Graham and the Emergence of Victorian Sexual Theory in America, 1830–1840," Ph.D. dissertation, University of Wisconsin, 1968. Nissenbaum's bibliography of primary sources is on pp. 279–94.

4. A copy of this pamphlet could not be obtained. Gregory quotes himself from this pamphlet in his Annual Report of the Female Medical Education Society (1852), p. 13. See also the manuscripts of the Director's Meetings, BU-A.

described himself as a former medical student, advocated a school for female midwives in his book, *Man-Midwifery Dissected: or the Obstetric Family Instructor* . . . *Containing a Display of the Management of every Class of Labours by Men and Boy-Midwives; also of their cunning, indecent and cruel practices* . . . *proving that Man-Midwifery is a personal, a domestic, and a national evil.*[5] Similarly, in the United States in 1817 Thomas Ewell called for government-sponsored midwifery schools. Ewell charged that the rampant immorality of the day was in part connected to the prevalence of male midwives in the larger cities. Ewell left little to the imagination as he recounted lurid tales of doctors "inflamed with thoughts of the well-shaped bodies of the women they have delivered, handled, hung over for hours, secretly glorying in the privilege, have to their patients, as priests to their penitents, pressed for accommodation, and driven to adultery and madness, where they were thought most innocently occupied. In one case . . . a physician in Charleston, infuriated with the sight of the woman he had just delivered, leaped into her bed before she was restored to a state of nature." [6]

The twin themes of female modesty and male prurience found fertile ground in the 1840s when women's magazines and books were saturated with the idea that "the purity of women is the everlasting barrier against which the tides of man's sensual nature surge." [7] Large male audiences flocked to hear Gregory in Boston in the fall and winter of 1847. It is impossible, of course, to determine how many came to protect their own marital situation, for cuckoldry was a popular

5. Fores recommended that husbands be present during deliveries requiring instruments to insure against doctors "making too free with women's persons, manually, ocularly, and instrumentally" (p. 143). Cited by Jane Donegan, "Midwifery in America, 1760–1860: A Study in Medicine and Morality," Ph.D. dissertation, University of Syracuse, 1972, p. 123.

6. Cited by Samuel Gregory, *Man-Midwifery Exposed and Corrected* . . . (Boston, 1848), p. 16.

7. Barbara Welter, "The Cult of True Womanhood: 1820–1860," in Jane Friedman and William G. Shade (eds.), *Our American Sisters* (Boston, 1973), p. 211.

theme in anti-male midwifery literature. Others may simply have been lured by the promise of illustrative material. It is likely that the slide show which Gregory promised his audience included the pictures that were prominently displayed in his brother George Gregory's *Medical Morals,* published in 1852 (see figs. 1 and 2).

Certainly those who came to be titillated must have left satisfied. Gregory described male-midwifery "with other 'indecencies' [as] a form of fashionable prostitution; a primary school of infamy—as the fashionable hotel and parlor wine glass qualify candidates for the two-penny grog-shop and the gutter." He exclaimed: "Who wonders at the present rage of women for exhibiting themselves upon the stage, in a state of semi-nudity, so that the public generally may be entertained, without the trouble and expense of studying medicine!" Gregory then went on to liken male midwives to bank clerks, who, as a result of handling so much money, were tempted to make unlawful appropriations. "So the physician, by constant familiarity, comes to consider female delicacy and reserve as not worth preserving." Capitalizing upon the public response to his lectures, Gregory published them as *Man-Midwifery Exposed and Corrected together with Remarks on the Use and Abuse of Ether and Dr. Channing's "Cases of Inhalation of Ether in Labor";* it sold 18,000 copies in six months.[8]

Gregory saw the possibilities of exploiting the public controversy surrounding Channing's use of ether in obstetrical cases. He declared that the use of male midwives with unconscious women was a wicked and unnecessary addition to the biblical injunction: "In sorrow shalt thou bring forth children." The only advantage of ether, Gregory argued, was that it put a woman's "modest sensibilities asleep, thus allowing the physician to give full reign to his passions." [9]

Gregory's concept of a school for women doctors derived further strength from the physiological movement of the 1840s. In 1837 Sylvester Graham and William Alcott had founded the

8. Gregory, *Man-Midwifery,* p. 48.
9. Ibid., p. 11.

American Physiological Society, which was dedicated to a
scientific knowledge of the human body. Of the 206 members

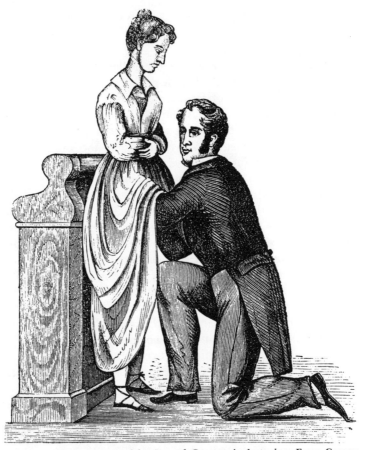

FIGURE 1   Illustration used by Samuel Gregory in lecturing. From George
Gregory, *Medical Morals* (Boston, 1852), p. 21.

of the Boston Physiological Society in 1837, more than one-
third were women.[10] Many of the female members felt that

10. Hebbel E. Hoff and John F. Fulton, "The Centenary of the First
American Physiological Society Founded at Boston by William A. Alcott

some of the lectures were too delicate to be discussed before mixed audiences and Mrs. Mary S. Gove of Lynn, Massachusetts, was engaged to lecture to the women in the fall of the following year.[11] The series proved immensely popular with between 400 and 500 women turning out to hear lectures on physiology, anatomy, menstrual difficulties, and the horrors

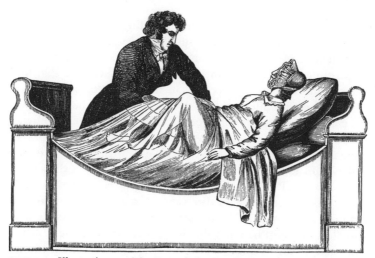

FIGURE 2   Illustration used by Samuel Gregory in lecturing. From George Gregory, *Medical Morals* (Boston, 1852), p. 25.

of self-abuse. The *Graham Journal* published synopses of them all, except "of course" the tenth and eleventh, which were given to unmarried and married women separately. When Mrs. Gove repeated, free, her lecture on tight lacing, the audience numbered 2,000.[12]

---

and Sylvester Graham," *Bulletin of the Institute of the History of Medicine* 5 (October 1937), p. 696.

11. Ibid., p. 702.

12. John B. Blake, "Mary Gove Nichols, Prophetess of Health," *Proceedings of the American Philosophical Society* 106, no. 3 (June 1962), p. 221. *Graham Journal of Health and Longevity* 2 (1838), pp. 325–30, 337–52, 357–75, 385; ibid., 3 (1839), pp. 20, 37, 69; *Library of Health, and*

There is no doubt that many nineteenth-century women, out of a sense of indelicacy, either avoided medical attention entirely or concealed difficulties from their doctors.[13] This embarrassment over sexuality affected many doctors as well. One Massachusetts Medical Society president proudly declared that he always delivered women "under their bedclothes" and that he never found it necessary to uncover a patient for a gynecological examination.[14]

Most doctors had little understanding of physiology and anatomy, a situation which should have called for caution, but which, in fact, allowed many physicians to spin out their own untested theories. Not surprisingly in a climate that produced the woman's rights movement, many women sought to gain a better understanding of their bodies. The result was the creation of a large number of independent female physiological societies in the 1840s in various urban centers. One of the most active of these was the Ladies' Physiological Institute of Boston founded in 1848. For their first meeting the society chose Dr. C. P. Bronson, an itinerant lecturer, to speak. Later, over 300 members paid Bronson a total of $1,000 for his course of lectures with the proviso that the professor's anatomical manikin be left with the society. By 1851 the institute boasted of an extensive collection of medical demonstration models in addition to the manikin. These included a full-size female anatomical model, a model of the heart and lungs, and models of the embryo from twelve days to nine months.[15] This

Teacher on the Human Constitution 2 (1838), pp. 357–58; M. S. G. Nichols, Mary Lyndon or, revelations of a life. An autobiography (New York, 1855), pp. 155, 159.

13. Richard H. Shryock, "Women in American Medicine," JAMWA 5 (1950), p. 373.

14. Alfred Worcester, "Reminiscences," p. 14, HWL-A. Worcester is describing a phenomenon which was much more prevalent in the 1840s. See James Ricci, One Hundred Years of Gynecology, 1800–1900 (Philadelphia, 1945), pp. 28–32.

15. BMSJ 41 (September 1849), pp. 201–03; Proceedings of the First Annual Meeting of the Ladies' Physiological Institute of Boston and Vicinity with Secretary's Report (1849) Boston, pp. 2–3. Harriot Hunt claims she helped found the Charlestown Ladies' Physiological Society,

equipment played a prominent role in the weekly lectures on anatomy held in the institute's quarters in Washington Hall on Bromfield Street, Boston. The hall also had a sizable library of medical books including *Diseases of Women, Lectures on Midwifery, Physiology of Women,* and *Principles and Practice of Obstetric Medicine and Surgery.*[16]

Although the institute was devoted to the study of all things scientific, its medical models and its library indicate that its members were especially interested in obstetrics. Mrs. F. A. M. Baldwin in the annual secretary's report in 1851 summed up the advantages of the institute: "Is not the knowledge here attained invaluable? What mother among us does not recur to the period of her first maternal responsibilities, with regret that the knowledge which has been here acquired, was not possessed at that time, thereby preventing much physical suffering and mental anxiety." [17]

During its early years, local doctors ignored the institute, forcing its members to rely on their own talents and on the services of medical lecturers who visited Boston. One woman who described herself as an "enthusiast upon the rights of women," complained to the *Boston Medical and Surgical Journal* that the medical profession had done nothing to prove "their sincerity by giving these ladies truly scientific lectures upon physiology and the means of preserving health." Significantly, the writer defined the rights of women not as "their right to legislate or rule the nation, but their right to fully understand the physical laws which govern their own organization." [18]

April 25, 1843. See Harriot Kezia Hunt, *Glances and Glimpses; or Fifty Years Social, Including Twenty Years Professional Life* (Boston, 1856; reprinted, 1970), p. 177.

16. Ladies' Physiological Institute, "List of Apparatus Belonging to the Institute," pp. 12, 20–27. See also *Synopsis of the Proceedings of the Second Annual Meeting of the Ladies' Physiological Institute of Boston and Vicinity with the Secretary's Report and the Constitution and By-Laws of the Society, with Catalogue of Library* (Boston, 1851).

17. Ibid., p. 9.

18. Martha A. Sawin, letter to the *BMSJ* 41 (1849), p. 202.

Such a definition of feminism reflects the diffuse nature of the woman's movement in the antebellum period. There were few hard-core feminists during those years; only 300 persons had met at Seneca Falls in 1848. The small numbers that met regularly in the following years devoted most of their time to changing state laws to protect woman's rights, converting legistatures to support of the suffrage, and publicizing the feminist cause.[19] Many more women, however, were involved in less dramatic approaches to their personal emancipation. Self-help educational facilities such as the physiological societies were part of a general drive by women to expand their knowledge.

Samuel Gregory's decision to open a women's medical college in the fall of 1848 was based on his conviction that it was an idea whose time had come. The success of the women's physiological societies, combined with the distrust that some women harbored toward male physicians, seemed to assure female physicians a guaranteed source of patients, especially in the area of obstetrical and gynecological care. In the absence of any supporting data, it is difficult to determine whether Gregory had a real commitment to women or whether he saw the school merely as an opportunity to improve his own situation.

The establishment of any medical school in mid-nineteenth-century America was, of course, a relatively simple matter compared to today. All that was needed was a faculty of four, a classroom, a dissecting room, and a few educational supplies. The typical course of instruction consisted of two four-month terms, usually taken in successive years. The second term was merely a repeat of the first term's lectures, thus minimizing the work of the faculty while maximizing the profits of the school. The net result was a proliferation of medical schools in the last half of the nineteenth century. By 1848 Boston could boast of three medical schools in addition to the women's medical college: Harvard Medical School and two proprietary

19. Anne F. Scott and Andrew M. Scott, *One Half the People: The Fight for Woman Suffrage* (Philadelphia, 1975), p. 12.

institutions, Tremont Medical School and Boylston Medical School.[20]

Women were, of course, not welcome at any of these three schools. Ironically, those who were in greatest need of certification were least able to obtain it. There were numerous young men like Dr. Dio Lewis who entered Harvard Medical School in 1845 and then dropped out after a few months because of financial problems. He immediately entered practice with an established doctor and later wrote a number of popular books on health problems. According to contemporary accounts, this practice was not uncommon, and the male medical school dropout, depending on his personal qualities and ability to inspire confidence, had little difficulty declaring himself an M.D. and establishing a medical practice. It was also relatively easy for a male practitioner to obtain an honorary M.D. degree if he needed the credentials. This was the case with Samuel Gregory's 1853 honorary degree from Penn Medical College. In some places, in fact, medical societies were given permission to grant M.D. degrees instead of licenses to new members who lacked them. Although attendance at a medical school and a degree became increasingly important in the nineteenth century, it was still possible for a man without a degree to make his mark in the profession.[21] This was not the case with a woman. Significantly, there are no examples

20. Seymour E. Harris, *Economics of Harvard* (New York, 1970), pp. 465 ff.; Thomas Francis Harrington, *The Harvard Medical School: A History, Narrative and Documentary, 1782–1905* (New York, 1905) vol. 2, pp. 489–505; William G. Rothstein, *American Physicians in the Nineteenth Century: From Sects to Science* (Baltimore, 1972), pp. 88–100.

21. Mary F. Eastman, *The Biography of Dio Lewis, A.M., M.D., Prepared at the Desire and with the co-operation of Mrs. Dio Lewis* (New York, 1891), p. 36. Biographical information on physicians is available in a number of sources including: Irving A. Watson (ed.), *Physicians and Surgeons of America. A Collection of Biographical Sketches of the Regular Medical Profession* (Concord, N.H., 1896); Howard A. Kelley and Walter L. Burrage (eds.), *American Medical Biographies* (Baltimore, 1920); and James Grant Wilson (ed.), *Appletons' Cyclopedia of American Biography* (New York, 1888), in several volumes. See also Rothstein, pp. 104–06.

of nondegreed female physicians who were taken seriously by the medical world.[22]

A woman was automatically doubted when she announced that she was a physician. One gauge of the problems women encountered is that of the *Boston City Directory*. Before 1847 only members of the Boston Medical Association were listed under the category of "Physicians and Surgeons." Female physicians were not allowed to apply for membership in the association, so Harriot Hunt and other women pioneers had to be satisfied with adding "female physician" to their names; thus their advertisements were effectively lost in the regular listing of many thousands of the city's inhabitants. When the Massachusetts Medical Society reorganized in the late 1840s, the Boston Medical Association was supplanted by the Suffolk District Medical Society, and a new classification for physicians appeared in the city directory. Three categories were now used: "Members of the Massachusetts Medical Society," "Physicians," and "Physicians-Female." [23]

To be listed under this third category suggested to the public that the female was something less than a physician. It is significant that after 1849, when the first Boston women physicians were able to travel to other cities and graduate from medical schools, they began to advertise the fact they had an M.D. degree. At no point in Boston medical history did male

22. See medical biographies cited above and Frances E. Willard and Mary A. Livermore, (eds.), *American Women: Fifteen Hundred Biographies: A Comprehensive Encyclopedia of the Lives and Achievements of American Women during the Nineteenth Century* (New York, 1897); Edward James (ed.), *Notable American Women: 1607–1950*, (Cambridge, Mass., 1971). The generalization is also based on an examination of the Boston directories and Boston medical history. As early as 1863 only "graduated" female physicians were included in statistics—see Virginia Penny, *The Employment of Women: A Cyclopedia of Woman's Work* (Boston, 1863), p. 25; this was not true for male physicians.

23. Kelley and Burrage, p. 329; Boston city directories. The first woman to formally apply to the Massachusetts Medical Association was Nancy Clark in 1853. The entire topic of Boston women physicians unlocking the gates to the male medical societies and institutions will be dealt with in chapter 5.

physicians use the M.D. after their names in the Boston medical directories. The listing of the medical degree was a feminine attempt, however feeble, to fight the stereotype of the female physician as incompetent and unqualified (see table 1).[24]

Samuel Gregory recognized this problem when he began his first class for midwives at the Boston Female Medical College. He promised them certification of their proficiency, and the publisher of the Boston City Directory at first cooperated. Eight names were listed in the 1849–50 directory under the heading of "Midwives." Five of these had asterisks after their names, indicating they had "certificates of qualification from Enoch C. Rolfe, M.D. of the Female Medical School, Boston." Similarly, any female practitioner, whatever her training, could enter her name in the "Physicians—Female" category. In fact, the more ambitious women entered themselves under both categories in order to catch the public's eye. Doubtless such difficulties created problems for the women themselves. They were now pitted against each other, rather than competing freely with the male practitioners. To make things even more difficult, the double listings for midwives and female physicians disappeared after a few years. Soon, midwives joined clairvoyants, Indian doctresses, electropaths, homeopaths, and formally educated female physicians—the latter fighting for recognition with their M.D. emblazoned after their names.[25]

24. It is significant that women used the degree listing as a weapon to defend their expertise as soon as they legitimately could earn such degrees. I would argue that degrees gave women their first self-confidence in fighting professional discrimination. Harriot Hunt wrote in 1856 after she had been listing her honorary M.D. degree in the city directory as if it were an earned degree: "Courtesy and respect had led many of my patients for many years to address me as Dr., but the recognition of [the Female Medical College of Pennsylvania in 1853] was very pleasant after eighteen years practice. It led me to ask these questions: How many males are practising on an *honorary* degree? Did they wait as many years for it?" (Hunt, p. 272).

25. The "Midwife" and "Physicians-Female" double listings disappear in 1857. This undoubtedly reflects the fact that the New England Female

Table 1 Designations for Boston Women Physicians, 1846–60

Category in City Directory	1846–47	1848–49	1849–50	1851	1852–53	1853	1854	1855	1856	1857	1858	1859	1860
Physicians—Female													
M.D.	0	0	0	0	1	1	4	4	10	7	7	12	12
Clairvoyant	0	0	0	0	0	0	0	0	0	1	0	0	3
Indian doctress	0	1	0	0	0	0	0	0	0	0	0	0	0
Midwife	0	1	3	0	0	0	0	0	0	0	0	0	0
Electropathist	0	0	0	0	0	0	0	0	0	0	0	1	1
Homeo[path]	0	0	0	0	0	0	0	0	0	0	0	0	1
No designation	4	6	6	6	12	13	9	11	6	15	18	17	15
Total	4	8	9	6	13	14	13	15	16	23	25	30	32 *
Midwives													
Certificate †	—	—	5	5	6	0	0	0	0	—	—	—	—
M.D.	—	—	0	0	0	1	3	3	3	—	—	—	—
No designation	—	—	3	8	5	11	10	10	9	—	—	—	—
Total	—	—	8	13	11	12	13	12	12	—	—	—	—

* Includes one double listing of an M.D. with a homeopath designation.
† Included this statement "Those marked thus [*] have Certificates of qualification from the Boston Female Medical School."

Source: *Boston City Directory* for respective years.

Twelve women enrolled in the November 1848 class of the Female Medical College. They had responded to advertisements that promised a three-month course on midwifery. Some fifty students from the New England states, New York, and Ohio attended the sessions during the school's first two years.[26] The faculty consisted of two physicians: Enoch Rolfe, whose M.D. degree was from Bowdoin Medical College, and William Cornell, whose A.B. was from Brown and M.D. from Berkshire Medical College. Cornell had the added distinction of being a member of the Massachusetts Medical Society. The teaching load was divided: Rolfe lectured on obstetrics and on diseases of women and children; Cornell taught physiology and hygiene.

The internal discord that attended the history of the Female Medical College emerged at the end of the first term. Rolfe and Cornell at first declared that the brief period of instruction was inadequate and refused to grant certificates, declaring that the women were unqualified to practice midwifery. They finally agreed to compromise with Gregory and signed statements that the women had "attended lectures three months," and Rolfe's name was used as a reference in the city directory. A major complaint of both professors was the lack of obstetrical models, which forced them to discuss in the abstract what should have been presented under laboratory conditions. Rolfe later likened the first midwifery courses to "Latin taught in twelve easy lessons." [27]

Medical College was chartered to officially grant degrees in 1856. I detected fraudulent advertising of female M.D. degrees as early as 1856, so it is clear that the publishers of the directory did not check credentials. See, for example, the listing of Anna Goulding in that year. Since less than a handful of New England Female Medical College M.D.'s were practicing in the city and Goulding was a chief agent at that time for the college, her lack of a degree could have been verified immediately.

26. Enrollment figures are those cited by Gregory in his publications. Actual names of all early students are not available. See *Senate Document No. 70*, April 3, 1851, MSA.

27. E. C. Rolfe, "Reply to Dr. Gregory's Circular, April 26, 1866," pp. 7-8, MSA.

Lacking any medical training, Gregory devoted himself to the financial and organizational problems of the school. Three weeks after the opening of the school, he formed the American Medical Education Society to "promote the medical education of females." Three men were to direct the affairs of the school: Rolfe as president, Gregory as secretary, and Mr. Bela Marsh, a local businessman, as treasurer. From the very beginning, only men were permitted to make decisions. Women were allowed to become members of the society but as one female member put it in a letter to the *Liberator:* "As the Constitution now stands, ladies are deprived, in all coming time of having the management of an institution which belongs to us only." [28]

In an effort to ease the school's financial difficulties, Gregory hired Mrs. Helen M. Gassett in 1849 as a fund raiser, agreeing to give her 50 percent of all she raised. By the spring of 1850 the membership of the society had expanded substantially and the Massachusetts legislature incorporated it as the Female Medical Education Society "for the purpose of providing for the education of Midwives, Nurses, and Female Physicians." [29]

Although she became increasingly disturbed by what she considered to be misrepresentation by the school, Gassett continued to raise funds. A number of donors assumed that they were assisting the poor in securing a livelihood when, at this time, all of the students paid their own fees.[30] Even greater difficulties surrounded Gassett's attempt to secure a larger role for women in the society. As she toured New England, she began to organize the female subscribers into local groups. The women responded eagerly, and Gassett forwarded their requests to be recognized as auxiliary societies with a constitu-

28. Trustees Report, November 23, 1848, BU-A; *Liberator,* October 3, 1850.

29. *Act of Incorporation,* April 30, 1850, Female Education Society, Commonwealth of Massachusetts, MSA.

30. Helen M. Gassett, *Categorical Account of the Female Medical College to the People of the New England States* (Boston, 1855), p. 10. This book has been dismissed by Waite as "a comedy of errors" (p. 21) and ignored as a historical document.

tion and by-laws. But Gregory summarily dismissed their petitions, pointing out that what the school needed was not a more complex "machinery" but rather *"getting funds now."* He warned her that "we wish to simplify our business." Then, to discourage her feminism, he advised her to avoid the "ladies" and solicit among men only, noting, "I find that gentlemen give quite as readily, to say nothing about any society." [31] Differences between them mounted rapidly until, in October 1850, Gregory dismissed her abruptly. After fourteen months Gregory "discovered" that Mrs. Gassett was neither a widow nor ever legally married. "Her domestic history was such as to render her an unsuitable person to occupy the position she did in a public institution." [32]

Gregory's difficulties with Gassett were symptomatic of his inability to allow women any meaningful role in the affairs of the school. Consequently, that same year found him engaged on a separate front with another group of women. The students, anxious to strengthen the school's finances, had petitioned the mayor for use of Faneuil Hall in order to hold a "social levee." Infuriated, Gregory quickly inserted an advertisement in the newspapers declaring that "this use of the name of the school was by persons not connected with the Society and without consultation with its officers." Although the women pointed out that the money was to be used to purchase needed equipment, Gregory declared that this was "an undignified method of raising funds." Moreover, it was "not in very good taste for middle-aged matrons pursuing obstetrical and medical studies to get up a dance in the most public hall in the city." [33]

31. Gassett, p. 12.
32. Trustees Report, October 24, 1850.
33. Ibid., February 22, 1850; Gregory inserted ads in the *Boston Traveler* and *Journal* for February 23, 1850, and used the opportunity to advertise the fourth term of midwifery classes given by the college. All the directors (at this time, King, Sewall, Shipley, and Sears) signed themselves in agreement with Gregory. Rolfe, who was a faculty member, disagreed and did not sign the statement. In order for the women to hold the levee, they had to exercise considerable initiative. They had to obtain the signatures

During its first two years lack of finances forced the school to lead a nomadic life, and classes were held in the homes of different students. The problem was temporarily alleviated in July 1850 when the independent-minded Dr. Winslow Lewis, president of the Boylston Medical School, offered to rent his home at 75 Boylston Street for the two years he would be in Europe. Lewis's offer, which drew the criticism of other doctors, was a boon to the society.[34] The completely furnished house offered a real sense of stability, and Lewis's more than 3,000 medical books supplied a much-needed library. Taking advantage of the building's desirable location at the foot of Boston Common, Gregory ordered a sixteen-foot sign erected on one wall announcing the presence of the New England Female Medical College.

Spurred by the new charter and the Lewis windfall, the directors of the society developed plans at the end of 1850 to raise $100,000 to erect and equip a medical college building and a hospital. A full-fledged program would be established with *"medical gentlemen as permanent Professors . . .* and competent *female instructors* in departments more concerned and appropriate to them."[35]

These grandiose plans were quickly stymied. Since only $3,000 had been raised in the previous two years, a goal of $100,000 was completely unrealistic. Only adequate salaries, not promises, would attract a strong faculty. Furthermore, the

---

of 100 voters (necessarily men at this point in history), present the petition to the mayor and aldermen, which they did February 11, and insert an ad in the newspapers. The levee only came to the attention of Gregory through the ad on February 12 in the *Boston Traveller,* which included the petition.

34. Waite, p. 22; *JGSB* (July 1869), pp. 5–6. Unfortunately, Lewis was a medical dissident and therefore left no papers to the medical establishment in Boston for preservation. His rental to the Female Medical Education Society may very well have been an act of defiance toward his brethren. He went to Europe to study gynecology, which was at that time an unpopular specialty not recognized by Harvard.

35. *Annual Report of the Female Medical Education Society* (1852), p. 16. Italics are my own.

few established Boston physicians who contemplated joining the faculty reconsidered after pressure from their colleagues.[36]

At the same time, the recently formed Philadelphia woman's medical college was experiencing similar difficulties. The common plight of the two colleges led spokesmen for the Philadelphia school to propose a merger in 1851. The plan called for a single faculty that would move between the two cities giving a session in the fall at Philadelphia and one in the spring at Boston. Gregory, who opposed the merger, postponed action in a final effort to attract a Boston faculty. Gregory was unsuccessful, and the Boston directors agreed on November 3, 1851, to cooperate with Philadelphia on a trial basis.[37] Accordingly, on February 26, 1852, the first medical course at the Boston Female Medical College began. Five of the seven faculty members were from the Philadelphia College including the only woman, Dr. Hannah Longshore, a demonstrator of anatomy. The college rented a vacant house on Washington Street for use as a dissecting room to supplement the practical anatomy course.

The fall term was held in Philadelphia, but the two Boston faculty members, Rolfe and Cornell, did not participate. Their decision to remain in Boston reflected both the continued

36. Direct evidence for this is lacking since there are no letters of resignation. The hostile editorials in the *BMSJ*, the official Boston Medical Society publication, suggest indirect evidence for such pressure. Gregory attributes the difficulty of getting well-qualified faculty to simple male prejudice. See, for example, his most explicit statement on this in the "Resolves," chap. 101, 1866, MSA, where he outlined the college's problems with the Boston medical profession. He claimed that a doctor's standing in the profession would be ruined or he would sabotage the female medical education movement, so strong was male prejudice against the advancement of women physicians.

37. Trustees Report, November 3, 1851, for the Boston college. See also the "Announcement to a Course of Medical Lectures to Women in the City of Boston by the Faculty of the Female Medical College of Pennsylvania to Commence Feb. 16, 1852," WMC-Pa. The course began ten days after the projected date. Very little source material on the Philadelphia college has been preserved, compared to that for the Boston college. The little that exists says nothing about the proposed merger.

reservations over cooperation and an internal schism in Phila-delphia. The Philadelphia faculty was divided over medical questions and several members resigned after the fall term to establish a rival coeducational institution, Penn Medical Col-lege.[38]

The Philadelphia schism ended the brief period of coopera-tion between the two colleges. Although Gregory had been opposed to the merger, its dissolution confronted him with the task of locating faculty for the spring term scheduled to begin on March 5, 1853. This came at a time when Gregory, as a result of Dr. Lewis's return from Europe, was busy trying to locate new quarters for the school. Letters appeared in the Boston newspapers inquiring about the whereabouts of Greg-ory's school and pointing out that public money had been raised for its support.[39] An angry Gregory responded in a letter to the *Boston Evening Transcript* that the school could be found on Cornhill Street and added that the previous letters were not honest inquiries, "but an attempt to excite prejudice and suspicion against the institution and its man-agers." [40] Gregory neglected to explain that the Cornhill Street address was that of a friend's store which he was using as a temporary base of operations. New floor space was finally rented over a carpet store on Washington Street in Boston. The last minute addition of a former member of Philadel-phia medical college who agreed to teach two subjects for double salary enabled the school to offer a medical course in the spring.

Despite their brave plan to raise $100,000, Gregory and the directors had been operating the college on an average annual income of $4,000, which was derived from donations and stu-

38. Frederick C. Waite, "Medical Education of Women at Penn Medical University," *Medical Review of Reviews* 39 (June 1933), pp. 255–60; Waite, *History*, p. 32.

39. *Boston Evening Transcript*, November 27, 1852; *Boston Traveler*, December 9, 1852.

40. *Boston Evening Transcript*, December 23, 1852.

dent fees.[41] Other Massachusetts medical colleges received state support and the society had applied unsuccessfully for aid in 1851 and 1852. Finally its efforts were rewarded, and the legislature agreed to award forty scholarships annually to Massachusetts women beginning in 1855. The society returned the following session and was able to secure an additional grant of $10,000 to be used for the purchase of equipment and a new building.[42]

Gregory had orchestrated the society's applications to the legislature. Appealing to their patriotism, he pointed out that Massachusetts women were forced to go to Philadelphia for a medical education. He argued that one could better gauge the qualifications of locally educated women: "It is certainly better to have our Commonwealth supplied with professional women of our own educating, in an institution of higher order, and under governmental supervision, than to have them furnished to us from irresponsible institutions abroad, or to have the community filled with uneducated and unauthorized women who are drawn into practice by the urgent demand for the services of female physicians." Gregory predicted that this demand was bound to grow and proudly informed the legislature that one of the school's recent graduates was serving as a medical adviser to the 300 students at the female seminary at South Hadley, Massachusetts. Reminding the legislators that they had passed an act in 1850 requiring physiology and hygiene to be taught in the public schools, Gregory recommended requiring female teachers to attend the medical college for at least one term. Of course, all of this would be accomplished with due respect for the sentiment of the day. Gregory was always careful to assure his readers that the women would limit themselves to the treatment of children and their own sex "in the delicate disorders and conditions peculiar to them." A proper division of duties between male

41. "Treasurer's Reports," New England Female Medical College, BU-A; Waite, *History*, p. 37.
42. Trustees Report, April 20, 1854.

and female physicians would be observed, and "that nice sense of delicacy which is the ornament of the female character, the soul of virtue, and the safeguard of morals" would be maintained.[43] Gregory also planted a number of favorable articles in small-town newspapers such as the one which appeared in Palmer, Massachusetts. The piece complimented the students at the college for being neither "upstarts nor old maids." The students were "true women" who did not wear "Bloomer costumes" or assert "women's rights, not wishing to encroach upon physicians, in the treatment of the other sex." [44]

In May 1856, fired by the state grants, the directors successfully petitioned the legislature for a new charter, officially changing the name of the corporation from the Female Medical Education Society to the New England Female Medical College. The charter named the seven former directors of the Female Medical Education Society as the original trustees. They in turn elected thirteen additional trustees. In an effort to gain scholarship funds from the other New England states, men of political prominence from the neighboring states were named to fill the vacancies on the board of trustees.[45] The seven trustees also voted to establish a board of twenty lady managers, equal to the number of trustees.

The lady managers were to elect an executive committee whose members would be allowed to attend but not to vote at the trustees meetings. The primary function of the lady managers was to solicit funds for the long-awaited women's hospital. The women were charged with nominating the officers of the hospital and with overseeing its "internal affairs."

43. Samuel Gregory, *Circular to the Members of the House of Representatives*, March 26, 1853, pp. 3, 5; *Senate Document No. 92*, March 30, 1855, *Senate Document No. 113*, March 24, 1856.

44. *Journal* (Palmer, Mass.), March 10, 1855; *Andover Advertiser*, December 29, 1855. These were pasted in Gregory's annotated scrapbook. Additional articles appear throughout the scrapbook.

45. Trustees Report, June 10, 1856, BU-A. See advertisements for this in Gregory's scrapbook. An 1866 investigation of the college found these trustees negligent in their duties; some never even attended one meeting. See "Resolves," chap. 101, 1866.

Unlike the trustees, the lady managers were expected to contribute personally to the upkeep of the school.[46]

A few months after the receipt of the new charter, an opportunity to purchase a hospital building emerged. In the fall of 1856 the directors of Boston Lying-in Hospital decided that the building was too expensive to maintain and closed the hospital. The City of Boston purchased the building in 1858 and then sold it to the medical college the following year for $50,000, to be paid in ten annual installments without interest. Dr. Marie Zakrzewska, a twenty-seven-year-old protégé of Elizabeth Blackwell, was appointed professor of obstetrics and diseases of women and children and resident physician in the hospital.[47]

No other event better illustrates Gregory's opposition to any meaningful female influence in the college than his treatment of Zakrzewska and the lady managers. From 1856 to 1859 the latter had been allowed to attend trustee meetings and raise funds for the hospital. In effect they were allowed to manage an institution that did not exist. But a real hospital was something else. In one of the first trustee meetings after the purchase, Gregory proposed that the women be prohibited from attending future meetings. The board initially refused to sup-

46. Although not stated in the *By-Laws of the New England Female Medical College* (1856), this was made clear to the women in their appointments. See "Records of the Lady Managers of the New England Female Medical College," BU-A. At every point in the history of the college, articulate women objected to their inferior leadership opportunities.

47. It is important to note that Boston Lying-in Hospital closed because of infection in the wards. The bad publicity scared away patients in the old building. The new building, which the New England College bought, was finished in 1854, but patients could not be obtained. By November 1856, despite advertisements in medical journals and eighty-five newspapers in eleven large New England towns, the empty beds forced it to close. See Frederick C. Irving, *Safe Deliverance* (Boston, 1942), pp. 121–23. No women physicians were associated with the Lying-in Hospital. After Zakrzewska began supervising the same building in 1859, such epidemics did not occur, suggesting that the infection resulted from conditions which could have been controlled earlier had the male physicians been more motivated.

port this motion; however, at the following meeting in October Gregory was able to get the trustees to take the more serious step of rescinding the power of the lady managers to appoint consulting physicians to the staff.[48] A number of the most influential lady managers resigned in disgust. As one disaffected member put it: "I must withdraw myself from all further action in the *so-called* management of the college." Meanwhile, Gregory's first objective was accomplished by simply failing to notify the women when trustee meetings were to take place. Consequently, within a year of the purchase of the hospital, the role of the lady managers had become largely ceremonial.[49]

Although the lady managers were easily vanquished, Gregory encountered a more formidable opponent in Dr. Zakrzewska. Almost immediately after arriving at the college, she had launched a campaign to raise the entrance qualifications and graduation requirements and to purchase scientific equipment. Gregory, who regarded the college as his own creation, objected to Zakrzewska's criticism of the facilities and organization. He openly attacked her, asserting that "foreigners" were not fit for American institutions because of their "pedantry

48. "Records of Lady Managers," July 29, 1859, BU-A; October 19, 1859; July 1, 1862.

49. S. R. Russell, Jamaica Plain, November 2, 1859 in "Records of Lady Managers." The women were both angry and helpless since Gregory officially had the power to determine what the bylaws meant. The first and apparently only "Annual Report of the Clinical Department" (1860) read: "What is the duty of the "Lady Managers . . . ? In answer we would say, that we have, so far, found the position to be merely honorary; conferring no voice or vote in the affairs of the college, and therefore no responsibility whatsoever in regard to it. The sphere assigned us is the Hospital . . ." (p. 4), New England Hospital Collection, SA. The successive minutes of the lady managers describe various strategies (all of which failed) used to attain a voice and power in the college. Finally, shortly before they were removed from office, they wrote: "As regards the college, the ladies can make no suggestions, their Delegates having received no notice of the Trustee meetings for the last three months, they are in entire ignorance of its state and action," "Records of Lady Managers," September 2, 1862.

and rudeness." When Zakrzewska asked for microscopes and other equipment, Gregory denounced this as "a new fangled European notion" and she in turn referred to him as "ambitious and narrow minded." [50] Zakrzewska claimed that the rest of the faculty secretly supported her: "My male-coworkers, men of education and experience, fully agreed with me and told me that in endorsing my election, they had hoped I would prevail upon the founders to elevate the standard of the school." [51] In February 1860, Zakrzewska refused to approve the graduation of two candidates, "who, excellent as nurses, were unfit to take the position as physicians." [52] Gregory protested, and the other members of the faculty compromised by allowing one of the candidates to graduate. One of the instructors rationalized his retreat by pointing out that her graduation would make little difference since "nobody in Boston would employ a woman doctor in serious cases anyhow." [53]

It is difficult to accurately evaluate the quality of the graduates of New England Female Medical College because no alumnae records were saved.[54] Dr. Mary Putnam Jacobi, who

50. Agnes C. Vietor, *A Woman's Quest; the Life of Marie Zakrzewska, M.D.* (New York and London, 1924), pp. 272, 284.

51. Ibid., pp. 276–77.

52. Ibid., p. 252.

53. Ibid. Faculty votes were not recorded individually. See "Faculty of New England Female Medical College," BU-A. The refusal of male medical faculty to take the education of women students seriously was a common complaint, apparently not unique to the Boston college. See Mary Putnam Jacobi, "Woman in Medicine," in Annie Nathan Meyer (ed.), *Woman's Work in America* (New York, 1891), pp. 174–75.

54. Even efforts to establish an alumnae club failed and Gregory alienated such powerful Boston graduates as Mercy Bisbee Jackson and Anna Goulding. When she graduated in 1860, Jackson was fifty-seven, twice widowed, and the mother of "several" children who required support. She was in active practice until her death in 1877. See *Boston Advertiser* obituary, December 15, 1877. Anna Goulding was an enormously successful fund raiser for the college for eight years beginning in 1850. She openly rebelled in November 1858 and founded a short-lived Ladies Medical Academy in November 1859. My own statistical analysis of the

studied under Zakrzewska in 1867 and who later became one of the most influential woman physicians of the nineteenth century, concluded that Gregory's school had performed a disservice to the cause of women in medicine. The failure, Jacobi charged, could be traced to the fact that no one at the school either knew or cared what a medical education should be. "It followed that, under the name of medical education, was offered a curriculum of instruction, so ludicrously inadequate for the purpose, as to constitute a gross usurpation of the name,—in a word, to be an essentially dishonest affair." [55]

Gregory, of course, claimed that the school had succeeded beyond expectation. In various advertisements for the college, he regularly singled out the more successful graduates: one who taught physiology at the Mt. Holyoke Female Seminary and another who performed the same task at the State Normal School; four who were teaching at New England Female Medical College; and one who was interning at New England Hospital for Women.[56] Significantly, all of the cases that Gregory cited were women who were not engaged in private medical practice. He did refer to some graduates who served "among their own sex," but the evidence indicates that they did so with little success. Several of the 1859 graduates com-

---

Boston city directories for the years beginning with 1854 (the graduates are not listed by name until 1854) indicates that of the ninety-eight graduates of the college, twenty-four practiced in Boston for some period of time. Of those thirteen graduates who were no longer listed in 1872, four had practiced ten to fifteen years, three had practiced four to seven years, and six had practiced one to two years. Of those graduates who were still listed in the directory in 1872, eight had practiced one to three years and three had practiced seven to thirteen years. In any given year from five to thirteen graduates of the college were practicing in Boston, approximately 16 percent of the total number of female physicians.

55. Jacobi, pp. 145-46.
56. Annual Report of New England Female Medical College (1869), pp. 15-16. Whenever Gregory mentioned the activities of the graduates of the college, names were not used. It is possible to check out individual names in Waite's useful list of graduates, History, appendix D., pp. 120-23.

plained that a dearth of cases had forced them to seek practical experience doing volunteer work among the poor, either as an assistant to a male physician or on their own." [57]

In all fairness, a few of the graduates did achieve some distinction as pioneers. Dr. Rebecca Lee, in 1864 the first black woman to receive a medical degree in the United States, established a successful practice in post-Civil War Richmond. Dr. Mary Harris Thompson, who graduated the year before, founded the first hospital for women and children west of the Allegheny Mountains in Chicago in 1865 and in 1870 founded the Woman's Hospital Medical College of Chicago, which was absorbed by Northwestern University in 1892.[58]

57. Vietor, p. 246. Some of the graduates of the college actually organized and tried to compensate for their inferior education by founding a Ladies Medical Academy in 1859. Of the twenty persons listing themselves as references for the new school, thirteen were students or graduates in the 1850s. The only existing brochure on this college is the first annual report and in it the writers stated that one of their principal objects "was to afford pupils facilities for studying disease by a personal examination of patients" (First Annual Report of the Ladies Medical Academy [Boston, 1860], p. 6). The evidence that women were able to establish lucrative medical practices by confining themselves to obstetrical deliveries is cited by Gregory without using actual names. Zakrzewska cites the case of a Mrs. Hassenfuss who claimed to be a graduate of the college and confined herself to midwifery: "Although she was never sought by the well-paying portion of the Boston community, she held a very reputable position among her patients and among such of the profession as had business with her" (Vietor, p. 246). Gregory's claim that female physicians could achieve economic and professional success through midwifery practice is unsubstantiated.

58. Waite, History, p. 88; it is more likely that these early pioneer women achieved success at least in part because they were first in the field and could make initial inroads. Some, like Rebecca Lee, were graduated and launched as pioneers because of peculiar circumstances in history. The faculty notes on Lee state: ". . . some of us have hesitated very seriously in recommending her . . . and do only out of deference to what we understand to be the wishes of the Trustees and the present state of public feeling" ("Faculty of the New England Female Medical College," February 25, 1864). There is no evidence that any other black women graduated from the college. Lee returned to the South immediately after

The quality of any student body is, of course, determined in part by the size of the pool from which it is drawn. The small number of applicants meant that anyone who applied to the college was almost automatically accepted. Dr. Ann Preston, president of Pennsylvania Female Medical College in the 1860s, believed that a combination of time and money discouraged most young women from pursuing a career in medicine. Estimates of costs ranged from $600 to $2,000, and even those New England College students who received state scholarships had to support themselves.[59] Thus, at this early date, female medical students came increasingly from privileged economic circumstances.[60] Yet even these women were victims of sexual stereotyping, and, as Dr. Zakrzewska discovered, they feared a loss of social caste. Most were convinced by society

---

graduation, according to Gregory, Annual Report of the New England Female Medical College (1864), p. 13; also Esther Pohl Lovejoy, *Women Doctors of the World* (New York, 1957).

59. Penny, pp. 28–29. This estimate is based on personal correspondence of the author with Preston and Dr. Elizabeth Blackwell. The responses of the writers are reprinted as excerpts.

60. Waite has drawn up lists of students who attended the New England Female Medical College but he found that the place of residency given by the student did not mean that she was a native of the town from which she entered. Altogether he found names for 197 students and birthdates for 31. Of Massachusetts students 67 percent were from Boston; 70 percent of all students were residents of Massachusetts. He claims that these percentages were roughly comparable to those of several male medical colleges, see *History*, pp. 86–87. No other studies have been done on female medical students in the nineteenth century which would give more than an impressionistic basis for judging social class origins. Rothstein cites a few studies on male medical students on pp. 113–14 and concludes that "many medical students were socially mobile." In an interesting essay, Gerald Markowitz and David Karl Rosner present evidence to show that some of those representing the medical establishment in the early 1900s were disturbed that members of the poor and working class were attending medical schools and earning degrees. See "Doctors in Crisis: A Study of the Use of Medical Education Reform to Establish Modern Professional Elitism in Medicine," *American Quarterly* 25 (March 1973), p. 95.

that the study of medicine would unsex them and they preferred to play "Lady Bountiful" among the poor.[61]

Ironically, Gregory, who had been rejected by Boston's male practitioners, succeeded in alienating what should have been his natural supporters: the students and the lady managers. The student reaction was touched off by Gregory's proposal to the trustees that the degree of "doctress" be conferred on all graduates in place of the "masculine term." Gregory's decision demonstrated a lack of sensitivity as "doctress" was usually used in a pejorative sense. Female abortionists such as the infamous Madame Restelle of New York were popularly referred to as "doctresses" and everywhere it meant something less than a qualified physician.[62]

Gregory's recommendation quickly ran into a wall of female opposition which included graduates of his college. Dr. Mercy Bisbee Jackson, a fifty-seven-year-old member of the class of 1860, wrote an angry letter to the Boston Evening Transcript. She pointed out that Webster defined a doctor as "one who has passed all the degrees of the faculty and is empowered to practice and teach it," whereas a doctress was merely described as "a female physician." She concluded on the basis of those definitions, that "a doctor, then, is something more than a doctress." As for Gregory, she caustically added that "he has not yet learned that women can elect for themselves the title of doctress, if they prefer it, and that women who have taken on the responsibilities of doctors, are not yet needing guardians, whose superior sense and judgment will select the proper title for them, and thus preserve the delicacy and feminine character necessary for their success." [63] Surprised by the resistance, the trustees voted to postpone any decision. Gregory, always a clever strategist, decided not to press the issue, but instead waited until 1864 when he was able to persuade the board to change the title.

61. Victor, p. 154.
62. Trustees Report, February 13, 1860; Samuel Gregory, Doctor or Doctress? (Boston, 1868).
63. Boston Evening Transcript, July 10, 1860.

Gregory also found himself besieged by the remaining lady managers who charged him with ignoring the needs of the hospital. Gregory had made no mention of the hospital in his annual reports and had made no effort to promote it. Frustrated by Gregory's unwillingness to cooperate, the managers wrote a letter to the trustees complaining that the hospital was suffering from a lack of publicity.[64]

The controversy surrounding Gregory led several of the trustees to consider dismissing him. It was clear to some of them that Zakrzewska would not remain if Gregory were retained; furthermore, some were convinced that Gregory's pamphlet attacks on a number of Boston physicians had severely handicapped the college's progress. Consequently, at their meeting in October 1860 the trustees decided not to reappoint Gregory as secretary and administrative officer. Gregory shrewdly offered to stay on as secretary until a replacement could be located. He spent the next several months mending fences and in June of the following year was able to get a majority of the trustees to rescind their previous vote. Angered by the reversal, four trustees (including the president of the board) immediately resigned.[65]

Not surprisingly, Zakrzewska decided in the same month that she would leave the college at the close of the 1862 spring term. Zakrzewska's decision alarmed Samuel Sewall, a wealthy Boston lawyer and later a pamphleteer for woman's rights,

64. "Records of Lady Managers," December 6, 1859; September 4, 1860. After the latter date, the women temporarily adopted the strategy of issuing their own annual report, independent of Gregory. This proved to be an insufficient measure.

65. Trustees Report, October 10, 1860, and June 5, 1861. Those resigning included: James Freeman Clarke, Gardner Drury, George Fabyan, William Thomas Minor, George Partridge Sanger, and Adam Wallace Thaxter, Jr. Enoch Rolfe described Gregory's strategy after his near defeat in 1860: "by coaxing some, getting the aid of some Trustees in the city, and some by a special effort from a distance, and by offering to do the work of the Secretary gratuitously, he succeeded in still holding the office" (Rolfe, p. 5).

who had been an influential trustee of the school since 1850. Sewall, whose daughter was currently studying under Zakrzewska at the college, asked her why she felt it necessary to take such a drastic step. Zakrzewska's response made it clear that she held little hope for the future of the school: "Not one of my expectations for a thorough medical education for women has been realized. . . . If it were the intention of the trustees to supply the country with underbred, ill-educated women under the name of physicians . . . I think the New England Female Medical College is on the right track." Zakrzewska went on to charge the college with granting medical degrees to women, the majority of whom could only be "good nurses . . . some . . . respectable midwives; and a very few, physicians." [66] This evaluation of the college alarmed Sewall, who appears to have been unaware of the educational problems at the school, and he wrote back to Zakrzewska to urge her not to mention these criticisms to the other trustees in her letter of resignation because it would "involve us all in a notoriety absolutely fatal to the whole cause." [67] Zakrzewska acquiesced; her letter of resignation simply stated that she was not happy with her position at the college and was therefore leaving it.[68]

Zakrzewska left to become the prime mover in the creation of the New England Hospital for Women and Children. Her resignation proved to be a catalyst as several of the medical

66. The only copy of the letter to Sewall is in Vietor, pp. 281–83. For a more detailed outline of Sewall's profeminist activities, see Nina Moore Tiffany, *Samuel E. Sewall: A Memoir* (Boston, 1898), pp. 127–46. After Sewall left the college he wrote a tract entitled "Legal Condition of Women in Massachusetts" (several editions: 1868, 1870, 1875); in 1870 he became a stockholder in the *Woman's Journal* Corporation and also president until his death in 1888.

67. Vietor, p. 283.

68. Ibid., pp. 283–84; "Records of the Trustees," June 1862. As earlier with Gassett, Waite ignores female versions of events in his *History*. On p. 52 he cites Zakrzewska's resignation as taking place in April 1862 and ignores the earlier letter she sent to Sewall even though he cites the Vietor biography in his footnotes.

college's faculty and trustees (including Sewall) withdrew to join Zakrzewska at her new hospital.[69] Gregory had won the battle against female influence, but he had lost the war. By 1862 he was in firm control of a college whose future looked bleak. When Zakrzewska left, the college lost not only its most capable faculty member, but also the only physician at the college who seemed aware of the growing trend toward hospital and clinical instruction as an integral part of medical education. In 1845, for example, most medical schools had either no clinical instruction at all or clinical instruction but no hospital instruction. But by 1865 two-thirds of the schools in the country provided both. In addition, Gregory's drive for personal power had alienated a number of the school's financial friends. Gregory was even willing to sacrifice the interests of the school to preserve that power. Consequently, when a benefactor offered to make a sizable donation to the college hospital, Gregory blocked the proposal. The lady managers noted that "Dr. Gregory opposed it so strenuously as to imply he would rather the college occupy hired rooms than to use a building paid for by a fund beyond his control." [70]

Two years of dissension had sapped the school's resources. The three faculty members who resigned in 1862 were forced to accept interest-bearing notes in lieu of their year's salary. Faltering finances made it impossible to meet the annual installment on the purchase of the hospital and it was closed on July 1, 1862, one week after the opening of Zakrzewska's Hospital for Women.[71]

Finally, in September 1865 a number of the school's benefactors demanded that the trustees investigate the problems.

69. Samuel Gregory Letterbook, August 22, 1863, New England Female Medical College Collection, BU-A. See also the annual reports of the New England Hospital for evidence of Sewall's continuing support of Zakrzewska.

70. "Records of Lady Managers," October 16, 1860; Rothstein, p. 282.

71. That the hospital could have become both self-supporting and an attractive clinical aspect of the college is evident from the history of the New England Hospital for Women and Children, which will be dealt with in greater detail in chapter 3.

When the board refused to act, Dr. Enoch Rolfe and Anna Goulding, a former agent of the college, gathered petitions asking the Massachusetts legislature to launch an inquiry. Significantly, 68 percent of the signatures were of women. Rolfe argued that the college was now financially worse off than in 1858 when the building program had been instituted. He put the blame squarely on Gregory's shoulders: "What a spectacle! Look! A man advocating the cause of female medical education, and yet not willing to trust women with business affairs." [72]

More serious charges of negligence and misapplication of funds were also leveled at Gregory and the trustees. The ensuing investigation demonstrated what was evident to anyone connected with the college. Gregory ran the college and the trustees were largely figureheads. More specifically, a number of trustees had been elected illegally, and one-quarter of the meetings had been conducted without a quorum.

The investigating committee also determined that funds had been used for other than their original purpose. The petitioners were rewarded by the finding of the committee that "the culpability for these acts rests chiefly with the Secretary and General Agent, Samuel Gregory." The legislature concluded its work by vacating all of the trusteeships and creating a new eight-man board. Then, inexplicably, the

72. Rolfe, p. 7. The statistic on the percentage of female signatures on the petition was obtained from the "Resolves," chap. 101, 1866, Waite, in *History*, incorrectly cites the percentage Samuel Gregory used on p. 3 of *The War Against the New England Female Medical College, Circular to the Members of the Massachusetts Legislature* (Boston, 1866). Gregory tried to diminish the size of the opposition. He claimed there were seventy-eight petitioners: twenty-nine men and forty-nine women. The actual petition shows ninety signatures: thirty-five men and fifty-five women. The text of the petitions read: "We, the undersigned friends and contributors of the NEFMC believing that it might and may take much higher rank among the institutions for which New England is so renowned and more fully secure the cooperation and approval of leading medical men and the confidence of the public generally hereby respectfully and earnestly pray that you would investigate the conditions. . . ."

legislators appointed three of the current trustees and one former member to the new board. Even stranger, the legislature did nothing when the new board reappointed Gregory to his old position of leadership.[73]

Once again, Gregory recovered from what had seemed certain defeat. But again the college paid the price. Sewall's advice to Zakrzewska in 1861 was soon shown to be sound. An investigation of the college had indeed proven "absolutely fatal to the whole cause." Newspaper stories of corruption and inferior education seriously damaged the school's reputation. The year after the scandal occurred, the school's enrollment dropped to a low of fifteen students and financial contributions dried up.[74]

Two major efforts were made during the final years of the decade to save the college. In 1868, in an effort to attract applicants, Gregory abandoned the use of the unpopular "doctress of medicine." Then, realizing that only a dramatic move could reverse the school's declining fortunes, the trustees began raising funds for a heavily mortgaged classroom facility which opened in 1870.[75] But it was too late. On March 23, 1872, Samuel Gregory died of consumption in his office at the college and with him went the last hopes of the school. Although Gregory's leadership had in no small part contributed to the college's decline, his enthusiasm had remained its only sustaining force. As secretary, chief administrator, and fund raiser, he had almost single-handedly run the college. His death left a vacuum difficult to fill.

Merger, a common solution for faltering medical colleges, appeared to be the only alternative to dissolution. Although the college was on the brink of collapse through mismanage-

73. "Resolves," chap. 101, 1866. Trustees Report, April 11, 1866.

74. Waite, *History*, p. 126. This appendix also contains a helpful summary of statistics on all the sessions of the college. See "Treasurer's Reports" and Waite, *History*, p. 61.

75. Trustees Report, February 4, 1867; "Brochure of New England Female Medical College, Laying of the Corner-Stone," Boston, June 9, 1870, BU-A.

ment, it did possess a number of attractive assets. In addition to the land, building, and equipment valued at $70,000, the school controlled $40,000 in endowments. Deducting the $43,000 in debts left the school with a net worth of about $67,000.

The only medical colleges in Boston at this time were Harvard and the recently founded Boston University Medical School, which was in the process of seeking a classroom building. Ironically, Harvard first expressed an interest in acquiring the Female Medical College. Its own medical facilities were completely inadequate; classrooms could not accommodate the students, and the laboratories had been designed for a student body one-third the size of the present class.[76] The situation had deteriorated to the point that President Charles Eliot in his annual report covering the academic year 1871–72 singled out the medical college for special criticism.[77] Previously Eliot had hinted in his 1869 inaugural speech that professional education for women at Harvard might be allowed.[78]

The records of the ensuing negotiations between Harvard and New England Female Medical College are brief and incomplete. A good deal appears to have been handled on an informal basis. The key figure in the bargaining was the Rev. Edward Everett Hale, a member of the Harvard Board of Overseers since 1866 and a friend of the Female Medical College. On May 29, 1872, Hale sent a letter to the trustees of the woman's college recommending the "uniting" of the two medical colleges.[79] A second letter was sent June 18 by Hale outlining the conditions for a transfer of the property.[80] Mean-

76. Jean A. Curran, "Charles William Eliot: Medical Messiah," *Harvard Medical Alumni Bulletin* (March–April 1971), p. 9.

77. Annual Report of the President and Treasurer of Harvard College (1871–1872), p. 36.

78. "Inaugural," Charles Eliot Papers, HCA; Hugh Hawkins, *Between Harvard and America: The Educational Leadership of Charles W. Eliot* (New York, 1972), p. 194.

79. Trustees Report, June 12, 1872, refers to the Hale letter of May 29, 1872, but the letter has not been preserved.

80. Ibid., refers to a letter of June 18, 1872.

while, the Female Medical College began negotiations with a committee interested in securing its building for the new medical school at Boston University.[81] By the fall of 1872 it appeared that the merger would take place with Harvard. On October 9 its overseers declared that it had no objections to the absorption of the woman's college as a separate department of the medical college, provided that its board of trustees supplied sufficient funds to implement the merger. They also stipulated that Harvard could discontinue the arrangement if the experiment should fail. Harvard's terms led Dr. Zakrzewska to oppose the merger on the grounds that it would provide the female students with separate and unequal education. Furthermore, she warned, Harvard could at some future date declare the experiment a failure and jettison the women.[82]

The appointment of the Rev. Edward Everett Hale on November 4 to a vacancy on the board of trustees of the Female Medical College appeared to herald the immediacy of the merger. Then disaster struck. Five days after Hale's appointment, the great Boston fire broke out, wiping out a large part of the city's business district. Thirteen of the sixteen trustees of the Female Medical College were businessmen and many of them sustained heavy losses in the fire. When Harvard demanded that an additional $50,000 be raised to implement the merger, the representatives of the Female Medical College broke off negotiations.[83]

The trustees, concerned with their own personal financial difficulties and anxious to free themselves of their responsibilities, shifted their attention to Boston University. Eager to

81. Ibid., July 12, 1872, reference to negotiations with Boston University; August 2, 1872, reference to negotiations with Harvard.

82. Vietor, p. 381. This is the only reference regarding Zakrzewska's position on the merger, although the *Boston Daily Advertiser*, February 12, 1874, has a brief reference indicating that she spoke against it along with Edward H. Clarke and Samuel E. Sewall. No petitions or transcripts regarding the testimony were preserved in the Senate documents; Trustees Report, October 9, 1872.

83. Trustees Report, March 1, 1873, and March 13, 1873.

acquire a building in order to commence operations, Boston University was willing to take over the Female Medical College in its present condition. Opposition to the proposal was raised by Dr. Zakrzewska, Samuel Sewall, a group of Boston woman physicians, and the executors of a number of the school's endowments.[84] However, their objections, which centered on the irregular nature of Boston University's medical curriculum—an unorthodox medical system known as homeopathy—were to no avail. On March 13, 1873, the trustees of the woman's college voted to transfer its property and interests on the condition that Boston University would assume its debts and guarantee that the college would be maintained "for all time, substantially in accordance with our charter." [85] Nevertheless, whatever the future held for women's medical education in Boston, the trustees' action guaranteed that a separate female medical school would not be part of it.

The failure of New England Female Medical College stemmed from a number of problems, some of which were rooted in society and others that were of Gregory's own making. Many of the school's failings can be traced to the resistance of the medical world to women. Few male physicians were willing to give the school a chance to prove itself. Doctors regularly turned out to oppose each new request for a charter change or for scholarship aid. According to one report, when a young doctor accepted an appointment at the college in 1865, "certain prominent physicians waited upon him and told him that if he wished to retain the friendship of the profession, he must not lecture." Another claimed that he had lost caste with his medical colleagues when he started teaching at the college. Whereas before taking the position he had been

84. *Boston Daily Advertiser*, February 12, 1874. On February 25, 1874, the *Boston Daily Advertiser* referred to testimony by Judge Thomas "representing some female physicians of the city [who] spoke against the proposed union contending that it was a judicial, not a legislative question." This testimony occurred in 1874 because the bill was introduced too late in the 1873 session to be heard.

85. Trustees Report, March 13, 1873.

treated with consideration, afterward "they would not appoint [him] a hog-reef!" When the school asked that its students be granted access to the female wards of Boston City Hospital, its twenty physicians summarily rejected the request.[86]

These reactions were not peculiar to Boston. As late as 1859 the Philadelphia County Medical Society passed "resolutions of excommunication against every physician who should teach in the [woman's medical college in the city], every woman who graduated from it, and everybody else who would consult with such teachers." Fifteen years later when the society issued a revision of its bylaws, it simply omitted all reference to its previous exclusion of women without any statement to the effect that both sexes were now eligible. The statewide Pennsylvania Medical Society was also reluctant to support women physicians: they adopted a formal resolution that stated specifically that though it did not bar women from admission to its ranks, there was nothing to commit the society "to acknowledge the right of women's medical colleges and associations of female physicians to representation in this society." [87]

86. "Resolves," chap. 101, 1866 (Approved May 30, 1866). In a handwritten document Samuel Gregory claimed that medical men in the legislature opposed efforts of the college in 1850, 1854, 1855, 1856. The City Hospital petition was refused in 1865. The physician who reneged on the appointment did so in the summer of 1865. See also: Gregory, *The War . . .* ; *BMSJ* 34 (1856), pp. 169–74; a copy of the latter, with the simple title "Female Physicians," was also distributed to the legislature by the medical profession in 1856 to oppose incorporation of the college. The reprinted article tried to link female physicians with abortionists: "That such persons [female physicians] should be unscrupulous in practicing the illegitimate arts of their calling, as well as its honorable duties, need surprise no one" (p. 172). The brochure singled out the three-month training period (which Rolfe himself criticized earlier) and noted that "the gross ignorance of two professedly educated females [in the city of Boston] had [recently] cost the life of one patient, and made another the subject of an infirmity which renders life a burden . . ." (p. 173).

87. *Boston Herald Traveler*, September 10, 1847; records on the Woman's Medical College of Pennsylvania, known as the Female Medical College of Pennsylvania until 1867, are very incomplete. Hiram Corson has drawn together the existing records for the period up to 1894 in regard to medical licensing in *A Brief History of Proceedings in the Medi-*

Nevertheless, Woman's Medical College of Pennsylvania did survive, while Gregory's college did not. Many considered New England Female Medical College's greatest handicap to be the image which Samuel Gregory had created for himself. While many doctors were naturally suspicious of his lack of medical training (although he managed to get an honorary M.D. degree by 1853), he infuriated obstetricians by his continued pamphlet attacks. The response to Gregory was as immoderate as he was in attacking the profession. One writer described Gregory's lecture against male midwives as "the smallest kind of potatoes, disgustingly affected with the rot; and was attended by a herd of human swine, such as might be expected to feed upon such kind of garbage." [88]

The net result of all of this was to make it impossible for the students to receive adequate training. Gregory's decision to sell the hospital facility in 1862 had denied the students what was fast becoming a necessary phase of medical education. By 1868 his school was the only one of five women's medical colleges in the country without its own hospital. In an effort to provide the students with some practical preparation, the school required them to study three years under a preceptor in addition to attending medical lectures. Many of the students, however, were unable to locate cooperative physicians, and the faculty was forced time after time to waive the preceptor requirement.[89]

---

cal Society of Pennsylvania . . . to Procure the Recognition of Women Physicians . . . (Norristown, Pa., 1894). In addition, records in the archives of the Woman's Medical College of Pennsylvania were examined, along with Clara Marshall, *The Woman's Medical College of Pennsylvania, An Historical Outline* (Philadelphia, 1897) and Guilielma Fell Alsop, *History of the Woman's Medical College, Philadelphia, Pennsylvania, 1850–1950* (Philadelphia, 1950). An extensive search has not turned up records for female medical colleges in other cities.

88. Samuel Gregory Scrapbook, n.p.

89. "Faculty of New England Female Medical College," February 19, 1856; February 20, 1857; February 15, 1858; November 15, 1859. No such notations appear after 1859, but this is not to say that the problem disappeared. Judging from the autobiographical writing of Zakrzewska for

In the final analysis, however, it was Gregory's inability to tolerate female participation that undermined the goals of the school. Ironically, an institution whose announced purpose was to give women a greater voice in medicine, was unwilling to give them even the smallest voice in its management. Gregory moved quickly to suppress even the slightest hint of independence by the lady managers, the students, and Zakrzewska. The result was the alienation of every source of female support. New England Female Medical College could possibly have overcome the animosity of the medical establishment, but it could not continue without feminist cooperation.

Furthermore, the patriarchal atmosphere at the college could not be anything but counterproductive. As important as the technical knowledge one acquired in medical school was the self-confidence necessary to implement it. As Gregory himself had noted, the profession would reward those women who possessed courage, independence, and perseverance.[90] Similarly, Dr. John Ware of Harvard Medical College advised his students to develop "an honest and well founded reliance upon [their] own judgment.[91]

But everything at New England Medical College worked against the development of these qualities. How could one build self-confidence when the instruction was so inferior?

1859–62, the problem seems to have worsened. When she left, standards rapidly deteriorated according to the 1866 legislative testimonials. See Vietor, pp. 249–87; "Resolves," chap. 101, 1866. Graduation statistics show that only about 35 percent of those who attended the New England Female Medical College between 1854 and 1873 received the M.D. degree. At least part of this high attrition may have been due to the difficulty of obtaining preceptors. Waite cites graduation rates for men's medical schools and these ranged from 48 to 51 percent for the period 1854 to 1873; he claims that this general trend held for all medical colleges in the United States at this time—See *History*, p. 86.

90. Samuel Gregory Letterbook, July 9, 1861, to Miss Annie Scanterbury, Charlestown, Prince Edward Island.

91. John Ware, "Success in the Medical Profession," *BMSJ* 43 (1851), pp. 496–504, 509–22. This speech was originally delivered on November 6, 1850, to the entire medical school class at Massachusetts Medical College (Harvard).

More important, how could a woman build self-confidence in a male-dominated school where women were deliberately excluded from decision-making? Even the male faculty members dealt with their students as their "handmaids" rather than future physicians. It is not surprising that Zakrzewska noted that the public treated the school's graduates more like well-trained nurses "than physicians who assume an authority which creates confidence." [92]

However, the passing of the school was an event mourned by a number of women. Although the merger with Boston University was marked by a celebration filled with speeches, music, and poetry, "a tinge of sadness was imparted to the closing, by a lady's singing 'Good night, my heart,' which showed too plainly," the *Boston Medical and Surgical Journal* noted, "that it was a match of interest rather than of affection." [93]

Yet, women had made significant progress since New England Female Medical College opened. Women had shown a disbelieving public that they could be trained as physicians. It was no longer a question of whether women could serve as physicians, but how competent they could become. What was necessary was a means by which women could prove they were as good as their male counterparts.

92. Vietor, pp. 251, 246.
93. *BMSJ* 89 (1873), p. 490.

3

Feminist Showplace

The disappearance of New England Female Medical College was due in no small measure to Gregory's failure to capitalize on the vast reservoir of female support that existed in Boston. Historians, by concentrating on the political side of feminism, have largely ignored the material and psychological support that the movement offered.[1] Nowhere is this better illustrated than in the case of the New England Hospital for Women and Children, established by Dr. Marie Zakrzewska, Gregory's old nemesis.

Zakrzewska has attracted relatively little attention from historians, although she was one of the most influential female physicians of the nineteenth century. In many ways she played a greater role in developing careers for women in American medicine than the more famous Blackwell sisters.[2] Born in

1. Books on political feminism include: Eleanor Flexner, *Century of Struggle: The Woman's Rights Movement in the United States* (Cambridge, Mass., 1959); Andrew Sinclair, *The Better Half: The Emancipation of the American Woman* (New York, 1965); Robert Riegel, *American Feminism* (Lawrence, Kansas, 1963); Aileen Kraditor, *Ideas of the Woman Suffrage Movement, 1890–1920* (New York, 1965); William O'Neill, *Everyone Was Brave: The Rise and Fall of Feminism in America* (Chicago, 1969); Anne F. Scott and Andrew M. Scott, *One Half the People: The Fight for Woman Suffrage* (Philadelphia, 1975).
2. Elizabeth Blackwell left America in 1869, spent most of her life in England, and died there in 1910. A recent, well-documented study is: Nancy Sahli, "Elizabeth Blackwell, M.D. (1821–1910): A Biography," Ph.D. dissertation, University of Pennsylvania, 1974. Emily Blackwell, who also died in 1910, was in many ways overshadowed by the fame of her older sister though she devoted her life to the practice of medicine in America. Both women have been the subject of many popular articles and biogra-

Berlin in 1829, her childhood experiences had a great deal to do with shaping her career. When Zakrzewska was ten, her father was dismissed from the Prussian army, forcing her mother to become a midwife and the family breadwinner. That same year Zakrzewska contracted an eye infection and was placed under the care of a physician who took a liking to her, allowed her to follow him on his hospital rounds, and loaned her medical books from his personal library. She quickly developed a keen interest in medicine and, as soon as she was old enough, began assisting in her mother's midwifery practice. At age twenty, after two years of petitioning the state authorities for a position in the government-sponsored midwifery school, Zakrzewska finally succeeded in gaining admission to the school at Charité Hospital, the largest hospital in Prussia. The fact that Zakrzewska was the youngest woman to have entered the school made her highly visible. In a short time, her medical aptitude and outstanding performance as a student won the admiration of Dr. Joseph Schmidt, the director of the hospital. A French midwife, Madame La Chapelle, had won international fame in obstetrics; Schmidt, in a burst of patriotic pride, predicted that Prussia, as well as France, might boast of "a La Chapelle" and, before Zakrzewska ever had an opportunity to earn the title, dubbed her "La Chapelle the Second." The name stuck and, like a self-fulfilling prophecy, Zakrzewska became his star pupil.

In 1852, a year after Zakrzewska's graduation, Schmidt, although critically ill, was able to overcome strong internal opposition against the appointment of a woman as his successor. Zakrzewska became the chief midwife and professor in the hospital's school for midwives with responsibility for more than 200 students, including men in the medical school. Unfortunately, the announcement of the appointment came only a few hours before Schmidt's death, and Zakrzewska was un-

---

phies. Zakrzewska's life, on the other hand, has gone relatively unnoticed except for two autobiographical memoirs cited in n. 3 below. Bibliographies of all three women are in Edward James (ed.), *Notable American Women* (Cambridge, Mass., 1971).

prepared for the jealousy and hospital politics that followed. Schmidt's protective sponsorship for three years had eliminated the necessity of her learning strategies for coping with competition in the hospital. Within six months, she found the job to be too burdensome and resigned, attempting for a time to establish a private midwifery practice. But an early taste of success in her field made it difficult for her to practice quietly and forget about assuming a larger role in medicine beyond that of an anonymous midwife. She recalled later: ". . . my education and aspirations demanded more than this." Not surprisingly, in view of the recent tide of emigration, her search for expanded opportunities turned to America. She remembered the positive reaction of Schmidt to the news of the establishment of the Female Medical College in Philadelphia: "In America, women will now become physicians like the men: it shows that only in a republic can it be proved that science has no sex." [3]

Convinced that she would find greater freedom to practice medicine in the United States, she sailed with her younger sister to New York in 1853. There she contacted a family friend, a German-American doctor, who quickly dispelled her illusions about American medicine. Pointing out that female physicians were of the lowest rank, even below that of a good nurse, he offered Zakrzewska a position as his own nurse, which she politely but firmly refused, unwilling "to be patronized in this way." [4] Handicapped by her difficulty in learning English and unsuccessful in attracting midwifery cases, she was soon forced to turn to the establishment of a cottage industry in her tenement apartment in New York. She and her sister began the production of worsted materials, employing as many as thirty girls at one time.

The success of her business in no way diverted Zakrzewska

3. Caroline Dall (ed.), *A Practical Illustration of Woman's Right to Labor or a Letter from Marie Elizabeth Zakrzewska* (Boston, 1869), pp. 60, 85; Agnes Vietor, *A Woman's Quest: The Life of Marie E. Zakrzewska* (New York, 1924), pp. 84–85.

4. Dall, p. 105.

from her goal of pursuing a medical degree, but her lack of contacts and difficulty in communicating made progress in this direction slow. Finally, a year after she had arrived in New York, she visited a Home for the Friendless and was able to describe her frustrated attempts to learn more about the Female Medical College in Philadelphia. The woman in charge introduced her to Dr. Elizabeth Blackwell, who, in addition to her regular medical practice, had opened a one-room dispensary on the East Side of New York for poor women and children. Blackwell not only offered to tutor the young immigrant in English in return for her aid at the dispensary, but also promised to help her gain admission to a medical college. Through Elizabeth Blackwell's efforts, Zakrzewska was accepted by the medical department of Cleveland Medical College (Ohio) from which Emily Blackwell had recently graduated. Up to this point, Zakrzewska had no sympathy for the woman's rights movement. The demands raised at one New York convention seemed so ridiculous that she found the caption in one newspaper, "The Hens Which Want to Crow," as "quite appropriate." However, when she received the news that ways and means had been found for her to attend medical school, she realized that she had been trying to crow as hard as any of the women without realizing it.[5]

A combination of Zakrzewska's neglect of her knitting business and changes in the fashions of the worsted industry had left her with little money for her education. Fortunately, Dr. Harriot Hunt had recently toured Ohio raising funds for female medical education in that state.[6] As a result of scholarship aid from this source, Zakrzewska's lecture fees were waived for an indefinite period, and since Elizabeth Blackwell supplied all the necessary medical textbooks, Zakrzewska only had to pay the twenty dollar matriculation fee. Furthermore, Caroline Severance, a friend of Blackwell's and president of a

5. Vietor, p. 134.
6. Ibid., p. 485.

ladies physiological society near Cleveland, agreed to pay for
her board out of a fund established by the society to assist
needy women medical students.[7] If one had attempted to construct a story revolving around the tangible benefit of sisterhood, one could hardly improve upon the example of Zakrzewska's early career.

It is impossible to exaggerate the importance of this web of
feminist friendship. One of only four women out of 200 students at the college, Zakrzewska encountered obstacles unknown to her male colleagues. It took several weeks for her,
even with the aid of a society woman's sponsorship (in this
case Caroline Severance), to locate a boarding house that
would accept a female medical student. Even here, the other
boarders would quickly leave when Zakrzewska and her room-
mate, another female medical student, entered the room.[8]
Upon completion of her medical education, Zakrewska returned to New York ready to hang out her shingle and begin
private practice. Once again, however, she encountered resistance unknown to a male physician. The ordinarily simple
task of securing an office elicited three types of negative response, all pointing out the stigma attached to being a female
physician in the 1850s. One group of landlords could not
accept the notion of a female physician and refused to rent
space to her on the grounds that she was probably masking
her real identity as a spiritualist or clairvoyant. The second
group accepted her credentials, but doubted that she would
be able to support herself and pay the rent. The third group
asked no questions, but demanded such expensive rents that
she could not afford to lease their quarters. After a month of
fruitless searching, Elizabeth Blackwell allowed her to open
an office in her back parlor.[9]

The burden of locating an office paled in comparison with
the difficulty of finding patients to develop a medical practice.

7. Ibid., pp. 119–21.
8. Ibid, p. 131.
9. Ibid., pp. 179–81.

Rothstein has described the necessary elements for success in the nineteenth-century medical world: "Family background and wealth, social standing, and friendships were paramount in gaining admission to a medical school, setting up a practice, obtaining appointments to hospitals, medical schools, and elite medical societies, and attracting a wealthy clientele." [10] A female physician began her pursuit of a career severely stigmatized because of her sex, and this fact hindered her in every step she took in establishing herself as a professional. Elizabeth Blackwell had already experienced every possible discouragement in her five years in New York. She was barred from practice in the city hospitals and dispensaries, ignored by her medical colleagues, and was the target of anonymous hate mail. She had solved the problem of office space by buying her own home and she had dealt with the loneliness by adopting a seven-year-old orphan in 1854. By the time Zakrzewska joined Blackwell, she was eagerly awaiting the return of her sister Emily who had been studying medicine for two years in Edinburgh.

In numbers there was strength as well as sociability. Both Zakrzewska and Elizabeth Blackwell were eager to reestablish the dispensary in which Zakrzewska had first assisted Blackwell and which failed for lack of funds. Zakrzewska, drawing

10. William G. Rothstein, *American Physicians in the Nineteenth Century: From Sects to Science* (Baltimore, 1972), pp. 206–07. Although there were important differences in the social stratification systems of England and America in the mid-nineteenth century, it is interesting to note how similar the plight of the beginning physician was in both countries—even without the added difficulty of sex discrimination. For an analysis of the problems of the male physician who started out alone in London, see M. Jeanne Peterson, "Kinship, Status, and Social Mobility in the Mid-Victorian Medical Profession," Ph.D. dissertation, University of California, Berkeley, June 1972, p. 153: ". . . for all the growth in medical education and licensing and the advancement of medical science, the basis on which Victorian medical men built their careers was not primarily that of expertise. Family, friends, connections, and new variations of these traditional forms of social relationships and social evaluation were the crux of a man's ability to establish himself in medical practice." Peterson uses statistical and biographical materials to substantiate this thesis.

on her business experience, drew up an operating budget for
the proposed hospital. She then threw herself into fund
raising and traveled to Boston to meet with Harriot Hunt,
Caroline Severance (who had moved to that city), and a number of other local women interested in woman's rights. She
was able to extract a promise of $650 to be paid over a three-
year period to the new hospital. This promise stimulated
donors in New York to raise an additional $1,000, enough to
open New York Infirmary for Women and Children on May 1,
1857; it was the first hospital staffed by women in the United
States.[11]

For two years Zakrzewska served without salary as resident
physician and general manager of the hospital, sharing with
the Blackwell sisters the responsibilties connected with a growing institution. By 1859, with the infirmary firmly established,
Zakrzewska felt that she had fulfilled her debt to the Black-
wells. Moreover, her own financial situation had improved as
a result of her private practice. In March of that year she
accepted an offer from Gregory's college to be professor of
obstetrics and resident physician of the proposed hospital. At
least three factors appear to have influenced her decision: the
conviction that achievement would add to a woman's personal
happiness; a desire for greater independence and leadership:
and a conviction that the women of Boston were intent in
"their desire to elevate the education of womankind in general and in medicine especially." In a letter to Harriot Hunt,
Zakrzewska revealed how depressing she found working with
the Blackwell sisters, especially after opening New York
Infirmary. The two women had such gloomy outlooks on life
that Zakrzewska found them bewildering: ". . . these two
women for instance have all right to be satisfied with their
efforts as it resulted . . . but they won't acknowledge it either
to each other or to themselves. . . . I feel sad that nothing
can cheer them up . . . they do wrong not to reward their
friends by showing them a pleased countenance." Zakrzewska's

11. Vietor, p. 211.

letter was filled with good wishes for all her friends in Boston, especially Hunt, whose pleasure in personal achievement was uninhibited and who had been hostess to Zakrzewska for several of her visits.[12]

As we have seen, Zakrzewska failed to realize her second objective in coming to Boston and resigned in 1862 after repeated clashes over school policy with Gregory. Yet, despite the problems connected with the Female Medical College, her experience there only reinforced her original convictions that a supportive body of women shared her belief in medical education for women: "I decided to work again on the old plan, namely to establish the education of female students on sound principles, that is to educate them in hospitals." [13] Hospital training was increasingly becoming recognized as an essential ingredient in a complete medical education,[14] yet the only American hospital open to women was the New York Infirmary. Fundamental to Zakrzewska's plans for a training hospital was her conviction that medical colleges such as Harvard would accept women students once pioneers like herself had demonstrated that women could perform a meaningful role in medicine.

Sound principles for Zakrzewska also meant uniting with the regular physicians and avoiding any association with the irregulars, particularly the homeopaths. In an effort to counter

12. Ibid., pp. 237–39, 149, 186, 192, 197; Marie Zakrzewska to Harriot Hunt, May 14, 1857, Caroline Dall Collection, MHS.

13. Vietor, p. 292.

14. Rosemary Stevens notes that the first use of the term "intern" in American hospital records was apparently in the Boston City Hospital Board of Trustees Report for 1865 (*American Medicine and the Public Interest* [New Haven, 1971], pp. 116–17). See also "Background and Development of Residency Review and Conference Committees," *JAMA* 165 (1957), pp. 60–64. By 1904 the AMA Council on Medical Education found that as many as 50 percent of new medical graduates went on to hospital training; by 1914 it was estimated that 75 or 80 percent of graduates were taking an internship (see Stevens, p. 118). Rothstein claims that by 1865 about two-thirds of medical schools made arrangements for some hospital and clinical instruction of students—see p. 282.

the conventional medical histories which dismiss the irregulars as quacks, recent historians have supplied us with a useful reinterpretation by focusing on the positive contributions of the irregulars. No doubt a thorough analysis of the irregulars will contribute to a new understanding of one particular strand of feminist ideology. Similarly, in order to understand the difficulties that have beset women seeking professional medical careers, we must study the pioneer women (such as Zakrzewska) with a view to understanding why they chose not to identify with the irregulars.

From both a political and a medicoscientific point of view, Zakrzewska was convinced that women must follow the regular medical path. Formally trained as both a midwife and a physician, she had little patience with those whose remedies verged more on mind cure than body cure. Her experience with the male-dominated medical world of Europe coupled with her initial experiences as a struggling immigrant made her a realist about the significance of professional power. For her, the only solution for medical women was to force men to deal with them as equals.

Accordingly, New England Hospital for Women and Children, a "sunny, airy house" at 60 Pleasant Street in Boston's South End, was rented for $600 and opened July 1, 1862. When it was incorporated the following March, its charter spelled out the two primary goals of the hospital: to furnish women with medical aid from competent physicians of their own sex, and to provide educated women with an opportunity for practical study in medicine. Significantly, two-thirds of the first board of directors were the same women who had served on the board of lady managers of Gregory's college.[15] There was no qualified woman surgeon available, so Zakrzewska was forced to employ a leading male gynecologist, Dr. Horatio Storer in 1863; when he resigned three years later, he was re-

15. Vietor, pp. 486–87. See also the "Records of the Lady Managers of the New England Female Medical College," BU-A, and the first Annual Report of the New England Hospital (1864).

placed by a female specialist, making the hospital the first in New England to be entirely staffed by women physicians.

In the first few years these women physicians were a union of the weak, rather than a combination of the strong. For example, Zakrzewska recalled how she felt in 1863: "My co-workers were young and inexperienced, looking up to me for wisdom and instruction while the public in general watched with scrupulous zeal in order to stand ready for condemnation." Fortunately, there were a few male physicians who were willing to cross the sexual boundary. Samuel Cabot and Henry I. Bowditch, both Harvard educated, had told her they would "refuse all aid" so long as she remained at Gregory's school; they readily came to her assistance when she left.[16]

Cabot became the first consulting physician at the hospital, offering his advice in difficult cases. He also provided Zakrzewska with important psychological support. She recounted in a letter to Dr. Lucy Sewall that Cabot did not feel it necessary for her to call him for forceps deliveries. "You see," she wrote proudly, "he rightly supposes we use the forceps *skillfully*." Bowditch had initially befriended Zakrzewska when she came to Boston in 1856 to solicit funds for New York Infirmary. She later recalled: "He remained the steadfast champion of medical women and continued as consulting physician to the New England Hospital until his death in 1892." Another physician, Benjamin Cotting, was especially helpful in sending both rich and poor patients to the hospital. Both were welcome: one group contributed much-needed fees as private patients; students treated the others in the dispensary. Such gestures, infrequent as they were, were a welcome tonic to someone generally treated as a pariah by the city's medical establishment. As Zakrzewska noted: "Every slight word or act of endorsement, even though with reservations, was like a ray of hope that at last the dawn was breaking. . . . Such consolations helped to uphold me." [17]

16. Vietor, pp. 330, 256.
17. Ibid., pp. 301, 336, 256, 332, 330–31.

Although Zakrzewska praised the early male consultants, except for Henry Bowditch they were for the most part fair-weather friends who withdrew support temporarily whenever there was too much pressure from the Boston medical establishment. Thus, when Zakrzewska took their advice and applied for membership in the Massachusetts Medical Society and was turned down because of her sex, Cabot and Cotting severed their ties with the hospital until the issue faded. Nevertheless, Zakrzewska felt their presence served to quiet those in the profession "who wanted to find fault but did not dare to do so openly so long as the two or three professional men stood as a moral force behind me." [18]

Finances were a problem of another dimension and, in the early years at least, were a major difficulty, even threatening the hospital's existence. The combined assets of the new institution in 1862 consisted of some $150 worth of hospital furniture brought from New England Female Medical College after Gregory evicted the lady managers and Zakrzewska. As the secretary of the board described the situation: "Our possessions were a few iron bedsteads, a few chairs, and bookcases, some straw, etc., our earnest purpose and our admirable Dr. Zakrzewska." [19] No gifts, however small, were refused, and the early annual reports are filled with lists of donations ranging from scissors and bandages to tea and cornstarch.

An important source of income during the hospital's first decade was an annual grant of $1,000 for maternity patients from the trustees of Boston Lying-In Hospital Corporation, which did not operate from 1856 to 1873 because it could not obtain patients.[20] In 1864, supported by a $5,000 grant from the Massachusetts legislature and matched by a number of

18. Ibid., pp. 277–78, 330.
19. Cited by Alice B. Crosby, *The Fiftieth Anniversary of the New England Hospital for Women and Children, October 29, 1912* (Boston, 1913), p. 17.
20. See the annual reports of the New England Hospital for Women and Children (AR-NEH) from 1863 to 1871; the 1871 report indicates final payment from the Lying-In Hospital Corporation, November 7, 1871.

donors, the hospital moved to larger quarters at 14 Warren Street. The state also offered additional assistance in the form of $1,000 each year for four years beginning in 1868. Fairs were also important sources of revenue; in 1871, $12,000 was realized in this fashion. Sizable donations from women during these formative years played a crucial role in the hospital's development. Zakrzewska's reputation inspired confidence as evidenced by a $2,000 bequest from the estate of Mrs. Robert G. Shaw that same year "to be used by Dr. Zakrzewska in aid of any Hospital or Infirmary . . . which may be under her superintendence in the City of Boston at the time of my decease." This money, coupled with other gifts (notably a $5,000 bequest from Miss Nabby Joy), enabled the hospital to move again in 1872 to what was to become its permanent location in the highlands section of Roxbury. By 1872 New England Hospital for Women and Children had become, in just ten years, one of the largest hospitals in Boston.[21]

The financial situation was further aided by the fact that a number of the staff, including Zakrzewska, donated their services. Driven by her desire to improve the cause of women in medicine, Dr. Lucy Sewall, for example, served as resident physician of the hospital for three years beginning in 1863 without salary or vacation.[22] Zakrzewska supported herself through her private practice and by renting rooms in her home in Roxbury to invalid boarders. Even in her personal practice, Zakrzewska sought to expand the role of women. Thus, she regularly walked to night calls in any type of weather to prove "that a woman has not only the same (if not

21. AR-NEH (1871), p. 17; Vietor, p. 353. Francis H. Brown, M.D., *The Medical Register for the Cities of Boston, Cambridge, and Chelsea* (Boston, 1873) deliberately downplayed the importance of New England Hospital by omitting it from its otherwise comprehensive listing of Boston hospitals. The judgment of the comparative size of New England Hospital is based on 1872 statistics given for the other Boston hospitals listed in the directory. Significantly, New England Hospital is the only "hospital" listed in the "Other Institutions and Societies" category of both directories.
22. Vietor, p. 348; *WJ*, February 22, 1890, p. 61.

more) physical endurance as a man." Women physicians were
handicapped by more than inclement weather in their pursuit
of night calls. Zakrzewska always went with the messenger who
called her. If he was unable to accompany her on her return home, she walked with the local policeman to the limit
of his beat and traveled in similar fashion from one beat to
another until she arrived home. This problem was solved in
1865 when she bought a horse and a secondhand buggy, which
also enabled her to "uphold the professional etiquette and
dignity of a woman physician on equality with men." [23]

Nevertheless, it is doubtful that Zakrzewska and her hospital could have succeeded without the support of the feminist
movement. During its first fifty years, the hospital had only
three presidents; Lucy Goddard, Ednah Cheney, and Mrs.
Helen F. Kimball. Ednah Cheney exemplifies the close bond
between feminism and the hospital. One of the lady managers
of the Female Medical College, Cheney was active at every
stage of the hospital's development, beginning with her pledge
along with three other women in 1862 to pay the first year's
rent on the first building on Pleasant Street. A close friend
and later neighbor of Zakrzewska, she served on the board of
directors of the hospital for 48 years—including 15 as president. In addition to her hospital activities, Cheney helped
found the New England Women's Club, served on the executive committee of the New England Woman Suffrage Association, and actively campaigned for women's right to vote in
school committee elections. Cheney was not unique, and an
analysis of the early bequest lists show that the hospital donors
often left funds to suffrage associations. In 1887 over 80 percent of the donors to a $10,000 hospital fund were women.[24]

To view feminism as simply a struggle for woman's rights
and the vote is to ignore the support and companionship it

23. Marie Zakrzewska to Paulina Pope, October 28, 1901, New England
Hospital Papers, SSC–SC.
24. Vietor, p. 335; Ednah Dow Cheney, *Transcript of the Memorial
Meeting of the New England Women's Club* (Boston, 1905), SA; bequest
lists appear in the annual reports of the New England Hospital.

offered those women who had broken with their prescribed roles. It is clear that a female physician could not have functioned autonomously in nineteenth-century America. Zakrzewska's dependence on the woman's movement was total: she needed female supporters to help finance her education, to raise money, to promote the hospital, to help administer it, to serve as patients, and—probably most critically—to proffer their friendship during difficult times. It was Zakrzewska herself who had originally suggested an association of women which was translated into the New England Women's Club and which met initially in the home of Harriot Hunt. For many women, it was the first time they came together not because of family, neighborhood, or church, but as women. The club regularly supported the women doctors; for instance, it sponsored a "social levee" when Dr. Lucy Sewall went to Europe to study. The members also were active in running fairs to raise money for the hospital. In turn, female doctors regularly gave lectures to the women at the club and sponsored discussion groups.[25]

One of the most openly militant supporters of the woman physician was the *Woman's Journal*, which was edited by Lucy Stone and began publication in Boston in 1870. Zakrzewska had called for a such a journal as early as 1862 when she and another woman doctor, Mary Breed, inserted a notice for a *Woman's Journal* in the *Liberator*, but at that date they were unable to secure enough support.[26] Lucy Stone's *Woman's Journal* championed the cause of women doctors and challenged the right of society to erect barriers to stand in their way. The editors encouraged reader response to this problem and

25. Mrs. Walter A. Hall, Mrs. Joseph S. Leach, and Mrs. Frederick G. Smith, *Progress and Achievement: A History of the Massachusetts State Federation of Women's Clubs, 1893–1962* (Lexington, Mass., 1962), p. 16; Julia A. Sprague, *History of the New England Women's Club from 1868–1893* (Boston, 1894), p. 3; "Record Book of the Weekly Social Meetings, New England Women's Club, 1869–1871," and records of discussion groups for entire period of its history, New England Women's Club Collection, SA.
26. *Liberator,* June 27, 1862.

published in full the letters of angry women doctors who felt blocked in their careers. An 1871 letter to the paper cautioned: "Let [men] not feel too sure that they alone hold the key that unlocks the door to medical science. They bar and bolt the doors of their hospitals in Boston against all women medical students. They heap upon them undeserved ridicule. They hold up to the world their constitutional weaknesses in a manner to lead one to suppose that they possess no such weaknesses themselves. They scorn the very idea of holding a consultation with a woman physician. . . . True women physicians would be glad to have the men in the profession see the mistake they are making and become their friends as they ought, in this manner. They would be glad to see the city hospitals and dispensaries opened to women medical students. They blush for the city of Boston that this is not done." The writer concluded by warning: "But, aided or unaided, the day is not far distant when women will compel medical men to know that as physicians they are their equals, whether they have the magnanimity to acknowledge it or not." [27]

Each act of exclusion by the medical establishment brought the wrath of the journal down on the heads of the perpetrators. Pointing out that Boston's Free Hospital for Women was served entirely by male physicians, the editor noted: "This is a shame in a city where there are competent women physicians. It is a poor, empty and prating pretense, that of indelicacy of common study, by those men who clutch at and crowd for medical practice among women." [28] The journal also did a great deal in advertising the success of women in medicine. It was happy to report that a research article of Dr. Sara E. Brown, which had been refused by the *Boston Medical and Surgical Journal* "on account of her sex," was published by the *Archives of Ophthalmology and Otology* and reproduced in a number of international medical periodicals, thus gain-

27. *WJ*, July 29, 1871.
28. Ibid., November 8, 1879.

ing wider publicity than it would have received from the Boston publication.[29]

New England Hospital gained a great deal of free publicity in the pages of the *Woman's Journal*. Each year it published a lengthy report on the hospital's progress. Readers were reminded of their obligation to support this feminist project and urged to attend each fund-raising fair. Women doctors were especially hard hit by the medical strictures against advertising in the public press while at the same time their professional brethren refused to recognize their existence and include them in the directories put out by doctors themselves. For example, the *Medical Register of Boston* refused to list the names of the women physicians even after it began to include all manner of peripheral practitioners such as artificial limb makers, collectors, makers of optical instruments, vendors of patent medicines, and female nurses. In order to fight the prejudice confronting them, the women physicians had to advertise. Here the *Woman's Journal* was a valuable ally. It did all it could to right the balance by publishing testimonials about the competence of women physicians such as one from "M. W.," a schoolteacher, who described how she had been restored to health by Dr. Zakrzewska's "skill and kindness, a debt that words are feeble to portray." Similarly, the journal publicized each addition to the hospital staff. Thus, Dr. Fanny Berlinerblau was introduced in a typical report that told the story of her difficulties in securing a medical education, extolled her "admirable scientific training," and informed the readers that she had abbreviated her name to Dr. Fanny Berlin "to suit the American tongue."[30] But the *Journal's* public relations efforts on behalf of the hospital could only do so much; in the final analysis, the hospital's performance would be the ultimate arbiter of its fate.

The two primary objectives of the New England Hospital

29. Ibid., December 12, 1874.
30. Ibid., April 14, 1877; May 26, 1883; December 3, 1887.

were to provide women with medical aid from doctors of their
own sex and to contribute to the supply of competent women
doctors by providing them with an opportunity for practical
clinical experience. While specializing in obstetrics, gynecology, and pediatrics, the hospital also offered a full range of
medical treatment, including surgery on a bed patient as well
as a dispensary basis. Zakrzewska's hospital filled an important
void in Boston medicine. Boston City Hospital, which opened
two years after Zakrzewska's institution, did not provide gynecological treatment until 1873, and then only on an outpatient
basis. It did not create a gynecological department until 1892.
Massachusetts General Hospital, which had been operating
since 1822, did not provide obstetrical services until the
twentieth century. At the time of its inception, New England
Hospital was unique in its provision for both obstetrical and
gynecological treatment of patients. The only other hospital
in the city to have specialized in obstetrics, Boston Lying-In
Hospital, had closed its doors in 1856, "a white elephant of
mastodonic proportions." Every effort had been made to attract patients, including a massive advertising campaign in
eighty-five newspapers, but women, if they had any choice in
the matter, avoided using Boston Lying-In.[31]

The unwillingness of such women reflected an accurate as-
sessment of the dangers connected with most maternity hospitals. Puerperal disease, which frequently resulted in death,
stemmed from the unsanitary techniques that were character-
istic of midcentury hospitals. There were a few physicians
early in the nineteenth century who had suspected the cause
of the high mortality rates of women in childbirth. Dr. Oliver
Wendell Holmes, for example, had attended a lecture in Paris
in 1833 which suggested that doctors themselves may have
played a role in communicating the disease. In 1843 he read a

31. Frederick C. Irving, *Safe Deliverance* (Boston, 1942), pp. 122–23;
Frederic A. Washburn, *The Massachusetts General Hospital: Its Development, 1900–1935* (Boston, 1939), pp. 364–65; Committee of the Hospital
Staff, *A History of the Boston City Hospital from Its Foundation until
1904* (Boston, 1906), pp. 157–58.

paper on his research findings to his Boston medical colleagues
and published an article which demonstrated that the obstetrician, midwife, and nurse were active agents in transmitting
the infection from one mother to another. He was promptly
rebutted by Dr. Walter Channing who delivered a paper on
the noncontagious nature of the disease, although Channing
later reversed his position.[32]
Zakrzewska's work in the large Charité Hospital in Berlin
had given her far more opportunity than most American physicans to observe the unsanitary conditions which were condu-
cive to spreading puerperal disease. Her experience confirmed
Holmes's theory. She had observed that when the medical students appeared in the Berlin hospitals with their forceps,
"untimely rupturing the membranes or by other meddlesome
interference with nature," the cases of the disease soared.
During her appointment as chief midwife in Berlin in 1852,
not a single case of the disease occurred because of the pre-
cautions that she took in the administration of the hospital.
Zakrzewska's scientific acumen and her experience with the
advantages of cleanliness were enormous assets to the hospital
in its early years when bacteriology and asepsis were still
matters of debate. A number of leading Boston physicians,
including Walter Channing, C. P. Putnam, Henry I. Bowditch, and Samuel Cabot signed an 1864 circular attesting to
the hospital's success in preventing various contagious fevers,
so impressed were these men with Zakrzewska's leadership in
this matter.[33]

32. Irving, pp. 145–59; Eleanor M. Tilton, *Amiable Autocrat: A Biography of Dr. Oliver Wendell Holmes* (New York, 1947), pp. 169–76, 366,
409–10.
33. Marie E. Zakrzewska, "Report of One Hundred and Eighty-Seven
Cases of Midwifery in Private Practice," *BMSJ* 121 (1889), pp. 557–58;
ibid., "Report of the Attending Physician," AR-NEH (1868), pp. 9–21. An
excellent source of information on maternity practices in the New England
Hospital is Emma L. Call, "The Evolution of Modern Maternity Technic,"
American Journal of Obstetrics and Diseases of Women and Children 58,
no. 3 (1908), pp. 392–404. Call, whose association with the hospital began
in 1868, documents and analyzes the puerperal disease statistics of the

By contrast, Boston Lying-In Hospital, reopened in 1873, was forced to close three times in the next thirteen years because of puerperal epidemics within its wards. In 1883, at the height of a puerperal disease epidemic in Boston, only one of the patients in New England Hospital died from the fever. In contrast, over 500 women contracted the disease and 50 died from it at Boston Lying-In Hospital from 1878 to 1883. Whether women physicians offered medical care superior to their male counterparts remains speculative, especially in view of the dearth of evidence related to treatment and the difficulties connected with comparing different patient populations. One researcher, whose pioneering investigation of this question involved an examination of doctor's comments on patient records at four different nineteenth-century Boston hospitals, concluded that the male practitioners reflected a negative or even hostile attitude toward their female patients. Complaints that the maternity patients were too lazy to "work" in delivering their babies or that their infections were their own fault were quite common. On the other hand, she found that these remarks were absent from the patient records at New England Hospital.[34] While it is difficult to assess the effect of physician's attitudes on their patients, it would be wrong to underestimate it.

One can make a strong case that a good deal of New England Hospital's success can be attributed to the fact that the physicians there were also women with special insights and sensivitity toward the medical problems of their own sex. In an age when medical techniques were generally undeveloped

hospital from 1862 to 1907. Her article is an invaluable source of information on the hospital procedures of this period and it quotes from internal reports of the New England Hospital. For the earliest period there is a printed circular, 1864, with letter from John H. Stephenson endorsed by Drs. Horatio Storer, Walter Channing, C. P. Putnam, S. Cabot, and Henry I. Bowditch in New England Hospital Collection, SA; Irving, p. 143, and annual reports of Boston Lying-In Hospital.

34. Lauri Crumpacker, "Female Patients in Four Boston Hospitals of the 1890's," Paper delivered at the Berkshire Conference on the History of Women, October 26, 1974; on file in SA.

and often unsafe, the women physicians' restraint, coupled with compassion, may have done much to effect a healthier hospital environment. For example, unlike many male doctors, the women seem to have been more willing to let nature take its course in childbirth. Avoiding the temptation to demonstrate their virtuosity with scalpel and forceps, the female physicians also avoided the medical dangers these instruments caused to both mother and child.[35]

Much of the work of the hospital in the nineteenth century was given over to charity cases. A number of "Free Hospital Beds" were donated by friends of the hospital. The dispensary charged ten cents a visit and twenty-five cents to fill a prescription at the hospital pharmacy, but those who could not afford these modest fees were treated without charge. Zakrzewska, who supervised the dispensary during the early years, noted: "A crowd of women, some from towns miles distant, came every morning." [36] One of her difficulties was to persuade wealthy women not to use the dispensary but rather to visit staff members who maintained a private practice. In one letter, she urged a friend of the hospital to recommend the services of two women physicians on the staff who were just starting their private practices: "Be sure to send them all the rich patients by telling [the patients] plainly that I don't want them." [37] In fact, charity cases became such an important part of the hospital case load that Lucy Sewall complained that many of the sick poor supposed the physicians were paid by the city, "and that they had a legal right to their services." [38]

The large number of charity and obstetrical patients in the

35. Ibid. See also Virginia G. Drachman, "Women's Health Through Case Records," Paper delivered at the Third Berkshire Conference on the History of Women, Bryn Mawr College, June 10, 1976.

36. Alice B. Crosby, *The Story of New England Hospital for Women and Children Through Seventy-Five Years 1862–1937* (Boston, December 10, 1937), pp. 4 and 13.

37. Marie Zakrzewska to Caroline Dall, March 6, 1869; ibid., March 26, 1869, Caroline Dall Collection, MHS.

38. Crosby, p. 11.

early years led the hospital to establish the first social service department in an American hospital. Each patient was interviewed; for those women who had no family, places were found for them to board both prenatally and postnatally. Jobs were also found for those women who were the sole support of their children. The women who provided these counseling services were the same lady managers whom Samuel Gregory found so annoying at Female Medical College. At the hospital, Zakrzewska used their desire to serve in a way which she described as mutually enriching: "It is thus the privilege of the [lady manager] to round off and finish the large charity done by the physicians, while she herself has her sympathies quickened and her experiences enlarged by intimate acquaintances with life flowing in different channels from her own." [39] The number of patients serviced by the hospital grew steadily throughout the century. During its first sixteen months, the hospital treated 1,507 individuals; by the end of the century more than 19,000 patients annually passed through the dispensary doors. There were now specialized clinics for eye, ear, nose, and throat; maternity; and child health. The sophisticated turn-of-the-century hospital was a far cry from the single room that Zakrzewska supervised in 1862.[40]

By 1900 the hospital had made a great deal of progress. Most important, it had at least convinced its patients that women could be successful physicians. Far better than statistics in showing how far the hospital had come was Zakrzewska's encounter at the end of the century with an Irish immigrant, whose wife had been a charity case at the original

39. Vietor, pp. 497–98; Grace E. Rochford, M.D., "The New England Hospital for Women and Children," *JAMWA* 5 (1950), p. 497; Felicia A. Banas, M.D., "The History of the New England Hospital," *JAMWA* 10 (1955), p. 199; AR-NEH (1864), p. 4, and succeeding reports which annotate the social services rendered patients. A similar service was not established at Massachusetts General Hospital until 1905 and at Boston City Hospital until 1918. See Washburn, p. 570, and John J. Byrne (ed.), *A History of the Boston City Hospital 1905–1964* (Boston, 1964), p. 372.

40. Crosby, p. 13; AR-NEH (1863), p. 11; AR-NEH (1900), p. 23.

Pleasant Street location. He wanted to arrange an operation for one of his family, and he insisted on having one of the woman physicians at New England Hospital. When he noticed Zakrzewska's surprise, he explained: "Well, Doctor, when I came to this country with my wife, we were very poor and knew nothing. The good women of the Pleasant Street Dispensary attended to us and taught us to take care of ourselves. All our children were born under their care and they watched that we did right by them, all without any charge. Now that we can afford good pay, I am sure we want the same, for I swear by the woman doctors." [41]

The second objective of the hospital was to provide educated women with an opportunity for practical study in medicine. One of the most difficult obstacles to the advance of women in medicine during the latter half of the nineteenth century was the lack of adequate facilities for clinical instruction. When women sought to gain this practical experience to supplement their classroom education, they were rebuffed because of the alleged indecency of observing cases in the presence of men—despite the fact that very frequently the patients themselves were females. The existence of this deep-seated opposition to the participation of women in clinical situations is dramatically illustrated by the experience of women at Philadelphia's Pennsylvania Hospital in 1869. Some thirty female medical students were invited to clinical lectures, but the male students objected "with insolent and offensive language." During the last hour, despite the efforts of members of the faculty, the men showered the women with "missiles of paper, tinfoil, and tobacco quids." Thus ended the effort at coeducation at the Pennsylvania Hospital.[42] It was obvious that with the exclusion of women from existing hospitals, they needed their own institutions in order to obtain clinical instruction. Zakrzewska's hospital anticipated a need that was only sur-

41. Vietor, p. 469: AR-NEH (1911), p. 10.
42. Evening Bulletin, (Philadelphia), November 15, 1869. Cited by Clara Marshall, M.D., The Woman's Medical College of Pennsylvania: An Historical Outline (Philadelphia, 1897), p. 20.

facing in 1862. Luckily, only a small number of women doctors applied to the hospital in the 1860s, for the staff was inadequate and the facilities severely limited. Of the twenty-seven interns in the first ten years of the hospital's existence, twelve were graduates of a medical college before coming to the hospital and the other fifteen were stimulated by their experience to complete the academic requirements for the degree shortly after leaving the hospital. While it was fairly commonplace for Boston hospitals to accept male "House Pupils" who had not yet earned their M.D. degree, what was unusual about New England Hospital interns was the distance they had to travel to finish a degree or to obtain advanced training. Five young women went to Europe for medical study, two of whom were pursuing postdoctoral training; seven went to the University of Michigan; four to the Woman's Medical College of Pennsylvania; one to Howard University. The reason, of course, was that in the early years, there were few medical schools open to women students. Zakrzewska was never enthusiastic about Gregory's school when he was alive, and after the merger with Boston University she refused to recommend students to or accept applications from what was in its early years, the city's only coeducational medical school, because of its irregular curriculum.[43]

The actual training that the hospital provided appears to

43. AR-NEH (1863). Statistics on the early graduates, even names and dates, are extremely unreliable if one uses the compilations in the New England Hospital "fact sheets" published in the twentieth century, for example, one entitled "Former Interns of the New England Hospital for Women and Children," c. 1934, New England Hospital Collection, SSC-SC. To insure an accurate portrait of the 1862–72 interns, I cross-checked information and verified it in a number of sources: New England Female Medical College graduate list; *Medical and Surgical Register of the United States* (Polk's) beginning with the first edition in 1886; *Woman's Medical College Graduates List;* and several listings in the AR-NEH to eliminate printing errors. There are eight women for whom information could not be obtained because they either died, left no forwarding addresses, or were of foreign birth and could not be traced in U.S. sources. The total of interns from 1862–72 was twenty-seven.

have consisted of a minimum of formal instruction and a maximum of practical experience. The overtaxed staff had little time to devote exclusively to the students, and the education itself was on a learn-as-you-go basis. The hospital kept no intern records, and the only picture of the training is based on the variegated reactions of the students themselves. While some found all they had hoped for and others were disappointed, one is struck by how many influential women doctors passed through the hospital during its first decade:

Most notable of the hospital's "alumnae" of the 1860s was Dr. Mary Putnam Jacobi who, although twenty-one years old when she arrived, was a graduate of both New York College of Pharmacy and Pennsylvania woman's medical college. She entered New England Hospital in 1864 but instead of the specialized training she expected, Jacobi found herself thrown into the work of the dispensary where close to 2,000 women were treated during the year. No bed remained empty and many patients had to be treated in their homes. During one two-week period, Jacobi counted eleven nights when Zakrzewska was called out on emergencies. Seeing so many patients suffering from such a variety of ailments day after day temporarily persuaded Jacobi that she was not cut out for a regular medical practice. Convinced that she was destined for a career in medical research, she went to Paris, where in 1868 she became the first woman to be admitted to the Ecole de Medicine. After her return to America, she embarked on a career of research and medical school teaching which made her the leading woman physician in America in the late nineteenth century.[44]

44. Jacobi was at New England Hospital for a few months during the summer of 1864. Neither her personal papers, her two-volume edited autobiography and articles, nor her later published works refer to her internship at New England Hospital. The reference to the busy schedule of Zakrzewska is taken from Rhoda Truax, *The Doctors Jacobi* (Boston, 1952), p. 36. Truax refers to private Putnam collections in writing her popular biography of Jacobi. See the complete bibliography on Jacobi in James.

Unlike Jacobi, Susan Dimock entered New England Hospital as the very first step in her medical career. Although only eighteen years old when she arrived in January 1866, her ability and prodigous capacity for work attracted the special attention of Zakrzewska and Sewall. With their encouragement, she and another student at the hospital, Sophia Jex-Blake, applied to Harvard Medical School the following year and were both turned down. Despite this rejection, New England Hospital was able to temporarily arrange for a limited amount of clinical instruction for the two at Massachusetts General Hospital when the Harvard students were not at the hospital. The 1867 Annual Report of the New England Hospital proudly announced: "They have availed themselves of all the opportunities offered them." [45]

Meanwhile Zakrzewska and Sewall persuaded Dimock to apply to the University of Zurich, which had been accepting female medical students since 1864. Two Boston women paid Dimock's expenses with the only stipulation that she return to New England Hospital for three years and assist some other struggling woman medical student in the future. After graduating with high honors from Zurich and then spending an additional year in Paris and Vienna, Dimock returned in 1872 to become the most skilled surgeon on the staff.[46]

Sophia Jex-Blake, Dimock's companion in the attempt to enter Harvard in 1867, first exhibited at the hospital the spirit that would eventually make her the spokeswoman for a woman's right to a medical education in Great Britain. Unwilling to accept Harvard's refusal, she embarked on a per-

45. AR-NEH (1867), p. 7; their letter of application to Harvard is in the Harvard Medical School Dean's Records, 1867, and in Chadwick Scrapbook, HCL-A.

46. Dimock's correspondence with Samuel Cabot about her Zurich experience is in the New England Hospital Collection, SSC-SC. *Notable American Women* contains a complete bibliography on Dimock. Dimock's reputation as a surgeon is demonstrated in a research article and obituary published simultaneously in "The Death of Dr. Dimock," *Medical Record* (1875), pp. x, 357–58.

sonal campaign while at the hospital to build up support to break this barrier. She arranged interviews with each member of the Harvard faculty and the Massachusetts General staff. Some, like Oliver Wendell Holmes, expressed a willingness to lecture to women "always provided that any special subject which seemed not adapted to an audience of both sexes, should be delivered to male students alone." A more representative response was recorded in Jex-Blake's diary: "Dr. A. 'not afraid of responsibility, of course'—only—he'd rather not admit us till other people do!" [47]

Georgia Sturtevant, an assistant nurse at the time the young women medical students were being permitted at Massachusetts General Hospital, noted in her memoirs that Dimock and Jex-Blake, "though championed by some of the most popular of the visiting staff, were really allowed this privilege under protest, and were under many restrictions, and were only allowed to visit in certain wards." [48] Jex-Blake, particularly, felt a constant sense of insecurity as one member of the staff was bitterly opposed to the presence of women and constantly searched for mistakes to bolster his prejudices. Such tensions took their toll as Jex-Blake wrote in her diary: "July 5th. Rest yesterday, but altogether weighed down yesterday and today with the fear and horror of this irritability which seems so fatally unconquerable." Dissatisfied with the situation at Massachusetts General and convinced that she had received enough practical experience, Jex-Blake went to New York where she was able to obtain private lessons in anatomy from the head demonstrator at Bellevue Hospital. A month later she left for home where she won fame as the leader of the movement to admit women to the medical profession in Great

47. Margaret Todd, *The Life of Sophia Jex-Blake* (New York, 1918), p. 192.

48. Sara E. Parsons, *History of the Massachusetts General Hospital Training School for Nurses* (Boston, 1922), p. 15. Sturtevant's memoirs are reproduced on pp. 4–18 of Parsons; they originally appeared in "Personal Recollections of Hospital Life Before the Days of Training Schools," *The Trained Nurse* (Boston, 1895).

Britain and the founder of the London School of Medicine for Women.[49]

Elizabeth Mosher, whose only previous medical experience involved nursing her tubercular brother, entered New England Hospital in 1869. After a successful internship and a year of assisting Lucy Sewall in her private practice, Mosher left for the University of Michigan where she received her M.D. degree in 1875. She went on to a number of important medical posts which culminated in her appointment as the first dean of students and professor of physiology at the University of Michigan. She later credited her year at New England Hospital as the turning point in her career: "I believe I voice all of the women . . . when I say I feel I largely owe to the teaching, the spirit of devotion, and the high standard maintained by this hospital whatever of success I may have been able to achieve in medicine." [50]

With each year the hospital raised the quality of its training. By the mid-1870s the staff of the hospital began debating the problems of selecting from the large number of qualified applicants for the internship positions and by 1879 they accepted, with reluctance, the solution of taking only those women who already possessed the M.D. degree.[51] Increasing numbers of women were also coming to the hospital for experience after having attended a liberal arts college as well as receiving the medical degree. This was the case with Dr. Minerva Walker, who attended Cornell University before receiving the M.D. from the Woman's Medical College of Pennsylvania in 1879.[52] The larger, more specialized staff of

49. Todd, p. 201. See also Edythe Lutzker's pioneering studies: "Medical Education for Women in Great Britain," M.A. Thesis, Columbia University, 1959; and *Women Gain a Place in Medicine* (New York, 1969).

50. *The Fiftieth Anniversary of the New England Hospital for Women and Children, October 29, 1912* (Boston, 1913), p. 11.

51. AR-NEH (1880), p. 13; Marie Zakrzewska, address to students (April 1, 1876), p. 3, New England Hospital Collection; SSC-SC.

52. Frances Willard and Mary Livermore (eds.), *American Women* (Buffalo, 1897), vol. 2, p. 741.

the last decades of the nineteenth century provided a far more intensive training period than had been possible in the 1860s. Dr. Kate Hurd-Mead, who interned at the hospital in the 1880s, described her experience there as highly structured: "Life was indeed serious to the young doctors under the watchful eye of resident and visiting physicians. If, in an unguarded moment, the intern was heard humming a little air or whistling softly at her work, or even if her shoes squeaked a trifle, she was taken to task by one of these dignified censors and questioned as to her reasons for studying medicine and for her unseemly deportment." [53]

By 1887, on the twenty-fifth anniversary of New England Hospital, Zakrzewska's original goal of a hospital run by women for women had been realized. From the board of directors to the delivery of health care to patients, women held full responsibility and authority, though, as the anniversary report pointed out, "the counsel and help of the other sex is gladly welcomed." This was especially true in regard to the consulting physicians, men who were selected not as mere status symbols but because "they have taken an active interest in the Hospital, and have been chosen for special eminence in some department." [54] As a result of the vision of Zakrzewska, an increasing number of trained doctors were being turned out to meet the rising patient demand. But the hospital was more than an institution where women absorbed the technical knowledge and skills of their profession. Equally necessary in the sexually-polarized world of the late nineteenth century was the psychic support and energy which they needed to enable them to practice in a profession that did everything it could to discourage them. Herein lies the significance of the hospital. It was not only a showcase in which women physicians could prove themselves; it was also an island of feminist strength and sisterhood in a society only familiar with brotherhood.

53. Kate Hurd-Mead, *Medical Women of America* (New York, 1933), p. 34.
54. AR-NEH (1887), pp. 9–11.

Consequently, when a group of twelve Greater Boston women physicians, ten of whom had been associated with the hospital, gathered in 1878 to form the first female medical society in the United States, they named the organization the "New England Hospital Medical Society." At a time when the Massachusetts Medical Society was closed to women, this separate group offered its members both a sense of colleagueship and a common voice. One of its first steps was to pressure the editors of the *Boston City Directory* to list its members under the heading of the society, a service which the directory had always rendered to the members of the Massachusetts Medical Society and any other local male medical group. The separate listing was important, for while the Massachusetts Medical Society members had been divorced from the other sectarian and irregular physicians, including patent medicine promoters, the women physicians had been indiscriminately lumped under the heading of "female physicians," which included phrenologists, magnetists, Christian Scientists, and electricians, as well as midwives and nurses. Zakrzewska was particularly eager to dissociate her hospital from any taint of homeopathy and sectarianism. Graduates of Boston University Medical School as well as other irregular schools were excluded from the New England Hospital Medical Society and interns from such schools were likewise barred from the hospital. The women hoped that by not confusing the issue of women's competence in regular medicine with the sectarian controversies in the profession at large, they would advance the cause of women more directly.[55]

Thus, New England Hospital fought for the causes of medical women and, indirectly, feminists, on a variety of fronts. Its separatism was a means to an end; ironically, that end was the elimination of separatism and the movement of women

55. Margaret Noyes Kleinert, "Medical Women in New England: History of the New England Women's Medical Society," *JAMWA* 11 (1956), pp. 63–64, 67; "Memoirs of Dr. Emma Call, June, 1928," SA; *New England Women's Medical Society Directory of Members 1878–1928*, SSC-SC. *Boston Directory* (1846–1910, annual editions).

into the mainstream of medicine. Whenever Zakrzewska spoke publicly about women physicians and particularly when she addressed her student interns, she always expressed the hope that the hospital would convince the medical profession of the ability of women physicians, "and shall thus force them to open Harvard College to such women as desire entrance there." [56] She believed that the presence of male consultants on the staff would demonstrate that men and women physicians could work side by side to the advantage of both sexes and society as a whole. In this spirit, the New England Hospital Medical Society even invited male physicians to membership, an invitation that the men chose to ignore, though a few did toy with the idea briefly.[57]

Quite clearly, many female physicians believed that as women they brought a much-needed dimension to the practice of medicine. But it was equally obvious that these benefits would not accrue to the profession as long as women were isolated. In nineteenth-century Boston, the mainstream of medicine had two major tributaries, the Massachusetts Medical Society and Harvard Medical School. With the progress of New England Hospital seemingly assured, the attention of the women physicians increasingly turned to these other institutions.

56. Marie Zakrzewska, address to students (April 1, 1876), p. 7; Marie Zakrzewska, address to students (October 30, 1891), New England Hospital Collection, SSC-SC.

57. Vietor, p. 336; *WJ*, January 6, 1872; for a discussion by a male physician (Dr. Derby) of whether or not the men should accept the women's invitation, see H. Derby to Dr. J. R. Chadwick, June 14, 1882, Chadwick Scrapbook.

4

Male Backlash

The efforts by women to gain entrance to Harvard Medical School and the Massachusetts Medical Society touched off a major debate concerning the role of women in medicine. The issue was, of course, only one part of the larger controversy that had developed in reaction to the feminist movement. Nevertheless, the arguments raised by the more articulate of the male physicians warrant detailed examination because they formed a major barrier to women's advancement in medicine and because the effects of their opposition are still being felt today. Further, these arguments furnished the antifeminists of that era with a major source of ammunition. Although historians have recently begun to examine the scientific and medical rhetoric about appropriate sexual spheres, no one has looked at the highly charged medical context out of which it arose.[1] Not surprisingly, many of the arguments having the greatest impact on the national level first unfolded in Boston, where medical women were making significant progress.

During the last third of the nineteenth century, in the

1. Studies on rhetoric include: G. J. Barker-Benfield, *The Horrors of the Half-Known Life* (New York, 1976); Carroll Smith-Rosenberg and Charles E. Rosenberg, "The New Woman and the Troubled Man: Medical and Biological Views of Women in Nineteenth-Century America," *Journal of American History* 60, no. 2 (September 1973), pp. 332–56; and Charles E. Rosenberg, "Sexuality, Class and Role in 19th-Century America," *American Quarterly* 25 (Spring 1973), pp. 1–23; Vern Bullough and Martha Voight, "Women, Menstruation, and Nineteenth Century Medicine," *Bulletin of the History of Medicine* 47 (January–February 1973), pp. 66–82; John Burnham, "The Progressive Era Revolution in American Attitudes Toward Sex," in *Journal of American History* 59, no. 4 (March 1973), pp. 885–908.

United States as in several other countries, the age-old question of woman's place became a central issue. Moreover, the appearance of feminists and educated women meant that the discussion was no longer merely academic. Women were knocking on doors marked "men only" and demanding to be admitted. Medical men in Boston as elsewhere in the nation found themselves confronted with some of the same problems and questions that their colleagues in politics, business, and the other professions faced. Unlike their peers, however, male physicians were in a profession that appeared more vulnerable to the female onslaught because if women were to enter any profession, their "special" talent for nurturing seemed to dictate a career in medicine.[2] Earlier, Catherine Beecher had successfully used a similar argument to defend the role of women in primary school teaching. Certainly, it was easier in the nineteenth century to envision a woman pursuing a career at someone's bedside, than in a courtroom, brokerage house, or political club. As early as the 1860s, feminists like Caroline Dall and Susan B. Anthony insisted that a woman's nature was her most important asset in treating female patients.[3] Whether true or not, their progress in medicine in the last half of the nineteenth century seemed to bear this out. The 6 female doctors listed in the *Boston City Directory* in 1850, a mere 2 percent of the total medical listings, had expanded to 210 by 1890—18 percent of the city's medical population. There were, in fact, more women

2. Ross Evans Paulson, *Women's Suffrage and Prohibition: A Comparative Study of Equality and Social Control* (Glenview, Ill., 1973) provides an excellent introduction to the feminist debates in the U.S. and Europe. Joan Burstyn, "Education and Sex: The Medical Case Against Higher Education for Women in England, 1870–1900," *Proceedings of the American Philosophical Society 112*, no. 2 (April 1970), pp. 79–89, demonstrates that medicine was the first occupation to be assailed by women in an attempt to enter the professions and it was the gynecologists and obstetricians who made the strongest attacks against higher education for women, probably because they were the first to feel the competition—see especially p. 81.

3. Caroline Dall, *Boston Daily Advertiser*, October 20, 1867; Caroline Dall, *New England Medical Gazette*, March 1869, pp. 87–90.

doctors in Boston alone that year than all the women lawyers (200) in the country.[4]

Whenever feminism has flourished, it has led to an intensification of assertions of male supremacy.[5] In order to prove their own superiority, the spokesmen for the opposition to women physicians had to demonstrate that a woman's nature, far from being an asset, was an insurmountable liability. Nowhere in the professions was there a greater urgency to promote this idea than among those men who specialized in gynecology and obstetrics, the areas where women posed the greatest threat.

Woman's unsuitability for medicine had first been raised in the late eighteenth and early nineteenth century in connection with midwifery. But the midwives' claim to professional status had been no match for the educated physicians, and they had been scattered by a few volleys. Similarly, the application of Harriot Hunt had produced little of what can be described as serious ideological opposition. She had been summarily rejected by Harvard on the grounds that her admission would be "inexpedient." It is little wonder that Zakrzewska, observing the Boston medical scene from New York in the 1850s, could have mistaken an absence of controversy as a sign of liberality. She was quickly initiated into the realities of anti-feminist hostility and later admitted that "the impression . . . which I had cherished and fostered as a belief, was not as well founded as I thought, and upon closer acquaintance I was soon convinced that here also it required a great deal of courage to advocate a new era in woman's sphere."[6]

4. Elva Hulburd Young, "The Law as a Profession for Women," *Association of Collegiate Alumnae Journal* 3 (February 1902), pp. 15–23. Young states that there were only nine women in active practice in the law in Massachusetts by 1902.

5. Steven Goldberg, *The Inevitability of Patriarchy* (New York, 1973); George Gilder, *Sexual Suicide* (New York, 1973); Lionel Tiger and Robin Fox, *The Imperial Animal* (New York, 1971) are examples of books stimulated by the woman's movement of the late 1960s and early 1970s. Some nineteenth-century books are discussed later in this chapter.

6. Agnes Vietor, *A Woman's Quest: The Life of Marie E. Zakrzewska* (New York, 1924), p. 245.

What Zakrzewska was witnessing was the first serious campaign in the struggle to check the advance of women in the Boston medical profession. In 1853 an editorial in the *Boston Medical and Surgical Journal* had observed the first female medical graduates and wryly commented: "It is not a matter to be laughed down as readily as was at first anticipated. The serious inroads made by female physicians in obstetrical business, one of the essential branches of income to a majority of well-established practitioners, make it natural enough to inquire what course it is best to pursue." The apprehension over Gregory's medical college turned to alarm with the successful establishment of Zakrzewska's hospital and the growing supply of educated women physicians. An editorial in the *Boston Medical and Surgical Journal* in 1866 went so far as to lump the hospital and New England Female Medical College together in its denunciation. When a reader informed the editor of his error, he unblushingly responded that the spirit that had given rise to the two institutions was essentially the same. The issue of women physicians was creating a chaotic situation in Boston medicine and the journal's editor announced that it was now time to bring the "unsettled question" into the open.[7]

The first response to this challenge came from a surprising source, Dr. Horatio Storer, the first and only male physician to be appointed to the New England Hospital staff during the nineteenth century. When Storer launched his full-scale attack on the women doctors, the reverberations carried far beyond the city itself. Part of Boston's medical establishment early in his career, Storer served as an assistant in the Harvard Medical School obstetrical department headed by his father, David Humphreys Storer. The younger Storer, a pioneer in separating the study of gynecology from obstetrics, was one of the founders and, later, president of the Gynecological Society of Boston. However, Storer found greater receptivity to his work nationally than in the more conservative professional atmo-

7. *BMSJ* 48 (1853), p. 66; ibid. 75 (1866), p. 504.

sphere of Boston. He served as secretary of the American Medical Association in 1865 and as its vice-president the following year.[8]

Storer's public attack came in the form of a letter of resignation from the staff of New England Hospital for Women and Children which was published in the *Boston Medical and Surgical Journal* immediately after it was submitted to ,the hospital authorities. What better evidence could there be? Here was a man who had observed female physicians, not from afar, but alongside them in the wards and operating rooms of their own hospital. Furthermore, he had been assisted for two years in his private practice by Dr. Anita Tyng, whom he described as "one of the very best woman physicans . . . as I suppose there is at present in the country . . . [whose] natural tastes and inclinations . . . fit her, more than I should have supposed any woman could have become fitted for the anxiety, the nervous strain, and shocks of the practice of surgery." Nevertheless, she and Marie Zakrzewska were described by Storer as "exceptions," for women "naturally" lacked the courage and the daring to aggressively pursue the dangerous and difficult decisions involved in gynecological surgery.[9]

But what else could one expect? How could women act freely and confidently when they were the captives of their own biology? Here, Storer turned to the subject to which every medical opponent of women was irresistibly drawn in the nineteenth century—the female reproductive system. "It was," another physician exclaimed, "as if the Almighty, in creating the

8. The only detailed biographical sketch of Storer is J. M. Toner, *A Sketch of the Life of Horatio R. Storer, a Memorial Volume of the Rocky Mountain Medical Association* (Washington, 1878). Frederick C. Irving provides an elaboration on oral traditions surrounding Storer in *Safe Deliverance* (Boston, 1942), pp. 109–19. Although Irving provides no documentation, he was associated with Boston Lying-In Hospital beginning in 1910 so it is likely he absorbed much of the local history of its staff. A few Storer letters are at Countway Library and the National Library of Medicine. The *Journal of the Gynecological Society of Boston (JGSB)* is an excellent source since Storer was editor.

9. *BMSJ* 75 (1866), pp. 191–92.

female sex, had taken the uterus and built up a woman around it." To Storer, woman was "what she is in health, in character, in her charms, . . . mind and soul because of her womb alone." Who could trust the great questions of life or death to one whose equilibrium varied from "month to month and week to week . . . up and down"? Storer claimed he did not object to women physicians per se, for they would make "most agreeable and charming attendants [but,] . . . to their often infirmity during which neither life nor limb submitted to them would be as safe as at other times." It was clear from Storer's description of menstruation as "periodical infirmity . . . mental influences . . . temporary insanity," that women were crippled, certainly more in need of medical aid than able to furnish it. But if women remained in their proper sphere all would be well with the world. Storer's view of a woman's place coincided with those of another widely quoted physician of the era, Dr. Charles Meigs, who wrote in his textbook on obstetrics that woman "has a head almost too small for intellect but just big enough for love." [10]

Storer's argument, however, was much more persuasive. As a leading physician, a man of obvious good will who had risked his reputation to conduct an experiment in the opposition's own laboratory, Storer's pronouncement that the experiment had proven to be a failure was not to be taken lightly. Yet it must be asked if the experiment and Storer's findings were as objective as he had intimated. Eighteen sixty-six had certainly

10. Ibid., p. 191. In every published article which dealt with the topic of female physicians after 1866, Storer made it a point to footnote his New England Hospital experience. He also did this at medical meetings; see, for example: *JGSB*, passim; *BMSJ* 84 (1871), pp. 371–72 (debate at an AMA meeting); Stephen G. Hubbard, quoted by M. L. Holbrook, *Parturition without Pain: A Code of Directions for Escaping from the Primal Curse* (New York, 1882), pp. 14–15; Horatio Robinson Storer, *The Causation, Course and Treatment of Reflex Insanity in Women* (Boston, 1871), p. 79; Horatio R. Storer and F. F. Head, *Criminal Abortion: Its Nature, Its Evidence, and Its Law* (Boston, 1868), p. 101; C. D. Meigs, *Lecture on Some of the Distinctive Characteristics of the Female, delivered before the class of the Jefferson Medical College, Jan. 1847* (Philadelphia, 1847), p. 67.

been a difficult year for Storer. His disagreement with senior
faculty members had led to his dismissal that spring from the
position he held as assistant in obstetrics and ended permanently his connection with Harvard Medical School. And
tucked away in his letter of resignation to New England Hospital was a brief reference to his immediate reason for leaving:
his objection to a new requirement that surgeons must consult
with their colleagues before performing high risk surgery.[11] On
August 13, 1866, the Board of Directors of New England Hospital had voted to accept the following resolution:

> WHEREAS: The Confidence of the Public in the Manage-
> ment of the Hospital rests not only on the character of the
> Medical attendants, having its immediate charge, but also
> on the high reputation of the consulting physicians and
> surgeons, and, Whereas, We cannot allow them to be re-
> sponsible for cases over which they have no control—
>
> RESOLVED: That in all unusual or difficult cases in medi-
> cine, or where a capital operation in surgery is proposed,
> the attending and Resident Physicians and Surgeons shall
> hold mutual consultations, and if any one of them shall
> doubt as to the propriety of the proposed treatment or
> operation one or more of the consulting physicians or
> surgeons shall be invited to examine and decide upon the
> case.[12]

The board's action was in response to the fact that all three
patient deaths during the previous year had occurred in the
surgical wards of the hospital, after what Dr. Lucy Sewall described as "hazardous operations." As Dr. Mary Putnam Jacobi,
who had been an intern while Storer was on the staff, later
recalled, the results of Storer's operations often failed to match
the boldness of his plans. And in 1866 the hospital's action came
as part of a double blow, following Storer's recent dismissal

11. *BMSJ* 75 (1866), p. 192.
12. Ednah Cheney's letter informing Storer of the hospital's new regulations can be found in Storer's uncatalogued correspondence, HCL-A;
Vietor, pp. 340–41; AR-NEH (1866), pp. 10–11.

from Harvard.[13] In addition, the requirement that he clear his operations with female physicians was no doubt galling to a man of Storer's stature. Of even greater significance was the fact that these restrictions blocked what had been the hospital's major attraction for Storer—a free hand to develop his skills as a gynecological surgeon. In 1863, when Storer first joined the hospital, none of the other hospitals in Boston allowed this type of surgery. In fact, the entire field of gynecology was treated with a great deal of suspicion by the conservative Boston medical establishment. Storer had even been warned that the profession in New England would never tolerate in its ranks an "avowed gynecologist." Storer's son, Malcolm, who also became a physician, later attributed the prejudice regarding gynecology to the low status associated with the treatment of women's diseases: "In the ears of conservative men, the very name of diseases of women savored strongly of quackery; and it was the honest belief of many a doctor of the old school that the preservation of a man's personal morality was highly dubious if he was constantly engaged in treating the female genitals." [14] Moreover, the few experiments in gynecological surgery in Boston had all failed. Six women had been operated on for ovarian tumors between 1830 and 1858 at Massachusetts General Hospital; after all six women died, gynecological surgery was not permitted inside the hospital until asepsis was fully established in the 1880s. The other major hospital, Boston City, had similar strictures against such operations, a not surprising fact since the medical leadership in Boston was closely knit and held tight reins on hospital affairs.[15]

13. Irving, p. 113; Malcolm Storer, "The Teaching of Obstetrics and Gynecology at Harvard," *Harvard Medical Alumni Association* 8 (1903), pp. 439–40.

14. Malcolm Storer, pp. 439–40. Vietor, p. 339; AR-NEH (1866), p. 14.

15. Grace W. Myers, *Massachusetts General Hospital, 1872–1900* (Boston, 1900), pp. 36–37. Her account is based on free access to the hospital's complete internal records (she had been a librarian at the hospital) and was accurate when I corroborated it with the Trustees Minutes, Massachusetts General Hospital, 1872–1900, to which I was able to obtain access (Count-

Although Storer was later able to continue his work at the newly opened, but less prestigious, operating rooms of the Carney and St. Elizabeth's hospitals, the more conservative medical atmosphere in Boston limited the extent of his experimentation as well as his publications. Nevertheless, Storer's later operations continued to exhibit some of the "boldness" to which New England Hospital had objected. Male surgeons have historically taken a cavalier view of operations on the female reproductive system, in sharp contrast to their protective attitude toward experimentation on the male organs. Thus, a later physician turned historian could describe a three-hour operation by Storer in 1868 as "the greatest feat" in his career. Similarly, Storer's assistant in the operation depicted it as "the most heroic of the bold procedures as yet resorted to." [16] Both

---

way Library is in the process of acquiring *all* of the internal records but only has records from 1904 to 1920 at present). See also histories of Boston City Hospital: Committee of the Hospital Staff, *A History of the Boston City Hospital From Its Foundation Until 1904* (Boston, 1906); John J. Byrne (ed.), *A History of the Boston City Hospital, 1905–1964* (Boston, 1964); and Irving, p. 112. A detailed article (based on a statistical survey) is Horatio R. Bigelow, "American Ovariotomies," *American Journal of Obstetrics and Diseases of Women and Children* 15, nos. 2 and 3 (1882).

16. Toner, pp. 7–14; Irving, pp. 114–16. After 1869, Storer had enough medical support behind him to found the *Journal of the Gynecological Society of Boston,* which lasted only as long as he was able to sustain it with his energy—until 1872. Storer's deliberate defiance of the Boston medical establishment became a frequent source of debate within the Massachusetts Medical Society. See, for example, the "Suffolk District Medical Society Minutes" for May 31, 1866, in HCL-A. The protectiveness of males toward experimentation on the bodies of their own sex is evident in the slow development of a medical specialty for the male reproductive system. See editorial, "Andrology as a Specialty," *JAMA* 17 (1891), p. 691; Hugh Young, *A Surgeon's Autobiography* (New York, 1940); William Niles Wishard, Jr., "Your American Board of Urology, Incorporated," *J. Urol.* 82 (1959), p. 178. Rosemary Stevens describes the slow development of the American Urological Association and then notes how the early period was marked by an effort "to protect patients from unprepared practitioners and to raise standards of education in urology" (*American Medicine and the Public Interest* [New Haven, 1971], p. 236. This did not occur in gynecology.

observers, however, glossed over the fact that the female patient died. What made Storer's lost or limited opportunities especially frustrating was his knowledge that freewheeling gynecological surgery was being performed elsewhere in the nation. During the late nineteenth century, Storer was easily outdistanced by his daring rival in New York, Dr. J. Marion Sims, who performed his operations in crowded amphitheatres. In one marathon display of surgical virtuosity, Sims performed a series of varied operations for four successive days, capped off by an entertainment dinner for the large audience of distinguished American doctors.[17]

Furthermore, whereas Storer had been thwarted by the New England Hospital women, Sims had vanquished the wealthy society ladies who had founded New York Hospital for Women in 1856. Sims had been appointed head surgeon with the expectation that he would engage a woman as his assistant, hopefully Dr. Emily Blackwell, who had just returned from study abroad and who was eminently qualified. Sims at first resisted, but when the women insisted, he derisively appointed a female acquaintance who had been serving at the hospital as matron and general superintendent. Needless to say she had no medical training whatsoever. Six months later, the board of lady managers of the hospital backed down and a male assistant was appointed to assist Sims in his surgery; the selection was not based on medical qualifications but on the fact that the man had married a friend of Sims's acquaintance.[18]

17. Barker-Benfield singles out J. Marion Sims as symbolizing the male lust for achievement in gynecological surgery. See "Sexual Surgery in Late-Nineteenth Century America," *International Journal of Health Services* 5, no. 2 (1975), pp. 284–85, and *The Horrors*, pp. 91–119. James Ricci, *One Hundred Years of Gynecology, 1800–1900* (Philadelphia, 1945) who cites gynecologists themselves who refer to their nineteenth-century history as one of a series of "crazes" when pelvic surgery "ran wild" (see pp. 36–37 and 46–47).

18. Vietor, p. 226; Mary Putnam Jacobi, "Women in Medicine," in Annie Nathan Meyer (ed.), *Woman's Work in America* (New York, 1891); J. Marion Sims, *The Story of My Life*, ed. H. Marion-Sims (New York,

Sims apparently recognized that female physicians might serve as a check on his aspirations. Now unhampered by the type of resistance Storer had encountered at New England Hospital, he performed an incredible variety of gynecological operations in the following years. Sims, who had previously made thirty experimental operations on a slave named Anarcha, now performed a similar number on an Irish woman, Mary Smith, in New York. His slashing scalpel dazzled the medical world, earning him the reputation of "one of the immortals" in gynecological surgery, and among the medical students at Harvard he was recognized as possessing "divinity." [19]

Physicians such as Storer and Sims, engaged as they were in gynecology and obstetrics, were especially apprehensive about women in medicine. Certainly if there was a "natural area" for women physicians it would appear to be in treating those problems peculiar to their sex. In fact, women physicians described these specialties as "the great opportunity, the main portal, through which women have passed, and are destined to pass, to general medicine." [20] To the male gynecologist and obstetrician, the increasing number of women physicians seemed bound to lead to a revival of the old charge of male immorality and insensitivity. Only this time the male physicians would have to do battle with trained professionals rather than unlettered midwives or publicists like Samuel Gregory. Significantly, at the first meeting of the Gynecological Society of Boston, founded by Storer in 1869, a resolution embodying one of the chief principles of the society was recorded: "That as in attending upon childbed, all impurity of thought and even the mental appreciation of a difference in sex is lost by the physician and an imputation of these would be resented as an in-

---

1885), p. 300; Seale Harris *Woman's Surgeon*, with F. H. Brown (New York, 1950), pp. 235, 272.

19. Harris, pp. 337, 339; Barker-Benfield, *The Horrors*, p. 100.

20. This statement was made by Mary Putnam Jacobi in 1891, but it seems generally accepted by women physicians in the earlier era; it was institutionalized in the founding of hospitals for women and children (see Jacobi in Meyer, p. 154).

sult by the profession, as the care of uterine disease tends to inspire greater respect in a patient for her attendant, and in him for her." [21]

Surprisingly, the women physicians in Boston did not react publicly to Storer's attacks. Throughout the 1860s and 1870s, Zakrzewska and those associated with New England Hospital continued to hope that their performance would, in the long run, be a more effective argument than words. Moreover, since they were seeking the professional respect of their male colleagues, they avoided involvement in what might become a public controversy. Consequently, their response to Storer's vituperative letter to the editor of the *Boston Medical and Surgical Journal,* in which he publicly announced that women doctors were disqualified by the biological defects of their sex from professional competence, was to turn the other cheek. The New England Hospital's annual report for 1866 simply announced Storer's resignation and offered him their best wishes for his future success. [22]

It must be remembered that Zakrzewska had the friendship and support of such leading male physicians as Walter Channing, Henry I. Bowditch, Edward Jarvis, Edward H. Clarke, and, later, Reginald Fitz, James Chadwick, and Francis Minot. The New England Hospital staff had a growing sense of security bolstered by their confidence in their own medical abilities, their feminist supporters, and this small but influential cadre of male physicians. The juxtaposition in their 1866 annual report of a laudatory letter from Dr. Samuel Cabot, a newly elected officer in the Massachusetts Medical Society, next to the announcement of Storer's departure may have been coincidental, but it was more likely a reminder to the hospital's supporters that the medical tide was turning in their favor. [23]

Convinced that part of Samuel Gregory's failure was due to

21. Horatio R. Storer, Secretary, "Report of the First Regular Meeting of the Gynecological Society of Boston, Jan. 22, 1869," *JGSB* (July 1869), p. 14.

22. AR-NEH (1866), p. 11.

23. Ibid., p. 10.

his polemical attacks on the medical establishment, Zakrzewska believed that she could enlarge her support by using the opposite tactics. Trained female physicians would sooner or later gain entrance to the medical societies and hospitals, and their record of performance would in turn lead schools like Harvard to open its doors to women.[24] Consequently, Zakrzewska objected to a letter by Caroline Dall to the editors of the *New England Medical Gazette,* a homeopathic journal, which argued that women could be best treated by other women. Although Dall, a leading spokeswoman for the Boston feminist movement and a close friend of Zakrzewska, echoed many of Zakrzewska's own sentiments, the tone and the timing appeared, to Zakrzewska at least, all wrong. In a personal letter to Dall, Zakrzewska expressed her distress over the course that Dall had taken and her own belief that the barriers to women physicians must be overcome "gradually and dignifiedly." [25]

Despite the professional silence by the women physicians, the increasing number of public letters in their defense, by Dall in Boston newspapers and by another close friend of Zakrzewska's, William Lloyd Garrison, in the *New York Independent,* convinced Storer that he was only seeing the tip of the iceberg. Bridling at statements concerning the "impossibility of any man's penetrating the mysteries of an organism which he does not share," Storer responded in separate articles on Dall and on "Mr. Garrison's slander." In his responses Storer returned to his favorite theme almost as if it were the chorus: the physical and mental disturbances induced by menstruation. Countering Dall, Storer claimed that women patients, recognizing the instability of their own sex, preferred the aid of a stable male physician.[26]

24. Marie Zakrzewska, letter (April 1, 1876) read at physicians' meeting, April 16, 1876, New England Hospital Collection, SSC-SC.

25. Marie Zakrzewska to Caroline Dall, October 26, 1869, Caroline Dall Collection, MHS.

26. Caroline Dall in *Boston Daily Advertiser,* October 20, 1867; Caroline Dall in *New England Medical Gazette,* March 1869, pp. 87–90; William Lloyd Garrison, *New York Independent* (supplement), Decem-

Storer's career demonstrates that a good deal of the pseudo-scientific opposition to women in medicine stemmed from what can hardly be described as dispassionate sources. Far from the picture that they sought to project of men passing judgments from a vantage point above the battle, the view of male physicians was often shaped by their own special conflicts with the opposition. When Horatio Storer was forced to withdraw from active medical practice in 1872 because of an almost fatal infection from an accident in one of his hazardous operations,[27] the opponents of women in medicine lost a vigorous spokesman.

It is testimony to the growing intensity of the struggle that his place was taken by an even more formidable figure, one who became a national spokesman for the antifeminists in America, Dr. Edward Clarke. Clarke had succeeded the distinguished Dr. Jacob Bigelow in 1855 as professor of materia medica at Harvard Medical School, but he resigned from the faculty in 1872 at the age of fifty-two and became a member of Harvard's board of overseers. Although Clarke was in no way a colleague of Storer's—he had, in fact, been a member of the faculty responsible for the gynecologist's dismissal from Harvard in 1866—the two men shared similar views on the need

---

ber 31, 1868; ibid., December 23, 1869; Horatio R. Storer (read before the society, March 16, 1869), "The Relations of Physicians to Invalid Women," *JGSB* (November 1869), pp. 284–88; Horatio R. Storer (read before the society, January 18, 1870), "The Gynecological Society of Boston and Women Physicians: A Reply to Mr. Wm. Lloyd Garrison," *JGSB* (February 1870), pp. 95–99.

27. The development of Storer's infection is described in successive reports in *JGSB* (1872). Frederick Irving, a Boston obstetrician writing in 1942, includes the following details in his tribute to Storer's "heroism": "He was the first surgeon to use rubber gloves, although he intended them to protect his hands from infection by the patient, not to guard the patient from infection by his hands. . . . Storer's gloves were so heavy that he could feel little through them; he therefore abandoned them and in so doing wrecked a brilliant professional career and almost lost his life. While operating on a septic case he acquired an infected finger, pyemia followed, and a desperate illness ensued which eventually left him so crippled that in 1872 he went to Italy in search of health and remained there five years" (p. 118). His permanent retirement followed.

for a masculine and "scientific" examination of the woman question. Like Storer, Clarke had been a liberal for several years on the question of women's advancement and had been one of Zakrzewska's earliest supporters.[28]

As early as 1869 Clarke had felt obligated to respond to the growing animosity shown by the male medical students in Philadelphia who had driven the women students out of the classroom with their tobacco quids and tinfoil. In an article published in the *Boston Medical and Surgical Journal*, he described the incident as "unfortunate" because of both the "unenviable notoriety" brought upon the young men involved and because "nothing advances any cause so much as the martyrdom or persecution of its disciples. In this way the Philadelphia medical class have given an unexpected impetus to the cause they opposed." Indeed, this is exactly what happened. That same year, almost directly linked to the incident, the Philadelphia County Medical Society proposed a resolution for the admission of women. Clarke apparently hoped to ward off both the brash activities of immature young medical students and also any premature action by his colleagues. He hoped that the publication of his remarks, originally presented to the graduating class the previous spring at Harvard, would contribute to an examination of the subject of women physicians "till a satisfactory solution is reached." There is little doubt that Clarke hoped that the discussion would proceed at a leisurely pace, without any catalytic incidents such as had occurred in Philadelphia.[29]

In his essay, he reminded his audience (who probably needed no reminding), that women were knocking loudly at the door

28. Vietor, p. 244.

29. *BMSJ* 81 (1869), p. 345. Hiram Corson, *Brief History of Proceedings in the Medical Society of Pennsylvania to Procure Recognition of Women Physicians* (Norristown, 1894); *Evening Bulletin* (Philadelphia), November 8, 1869; "Women as Physicians," *Philadelphia Medical and Surgical Reporter* (April 1867), p. 2; *The Press* (Philadelphia), November 18, 1869; Clara Marshall, *The Woman's Medical College of Pennsylvania* (Philadelphia, 1897), pp. 17 ff.

of medicine. Pointing out that whatever a woman can do, she
has a right to do, and eventually she will do, Clarke stated
that a priori she had "the same right to every function and
opportunity which our planet offers, that man has." Nor did
Clarke believe that there was anything in medicine that was
improper for women to study—"for science . . . may enoble,
it can never degrade man, woman, or angel." But, he warned,
the real question was not one of right but of capability or
possibility. If a woman were capable, no law, argument, or ridicule would prevent her success. Therefore, Clarke urged, neither the medical profession nor the community should stand in
her way: "Let the experiment . . . be fairly made . . . [and]
in 50 years we shall get the answer." Clarke even went so far as
to volunteer his guess that women could master the science of
medicine.[30]

The address was certainly a welcome contrast to Storer's repeated declaration that the experiment had in fact already
been tried and proven a failure. There were, however, a few
items in Clarke's talk that should have set off warning signals
in the feminist camp. Although he had stated that women
could master medicine, he also declared that except for a few
areas he doubted that they would become successful practitioners. But this appeared to be no real obstacle. All the women
physicians wanted was the fair test that Clarke had sanctioned,
for they were convinced that they would pass with flying colors.
More menacing was Clarke's insistence that the test should
take place in separate classrooms. Although Clarke felt that
there was nothing improper in the study of medicine by
women, some mysterious and dangerous element materialized
when the pursuit took place in a coeducational context. After
all, a bath was a necessary and even purifying process for all,
claimed Clarke, but he warned that it did not follow that the
two sexes needed to bathe "at the same time and in the same
tub." No narrow-minded reactionary, Clarke welcomed the
suffrage for women, but "God forbid that I should ever see

30. *BMSJ* 81 (1869), pp. 345–46.

men and women aiding each other to display with the scalpel
the secrets of the reproductive system; . . . or charmingly discuss together the labyrinthine ways of syphillis." [31]
But Clarke's most ominous note appeared in his outline of
the types of questions which should be included in any test of
a woman's fitness to be a physician. The heart of the matter
was the issue of whether or not a woman's nature would enable her to advance in medicine. The answer in the final
analysis would be found in the knowledge of the female physiology—"the facts which physicians can best supply." [32] Nevertheless, Clarke's address did not touch off any public criticism
from the women, who apparently chose to concentrate on the
positive notes.

Their optimism was in no small measure due to the advances
that women were beginning to experience. Elizabeth Mosher,
who interned at New England Hospital in 1869 and 1870, described this period: "I well remember the day we read in the
Boston papers that the University of Michigan had opened its
doors to women in all departments. We five young women
joined hands and danced around the table. We all went to that
college and graduated from there with a degree of M.D." [33]

31. Ibid., p. 346.
32. Ibid., p. 345. Although other Boston hospitals had their own medical
libraries, specially designed for staff use, the New England Hospital had no
such facility and therefore it is difficult to know whether the women
doctors there ever read this speech. Since Marie Zakrzewska's German was
fluent, it is more likely she regularly read German publications, which at
this time were in advance of American medical research. She lived with
a well-known German-American journalist and writer, Karl Heinzen, and
his wife. See Carl Wittke, *Against the Current: The Life of Karl Heinzen*
(1809–1880) (Chicago, 1945), pp. 104, 112, 134, 214. In 1889 she had her
first and only scientific article published in the *BMSJ* but this publication
dearth reflects the degree of male prejudice more than scientific enthusiasm of Boston women physicians. As the patients records of the hospital
indicate, Zakrzewska was in the vanguard of medical science, utilizing
thermometer charts, the metric system, and other innovations (see the
collection of New England Hospital patients records, HCL-A).
33. Eliza M. Mosher, "A Woman Doctor Who 'Stuck It Out,'" *Literary*
Digest (April 9, 1925), p. 67.

Likewise, the administration and staff of New England Hospital warmly applauded the forward movement of women in medicine in their annual reports. They were especially proud of the fact that the women interns did so well in their academic studies in medical school. Amanda Sanford, for example, who had studied at Woman's Medical College of Pennsylvania as well as New England Hospital, was able to complete her medical school program at the University of Michigan in only one year and to receive her M.D. degree with honors. What the women failed to mention was the fact that Dr. Sanford had been "hooted and showered with abusive notes" at her graduation in Ann Arbor.[34]

Women, quite clearly, were both eager and able to participate in Clarke's fifty-year experiment. In fact, they were too eager as it turned out—at least as far as Clarke himself was concerned. It is difficult to explain his sudden reversal and the disappearance of his liberality with regard to the advancement of women. It may have been because women were now pressing Harvard itself to open its doors to them. Clarke, after all, had been elected to the board of overseers to guard Harvard's male sanctity. It was one thing to talk nobly of a half-century test of time; it was something quite different to look out and see contestants preparing to storm the gates of one's own home. Although Clarke had received his M.D. at the University of Pennsylvania, he loved Harvard with the zeal of a convert.

Clarke spoke to all these issues—the immediacy of the women's petitions to enter Harvard, the proper role of women, and the sacredness of an all-male educational environment—at the New England Women's Club of Boston in December 1872.[35]

34. See AR-NEH and Dorothy Gies McGuigan, *A Dangerous Experiment: 100 Years of Women at the University of Michigan* (Ann Arbor, 1970), p. 38. McGuigan used the Michigan Historical Collection for her sources on this book but the Sanford incident is not footnoted. Presumably she used newspaper accounts.

35. A comprehensive article on Dr. Clarke's lecture and the immediate reaction appeared in the *WJ* on December 21, 1872, and it was followed by a series of articles in the next few years, culminating in a commentary

Although his own medical specialty was ontology, he picked up the challenge he had thrown out in 1869 and proceeded to discuss the relationship between the education and the physiology of women. Not surprisingly, for few male physicians could resist the temptation, he found women limited by their biology. Clarke was surprised by the furor that erupted after his talk in Boston and decided to review his statements carefully with the objective of publishing them in a more comprehensive form.

The result was *Sex in Education; or, A Fair Chance for the Girls,* published in the fall of 1873. Perhaps no other single book on the limitations of the female system evoked such controversy. Within thirteen years, Clarke's book went through seventeen editions, indicating that he had struck a responsive chord. As far away as Ann Arbor, Michigan, it was reported that everyone was reading Clarke's book. A local bookseller there claimed sales of 200 copies in a single day, chortling: "the book bids fair to nip coeducation in the bud." But neither the number of printings nor their geographical distribution reflect the full impact of the book. Years later, M. Carey Thomas, the first president of Bryn Mawr College, recalled that "we did not know when we began whether women's health could stand the strain of education. We were haunted in those days, by the clanging chains of that gloomy little specter, Dr. Edward H. Clarke's *Sex in Education.*" [36]

Despite the difference in impact between Clarke's 1869 ad-

---

on his will as it went through probate. As if to prove his loyalty to Harvard, his entire estate was left to Harvard Medical College (*WJ*, May 4, 1878).

36. M. Carey Thomas, "Present Tendencies in Women's College and University Education," *Educational Review* 25 (1908), p. 68; McGuigan, p. 56. Lilian Welsh cites the impact that Dr. Clarke had on young women patients she treated in 1894, see Lilian Welsh, M.D., *Reminiscences of Thirty Years in Baltimore* (Baltimore, 1925). See also *RCE* (1902), for an indication of how enduring Clarke's ideas actually were. As late as 1904, G. Stanley Hall wrote, "even though he may have 'played his sex symphony' too harshly, E. H. Clarke was right" (*Adolescence* 2 [New York, 1904], pp. 569–70).

dress at Harvard, which apparently fell on deaf ears, and his 1872 speech, which led to his overnight fame, there was a strong thread of continuity connecting the two: the question of coeducation. Whereas Clarke had originally opposed coeducation only in the sensitive area of medical instruction, he now reworked and expanded his thesis to encompass all post-puberty education. Clarke argued that unlike the male, whose development into manhood he viewed as a continuous growth process, the female at puberty experienced a sudden and unique spurt during which the development of her reproductive system took place. If this did not occur at puberty, or if some outside force interfered, this "delicate and extensive mechanism within the organism,—a house within a house, an engine within an engine" would fail to develop. The most dangerous threat, Clarke believed, stemmed from the mistake of educating females as if they were males. Since the uterus was connected to the central nervous system, energy expended in one area was necessarily removed from another.

Clarke cited the dramatic case of Miss D—— who entered Vassar College at the age of fourteen, a normal and healthy girl. Within a year, menstruation began and Miss D—— continued to follow what Clarke described as the normal regimen of a male student. The results were predictable. Fainting was followed by painful menstruation, but she persisted in her studies until at last she graduated with "fair honors and a poor physique." In the following year, the young woman was "tortured" for two or three days every month and left weak and miserable for several more days. Then, the flow stopped altogether and Miss D—— became pale, nervous, hysterical, and complained of constant headaches. On examining the girl, Clarke found evidence of arrested development of the reproductive system. Confirmatory proof was found in his examination of her breasts, "where the milliner had supplied the organs Nature should have grown." [37]

37. Edward H. Clarke, *Sex in Education; or, A Fair Chance for the Girls* (Boston, 1873), pp. 81–82.

In the pages that followed, Clarke went on to describe six
similar cases in which the women all experienced "those griev-
ous maladies which torture a woman's earthly existence: leu-
corrhoea [sic], amenorrhea, dysmenorrhoea, chronic and acute
ovaritis, prolapsus uteri, hysteria, neuralgia, and the like."
And, as if this were not enough, Clarke elaborated on the end
results of female education: "monstrous brains and puny bodies; abnormally active cerebration and abnormally weak diges-
tion; flowing thought and constipated bowels." [38] The wonder
is not that *Sex in Education* loomed so large in the thinking of
women like M. Carey Thomas, but that they dared to enter-
tain any thoughts of education at all.

The implications of Clarke's book went far beyond the field
of education; they extended into the sphere of population
problems. The increasing number of educated women would
mean that within fifty years "the wives who are to be mothers
in our republic must be drawn from trans-Atlantic homes." [39]
Clarke's study dovetailed neatly with the growing concern over
the shrinking size of the American family—especially among
the genteel classes. [40] As early as 1850, the Massachusetts census

38. Ibid., pp. 23, 41.
39. Ibid., p. 63.
40. As early as 1850, Jesse Chickering reported in a Boston census document that "the births, marriages, and deaths in [foreign born] families,
are far more numerous than with Americans" (see *Boston City Document
#42, Tabular Statement of Censors . . . State Census of Boston, May 1,
1850*, pp. 11–12. Chickering then went on to express his anxiety that the
American native was disappearing, an endangered species. His work was
followed by New England and national treatises on the subject. Of particular interest here is the large number of studies published by local doctors.
Horatio Storer, "On the Decrease of the Rate of Increase of Population
now Obtaining in Europe and America," *American Journal of Science and
Arts*, 2nd ser. 43 (March 1867), pp. 141–55 (first read to the American
Academy of Arts and Sciences in 1858 but delayed in publication to permit
revisions); Nathan Allen, M.D., *Changes in New England Population*
(Lowell, Mass., 1866). Nathan Allen's tireless advocacy of Puritan decline
is documented in a series of articles in Smith-Rosenberg and Rosenberg. Of
the recent research on this subject, Oscar Handlin's essay "The Horror,"
in *Race and Nationality in American Life* (New York, 1957) has been

indicated that the foreign-born had a considerably higher birthrate than that of the native Americans, a situation that would
later give rise to fears of race suicide.[41]
Once again women found themselves blocked by someone
who had originally appeared to be a friend. Five years after
having urged a fair test of women's capabilities, Clarke declared his dread of seeing "the costly experiment" tried.[42] His
only solution was to provide women with *"a special and appropriate education, that shall produce a just and harmonious
development of every part."* [43] Clarke was vague as to how to
construct this special education, except to recommend that girls
spend one-third less time on their studies than boys and that
they be given time off during their menstrual periods.[44]
During the public controversy that followed the publication
of Clarke's book, Zakrzewska and her associates at the hospital
continued to maintain a low profile. Intent on proving themselves, this small group of highly trained doctors continued to
seek the approval of their male colleagues. The Annual Report of the New England Hospital that year merely regretted
that Harvard remained closed to women, but went on to laud
the general progress of women in other medical colleges.[45]
Zakrzewska, in a letter to the *Woman's Journal*, even sought
to paper over any differences with Clarke by treating his book
as a manual designed to encourage better health for *both* boys
and girls. The only accurate item contained in her letter was
the prediction that the book would initiate a wide-ranging discussion of ideas on education.[46] No doubt the fact that Clarke

seminal. I am indebted to many of his suggestions for my own investigation.
   41. Theodore Roosevelt, *The Foes of Our Own Household* (New York,
1917), p. 257.
   42. Clarke, p. 145.
   43. Ibid., p. 140.
   44. Ibid., p. 156. Here he notes that a "growing boy" may study six
hours daily but a girl only four hours. On p. 159 he cites his approval of
girls taking a vacation of three days every fourth week.
   45. AR-NEH (1873), p. 6.
   46. *WJ*, February 21, 1874, p. 59.

and three other highly regarded doctors became consulting
physicians for the hospital that year (bringing the number of
Harvard medical staff members to eight), influenced her position.[47] Men who would permit their names to appear on the
hospital's roster of "officers," it was hoped, would bring
others behind them. It was just a matter of time.

But the public debate that followed Clarke's book turned
out to be less a discussion than an all-out battle. Counterattacks
came in the form of numerous articles, studies, and four books,
all published within a year: *Sex and Education, No Sex in
Education, Woman's Education and Woman's Health,* and
The Education of American Girls.[48] Each critic recognized the
dangers if Clarke's book remained unchallenged. As E. B. Duffey, editor of *No Sex in Education,* noted, Clarke's covert plan
"has been a crafty one and his line of attack masterly. He
knows if he succeeds . . . and convinces the world that woman
is a 'sexual' creature alone, subject to and ruled by 'periodic
tides,' the battle is won for those who oppose the advancement
of women." [49]

Opponents hammered away at each of Clarke's points.
Among them, there was unanimous agreement that his study
would fail any scientific test. As Thomas Wentworth Higginson pointed out, to take seven cases out of a physician's notebook, assuring the readers that there were a good many more,
was simply not enough.[50] Furthermore, Clarke had neglected
to present seven "representative" males for comparison, but
simply assumed that boys could withstand whatever educational pressures they were exposed to. Similarly, the resident

47. AR-NEH (1873), p. 2.
48. Julia Ward Howe (ed.), *Sex and Education. A Reply to Dr. Clarke's
"Sex in Education"* (Boston, 1874); Eliza Bisbee Duffey, *No Sex in Education; or, an equal chance for both girls and boys* (Syracuse, 1874); George
Fisk and Anna Manning Comfort, *Woman's Education and Woman's
Health: chiefly in reply to "Sex in Education"* (Syracuse, 1874); and Anna
Callender Brackett (ed.), *The Education of American Girls* (New York,
1874).
49. Duffey, p. 117.
50. Howe, p. 35.

physician at Vassar questioned Clarke's accuracy, noting that
the case of Miss D—— was not even possible since the college
had never had a girl as young as fourteen enrolled. She claimed
that an error of such proportion could not help but shake one's
confidence in the book's other cases and, indeed, its very
thesis.[51]

Critics generally agreed that whatever difficulties were experienced by female college students were environmentally
induced. Julia Ward Howe asserted that, if anything, a woman's
education should be more like a man's, in that she should be
given equal amounts of exercise and fresh air rather than being
confined to the home after school to perform domestic duties.
Furthermore, she argued, rather than suffering from the pressures of keeping up with the male students, women were, in
fact, victimized by the constant reminder that for them "education does not matter." [52]

Clarke's vague recommendations for a special educational
program for women was rejected as so impractical as to lead
to little or no education if it were implemented. Duffey
pointed out that Clarke's plan could only work if each student
were subject to a uniform menstrual period. "But each girl
has her own time; and if each were excused from attendance
and study during this time, there could be neither system nor
regularity in the classes." And what of the teacher, who probably also was a woman? "She too requires her regular fur-
lough, and then what are the scholars to do?" Duffey wondered
whether Clarke would extend his argument to the home so
that wives could leave children uncared for and dinners un-
cooked for three or four days each month. "I think a concerted
action among women in this direction," she wrote, "would
bring men who are inclined to agree with the doctor to their
senses sooner than anything else." [53]

Most of the critics, understandably, were unwilling to go as

51. Ibid., pp. 191–92.
52. Ibid., pp. 27–28.
53. Duffey, pp. 115–16; 97.

far as a general woman's menstrual strike and simply called for
scientific studies which would test Clarke's thesis. The first response to their cries came when Harvard Medical School in
1874 announced that one of the two topics that would be considered for its annual Boylston Medical Prize competition was,
"Do women require mental and bodily rest during menstruation and to what extent?" Since the applicants' names were not
revealed to the committee, it was possible for a woman to be
judged fairly in the competition, and Cambridge friends urged
Dr. Mary Putnam Jacobi of New York to apply.[54]

Jacobi had previously examined the question in "Mental
Action and Physical Health" in Anna Brackett's *The Education of American Girls,* one of the four books responding to
Clarke in 1874. That article had been written with the general
public in mind, and Jacobi had concentrated on causes other
than education which might explain female disabilities such
as "competition, haste, cramming, close confinement, long
hours, and unhealthy sedentary habits." [55] For the Boylston
competition, which she eventually won, Jacobi sent out 1,000
questionnaires concerning the relationship between rest and
general health. She received 286 responses to such questions as
how far young women walked, the presence or absence of uterine disease, and the degree and intensity of mental activity in
and after school. Tests were also run on a smaller number of
women at the New York Infirmary where scientific measure-
ments could be taken on biological responses during and outside the menses.

Her scientific findings were clearly at odds with the Clarke
thesis. Fifty-four percent did not experience any menstrual difficulties whatsoever; since most of those who did experience
difficulties suffered only moderate pain, Jacobi felt there was
nothing in the nature of menstruation to imply the necessity
or even the desirability of periodic rest for the vast majority of

54. Alice C. Baker to Mary Putnam Jacobi, Cambridge, Mass., November 7, 1874, folder 18, Jacobi papers, SA.
55. Brackett, p. 295.

women. In fact, proper physical exercise combined with better nutrition could do a great deal, in Jacobi's view, to prevent the development of menstrual pain. Rather than rest, Jacobi (striking a modern note) declared that most women could better tolerate moderate menstrual pain while continuing their normal work patterns. Equally important was her finding that mental activity was not dangerous. In those cases of severe menstrual pain the root cause was nearly always some anatomical imperfection.[56]

Jacobi's monograph was followed by a number of studies that appeared to clearly demonstrate that higher education was not injurious to the health of American women. Thus, one of the first acts of the Associated Collegiate Alumnae, formed in 1882, was to commission an examination of the health of college women. A list of questions was drawn up with the help of a group of physicians and mailed to 1,290 women college graduates in the United States. The 705 returns were analyzed by the Massachusetts Bureau of Labor Statistics. The bureau found that 78 percent of the respondents were in excellent health; 5 percent were classed as in fair health; and 17 percent were in poor health. If anything, college women appeared to enjoy better health than the national average. Similarly, L. H. Marvel in an article in the journal *Education,* found that college life, far from being deleterious to woman's physical adjustment, "has resulted in a stronger physique and a more perfect womanhood." In addition, Marvel's statistics demonstrated that the mortality rate for graduates of Mount Holyoke was substantially lower than that of graduates from Amherst, Bowdoin, Harvard, and Yale.[57]

It was one thing to study college women as a group, but what about those who undertook the strain associated with a

56. Mary Putnam Jacobi, *The Question of Rest for Women During Menstruation* (New York, 1877). Harvard did not publish the prize-winning monographs. Fortunately, Jacobi belonged to the wealthy and proud publishing family of G. P. Putnam which saw that the book got into print.

57. Louis H. Marvel, "How Does College Life Affect the Health of Women?" *Education* 3 (1883), p. 501.

professional career? In 1881 Emily Pope, C. Augusta Pope, and
Emma Call, doctors on the staff of New England Hospital,
published a study on women physicians. Their sample included
a group of 430 women doctors who had graduated from various medical schools since 1870. Only 13 of the respondents reported poor health and only 4 of these ascribed their illness to
the pressures of their practice. Furthermore, only 34 of the 307
who responded to a special question regarding menstruation
stated that they were periodically incapacitated. "We do not
think it would be easy," the authors declared, "to find a better
record of health among an equal number of women, taken at
random from all over the country." [58]

It is difficult to assess the effect of these studies. No doubt,
over the years, a number of medical men grudgingly accepted
the notion that women could be doctors. Others simply treated
each new investigation as one more exception to the rule that a
woman's place was in the home and not the hospital. But,
despite all of the studies, few were willing or able to grant the
woman doctors their ultimate objective: to be treated as equal
colleagues. Most male physicians were unable to comprehend
the professional meaning of young Susan Dimock's plaintive
letter, published in the *Boston Medical and Surgical Journal,*
in which she described her happiness as a medical student in
Switzerland because, in being able to study with the male
students "who will be her fellow practitioners, [she] had the
opportunity to make them her friends." [59] Even fewer could
have imagined how the women physicians traded confidences
about their progress in establishing such friendships on a colleagueship level. In 1863, for example, Zakrzewska happily
wrote to Dr. Lucy Sewall to describe how a Boston physician
"called on me and invited me to call upon him, as he is anxious
to extend colleague-ship to me." [60]

In the final analysis, the opposition to the women physicians
was more emotional than intellectual and thus impervious to

58. Emily F. Pope, Emma L. Call, and C. Augusta Pope, *The Practice of
Medicine by Women in the United States* (Boston, 1881).

59. *BMSJ* 84 (1871), p. 50.

60. Vietor, p. 310.

statistical studies. It was often motivated by unconscious forces that played tricks on those men who tried putting their ideas on the subject in print. Witness Edward Clarke, who had little difficulty in maintaining friendly relationships with women physicians, but whose prejudices were immediately apparent when he lectured and wrote on the subject of women. With this type of opposition, rational arguments about the capabilities of women, supported by mounting research data, might occasionally breach a barrier, but they could not turn the battle. Thus, a Horatio Storer could admit that some women were as well educated, had as much talent, were as courageous and "unflinching in the presence of suffering or at the sight of blood, as were many practitioners," yet go on to argue that they should not be allowed to practice medicine because of their biological makeup. The rigidity of the opposition's position is perhaps best illustrated in an editorial in the *Boston Medical and Surgical Journal* concerning the entrance of women into the Massachusetts Medical Society. The writer began by pointing out that there were simply not enough respectable female physicians to warrant a revision of the society's policy. Then, after a lengthy discussion of the subject and almost as an afterthought, he concluded with the question of whether women would qualify for membership when a considerable number of well-educated female physicians became a fact. His answer was succinct: "We think not." [61]

Although rarely stated as such, there is little doubt that part of the opposition to women physicians was economically inspired. Economists have shown that men experience lower wages and often higher unemployment rates in occupations with a large proportion of women. Unfortunately, American women first began knocking at the doors of medical institutions at a time when physicians were concerned about what they perceived to be the depressed state of the profession.[62]

61. *BMSJ* 98 (1878), pp. 676–77.
62. Richard H. Shryock, "Women in American Medicine," *JAMWA* 5 (1950), p. 375. Shryock makes this economic argument, which may be overly simplistic. He notes, for example, that the ratio of doctors to the population in America was higher than it was in Europe: "Had there been

"Never was the outlook so gloomy," the *Journal of the American Medical Association* complained, "the profession is overcrowded already to the starving point." [63] Physicians were obsessed with questions of supply and demand. Not only were doctors no longer able to support themselves, the *Boston Medical and Surgical Journal* pointed out, but each year brought a new invasion of "swarms of young men (and young women)." [64] The raising of standards and the successful organizational drive of the American Medical Association at the end of the nineteenth century were both responses to the physicians' fears.[65] Concerned as they were with their own survival, male physicians were hardly in a mood to welcome on board a group of women whose potential number could sink the already foundering ship.

---

a dearth of practitioners, opposition to women would doubtless have been less. . . ." In fact, European opposition to women was much stronger than it was in America if we are to compare the pre-World War I difficulties of women there to America. For the general argument on "overcrowding" see Francine D. Blau and Carol L. Jusenius, "Economists' Approaches to Sex Segregation in the Labor Market: An Appraisal," *Signs* 1 (Spring 1976), pp. 181–99.

63. *JAMA* 31 (1898), pp. 932–33. This complaint, however, was uttered throughout the period women were attempting to enter medicine. In Boston, Harvard opposed the establishment of any new medical schools with an economic argument. See, for example, references to Harvard opposition to a Tufts petition in 1866 to open a medical school (MSA). Tufts was not successful in its efforts until 1893. The data indicate that the doctors wildly exaggerated the growth in the number of practitioners, which, in fact, was matched by the population growth. Thus, there was one physician for every 572 people in 1860, and one for every 578, forty years later (B. J. Stearn, *American Medical Practice in the Perspectives of a Century* [New York, 1943], p. 363; N. S. Davis, *Contributions to the History of Medical Education and Medical Institutions in the U.S.A. 1776–1876* [Washington, 1877], pp. 42–44).

64. *BMSJ* 111 (1884), p. 90.

65. Two studies that document this in detail are Gerald E. Markowitz and David Karl Rosner, "Doctors in Crisis: A Study of the Use of Medical Education Reform to Establish Modern Professional Elitism in Medicine," *American Quarterly* 25 (March 1973), pp. 83–107; and Stevens, especially pp. 35–38.

There was also the latent fear that the men might be left to drown while the women took command of the vessel. As early as 1849, the *Boston Medical and Surgical Journal* had called attention to Samuel Gregory's preparation of women "for a department of practice considered quite lucrative." [66] Female patients made up a majority of a doctor's medical practice in the nineteenth century.[67] One hesitated to even think of what would happen to the size of that practice if they all defected to their professionally trained sisters. So concerned were medical men over the possible loss of this trade that Dr. John Ware, whose practice had made him one of the wealthier men in Massachusetts, felt compelled to caution a class of graduating doctors in Boston to couch their opposition to women physicians in terms other than those that would reflect a "mean jealousy of encroachment on a profitable field of labor." [68] It is little wonder that these anxieties periodically surfaced, as they did in the *Boston Medical and Surgical Journal* reprint of this Edinburgh ditty:

> An' when the leddies git degrees,
> Depen' upon't there's' nocht'll please
> Till they hae got oor chairs an' fees,
> An' there's an en/ o' you an' me.[69]

This fear of feminine competition can be illustrated in a variety of ways. In the case of Dr. Charles Ellery Stedman, recording secretary of the Dorchester Medical Society, it emerges from the sketches he made while taking notes at the meetings. Thus, appended to his report on a successful social meeting, attended by "beauteous damsels who flitted about the tables like

66. *BMSJ* 40 (1849), p. 505.
67. This generalization is based on the examination of nineteenth-century physician record books deposited in HCL-A.
68. John Ware, "Success in the Medical Profession: An Introductory Lecture, delivered at the Massachusetts Medical College (Harvard), Nov. 6, 1850," *BMSJ* 43 (1851), p. 520.
69. *BMSJ* 89 (1873), p. 23.

joys forever," we find his image of the ideal woman physician: feminine, demure, and passive (see fig. 3). The women physicians limned in later notes are anything but a joy. One woman physician is symbolically in the driver's seat of a carriage, from which she looks down at her "unsuccessful competitor" to say,

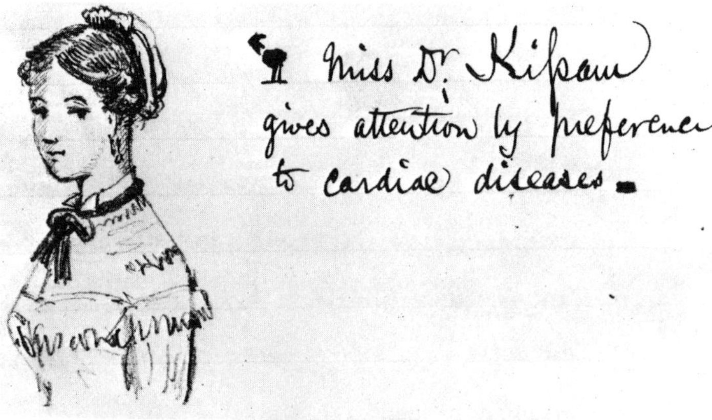

FIGURE 3   Charles Ellery Stedman notebook drawing, December 17, 1874. From the *Records* of the Dorchester Medical Club. Courtesy of the Boston Medical Library in The Francis A. Countway Library of Medicine.

"Doctor let me give you a lift" (see fig. 4). In another drawing, a well-dressed woman physician is seated on a fast-moving charger; behind is her black servant carrying her medical satchel with her competitors fading into the background. The caption tells us that the woman is "Alice Ethel Arlington, A.B., A.M., M.D, Harvard, 1888, Surgeon Massachusetts General Hospital, Boston Obstetrical Society, Boston Society of Medical Inspectors, Boston Society for Medical Science, Boston Dispensary, etc. etc. etc." (see fig. 5) [70]

Closely allied to the economic argument was the conviction that the introduction of women would impede all attempts to

70. "Records of the Dorchester Medical Club kept by Dr. Ellery Stedman (1874–78)," HCL-A.

raise the status of the profession.[71] For connected to the fear that medicine would defeminize women was a second apprehension, perhaps springing out of the failure of the first to materialize, that women would "feminize" the profession. In

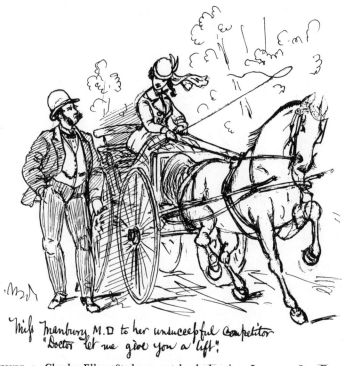

FIGURE 4   Charles Ellery Stedman notebook drawing, June 24, 1875. From the *Records* of the Dorchester Medical Club. Courtesy of the Boston Medical Library in The Francis A. Countway Library of Medicine.

the business and professional world outside the home, male and female have been synonymous with high and low status respectively.[72] So deeply entrenched is the notion that women

71. This is documented in the rhetoric used in the institutional battles described in chap. 5.

72. Epstein provides contemporary evidence for this in American professions; the problem, however, is widespread and ongoing. See, for ex-

lower the status of a professional field that mere mention of the fact that women may comprise a disproportionate number of the workers causes people to rate that field lower in prestige. Doctors took their status from the larger society, and there was

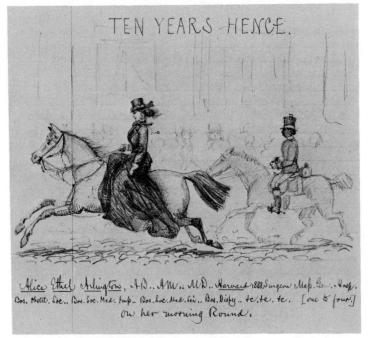

FIGURE 5 Charles Ellery Stedman notebook drawing, March 15, 1878. From the *Records* of the Dorchester Medical Club. Courtesy of the Boston Medical Library in The Francis A. Countway Library of Medicine.

no room for the incorruptible innocence of the "softer sex" in a world where competition, rationality, and strength spelled success.

---

ample, "Problems of Feminization of the Medical Profession in Slovakia," *Jancovicova J. Cesk. Zdrav* 20 (June 1972), pp. 218–22. John C. Touhey, "Effects of Additional Women Professionals on Ratings of Occupational Prestige and Desirability," *Journal of Personality and Social Psychology* 29 no. 1 (1974), pp. 86–89.

While doctors viewed themselves as essentially humanitarians, they saw nothing wrong with capitalizing on their talents, as demonstrated by books bearing such titles as *Dollars to Doctors, Large Fees and How to Get Them,* and *The Physician as Businessman.*[73] After all, the American Medical Association declared, the standing and influence of the profession depends on the "material success and financial independence of its members." [74] Sternness, control, efficiency, strength, and organization were terms late nineteenth-century doctors liked to use to describe themselves. Feminization, on the other hand, was the antithesis of all that led to achievement in the field. This explains why so many doctors were fond of describing their work in highly masculine terms. Thus, one Boston doctor could dismiss the women: "If they cannot stride a mustang or mend bullet holes, so much the better for an enterprising and skillful practitioner of the sterner sex." [75] No doubt mustangs and bullets played a major part in the day-to-day practice of the stern physicians who had their offices on Boylston Street.

The most deep-seated and persistent emotional resistance to women doctors, and hence the least subject to rational discourse stemmed from the male-female nexus itself. Male physicians subscribed to the same sexual stereotypes as other men and suffered from the same sexual tensions. Plagued by the divisive effects of civil war, territorial expansion, immigration, and industrialization, American society placed a high premium

73. Nathan E. Wood, *Dollars to Doctors* (Chicago, 1903); Albert V. Horman, *Large Fees and How to Get Them* (Chicago, 1911); J. J. Taylor, *The Physician as Businessman or How to Obtain the Best Financial Results in the Practice of Medicine* (Philadelphia, 1892)—the latter went through at least seventeen editions and authorship passed from father to son. These and similar titles occupy several shelves in the historical collection of the Countway Library, Harvard Medical School. The entire question of economic competition in medicine in the late nineteenth and early twentieth century deserves further study. A beginning has been made by Lloyd C. Taylor, Jr., *The Medical Profession and Social Reform, 1885–1945* (New York, 1974), esp. pp. 98–101.

74. *JAMA* 44 (1905), p. 1933.

75. Newspaper clipping in Chadwick Scrapbook, n.d., HCL-A.

on the stability that it believed stemmed from the family and
the rigidly defined sex roles which supported it. Consequently,
what appears to be a pathological resentment toward "un-
natural female physicians"—or the "third sex" as the Boston
Gynecological Society referred to them—was to nineteenth-
century society simply one response to a major threat to society. As a recent scholar has pointed out, men dreaded any
change in their sex roles because, as the century drew to a
close, they were finding it more and more difficult to "be a
man." The masculine role was becoming increasingly uncertain
as the work role of men grew more "feminine" in its characteristics. Many men, and women too, felt threatened by the
reforms prompted by the woman's rights movement.[76]

When male physicians thought of female physicians it was
within this context. Furthermore, the polarized sex roles of the
day made it impossible for most men to think of women as
colleagues. Communication between husband and wife was
strained and often nonexistent despite the fact that changes
in the structure of society were placing an increasing emotional burden on couples to be congenial and affectionate.
Emile Barbier, a traveler to the United States in the 1890s,
described women as living a life in which a "veritable abyss"
separated them from their husbands.[77]

This is illustrated in the diary of Susan Oliver, wife of Dr.
Edward Oliver, an editor of the *Boston Medical and Surgical
Journal* and a member of the Harvard faculty. The Olivers,
who had what can be described as a typical Victorian marriage,
spent little time together, shared almost no mutual interests,

76. Peter Filene, *Him, Her, Self: Sex Roles in Modern American* (New
York, 1975), p. 77.
77. Emile Barbier, *Voyage au Pays des Dollars* (Paris, 1893), p. 130.
More recently, Carroll Smith-Rosenberg has analyzed the correspondence
and diaries of women and men in thirty-five families between the 1760s
and the 1880s and drawn similar conclusions—see "The Female World of
Love and Ritual: Relations between Women in Nineteenth-Century
America," *Signs* 1 (Autumn 1975), pp. 1–29.

and, according to her diary, did not engage in even one meaningful exchange of ideas. They were separated by widely different worlds. While Edward Oliver spent his days active in his
professional field and his evenings pursuing his many interests
in historical studies, Susan Oliver appears as a passive witness,
weighted down by each illness of her several small children
and tired out by the constant round of visiting and shopping.
They were an affluent family, well supplied with servants and
household help, yet when they had an evening together, she
listened while he talked about his enthusiasms. By the standards of the day, each was in the proper "sphere." [78]

Yet, while this polarization left man dominant in his sphere
and woman in hers, it was a precarious bargain with man the
victor, at least temporarily. As William R. Taylor noted, men
were willing to give women the home if they would agree to
stay in it. But some women were beginning to reject the bargain. Consequently, male physicians uneasily contemplating
the female challenge in their own field, saw in the women doctors something more than professional competitors. Women
were competing for the power that had been a man's right in a
patriarchal society. It was more than coincidence that the
medical campaign to define women by their reproductive capabilities came at a time when they were seeking to define themselves in other ways. This fear of female power regularly surfaced when medical men gathered professionally. Thus, at an
1884 meeting of the Massachusetts Medical Society, one physician cried out that women already had enough influence "as
testified by three ex-presidents being now absent on account

78. Susan Lawrence (Mason) Oliver, "A Ms. Diary for 1878" Boston
Public Library Research Room. On the role of the doctor's wife, Ellen M.
Firebaugh (*The Physicians' Wife and the Things That Pertain to Her
Life* [Philadelphia, 1894]) wrote: "We, their wives, cannot do the good in
the world that our husbands have it in their power to do. Our sphere is
circumscribed; and so our real usefulness to those around us as compared
with theirs, may be likened, perhaps, as shadow unto form. But it is good
to know that shadows, too, have their mission in the world."

of their 'women-folks' dragging them away to some other arrangement." [79]
Nothing better illustrates this question of power than the physicians' attitude toward nursing. Significantly, those who opposed the entrance of women into medicine as doctors welcomed them as nurses. The nurse's uniform seemed to serve as a successful antidote to the biological limitations that had been the curse of the women doctors. Thus, the *Boston Medical and Surgical Journal* had objected to women doctors because their health would prevent them from enduring the strain of constant house calls, while their sensitivity would wilt before the "rough contact with the vulgar and vicious." [80] Yet, later in a glowing tribute to the nursing profession, the journal described the nurses as they went "into the slums of our city, through the dark alleys, among the ash barrels and swill, up the dark, dirty, rickety staircases of the tenements." [81] Health no longer seemed a problem, as the journal noted that eleven trained nurses had made 46,933 visits among the sick in the previous year alone.[82] Menstrual difficulties had apparently also been swept away because, according to the editor, characteristics that made for success in nursing were bodily strength, knowledge of symptoms, the ability to deal with emergencies, and mature judgment.[83]

Clearly, women as nurses, engaged as they were in a domesticated version of the doctor's role, posed no threat to the male physician. As the *Boston Medical and Surgical Journal* pointed out: 'The doctor's responsibility as to the nursing service is like that of the captain to his ship." [84] And, as everyone knew, mutiny was the greatest crime of all. Consequently, Dr. Edward

79. William R. Taylor, *Cavalier and Yankee: The Old South and the American National Character* (New York, 1963), p. 126; *New England Medical Gazette*, July 1884, p. 199.
80. *BMSJ* 76 (1867), p. 272.
81. Ibid., 136 (1897), p. 214.
82. Ibid., p. 216.
83. Ibid., p. 217.
84. Ibid., 130 (1894), p. 437.

Cowles, superintendent of Boston City Hospital, in recommending the appointment of a supervisor of nursing, made it clear that whoever filled the position, must stay within her "proper station" and in no way be allowed to work against the physician in charge. The *Journal of the American Medical Association* was always quick to complain of any tendency of nurses to stray from their station; in 1901 it charged that many doctors found the nurse "often conceited and too unconscious of the due subordination she owes to the medical profession, of which she is sort of a useful parasite." [85] The *Woman's Journal* accurately described the typical response of the male physician: "It's no argument at all to say that if we work with them as nurses we might just as well when they are doctors; that's a very different thing. Nurses are docile, submissive, and keep their proper place, while *once let a woman study medicine and she thinks her opinion is as good as a man's*." [86]

Finally, how much of the doctors' opposition arose from a fear of female sexuality? Historians are just beginning to investigate the nineteenth-century physician's obsessive concern with the female reproductive system. Writers of popular manuals on women's health, for example, often brushed over widespread, fatal diseases such as consumption and breast cancer in their eagerness to describe the myriad dangers emanating from

85. Frederic A. Washburn, *The Massachusetts General Hospital: Its Development 1900–1935* (Boston, 1939), pp. 443–44. The letter partially reproduced in Washburn is not available to scholars for examination. Washburn comments that failure to adhere to the principle involved in this letter "has many times caused trouble in hospital management" (p. 444). Contemporary writers are beginning to argue that the docile behavior of nurses has caused a different kind of trouble, an inferior kind of hospital care. See Leonard Stein, "The Doctor-Nurse Game," *Archives of General Psychiatry* 16, pp. 699–704. See Barbara Ehrenreich's excellent paper "The Status of Women as Health Care Providers in the U.S.," Paper delivered at the International Conference on Women in Health, Washington, D.C., June 16, 1975, p. 7. The *JAMA* quote is from an editorial, "The Unsentimental Nurse," vol. 37 (1901), p. 33, which she cites.

86. *WJ*, January 5, 1884, p. 6 (italics mine).

the womb.[87] As one woman physician noted, following what she termed the Marion Sims epoch, "the profession went mad in the direction of gynecological tinkering, womb prodding, and probing, and woman was rarely permitted to have an ache or a pain referable to any other part of her anatomy." According to another woman physician, there was a "wholesale onslaught upon those innocent organs . . . removing them for nervousness . . . because the husbands request it, removing them for everything but disease." Significantly few women physicians participated in this surgical craze.[88]

Certainly, a spate of books was published illustrating the growing concern with a cult of manliness: *Manhood: The Causes of Its Premature Decline* (1870), *Manliness in the Scholar* (1883), *Manhood Wrecked and Rescued* (1900), and *The Masculine Power of Christ* (1912).[89] Fear of sexuality was also expressed in the application of the term nymphomania to sexuality that would be considered quite normal today. Horatio Storer, for example, wrote extensively on this topic and even went so far as to refer to one of his patients as a case of "virgin nymphomania." [90] Oscar Handlin cites the writing of Storer as typical of the orthodox medical men of the nineteenth century and it is therefore likely that Storer mirrored the

87. Ann Douglas Wood, "The Fashionable Diseases: Women's Complaints and Their Treatment in Nineteenth-Century America," *Journal of Interdisciplinary History* 4, no. 1 (Summer 1973), pp. 28–29.

88. Lillian G. Towslee, M.D., *WMJ* 13 (1903), p. 121. Editorial by Mary A. Spink, M.D., Associate Editor, *WMJ* 2 (1894), p. 18.

89. E. De F. Curtis, *Manhood: The Causes of its Premature Decline: With Directions for Perfect Restoration* (1870); Richard Salter Storrs, *Manliness in the Scholar* (New York, 1883); William John Hunter, *Manhood Wrecked and Rescued: How Strength or Vigor is Lost, and How it May be Restored by Self-Treatment* (New York, 1900); Jason Noble Pierce, *The Masculine Power of Christ; or, Christ Measured as a Man* (Boston, 1912). For an extensive bibliography of books of this type see, Joseph H. Pleck (compiler), "Male Sex Role and Personality: Historical Materials," (November 1972); this bibliography is available from the author at the Institute for Social Research, University of Michigan, Ann Arbor.

90. Horatio Storer, *Causation, Course and Treatment of Reflex Insanity in Women*, pp. 211–12.

views of many physicians when he wrote of the powers that were associated with puberty: "Passions . . . are now established, unrecognized though it may be by the girl herself; yet like the smoldering fires of a volcano, ready to burst forth at any exciting moment." [91] Were the doctors who constantly called attention to the diseases associated with the womb unconsciously seeking to neutralize this potential power?

Although most men seem to have preferred sexually responsive wives, the nineteenth century witnessed an increasing fear of "excessive" female sexuality. For the first time the dangers of sexual intercourse within marriage became widespread, as evidenced by the concern over the proper frequency of intercourse. This fear of excessive female sexuality may have stemmed in part from a fear of infidelity. But one also suspects that there may have been an unconscious fear that excessive demands might be made on male abilities to perform adequately.

Many of these anxieties—the fear of female sexuality, the decline in the birthrate, and the loss of male control—came together in the general consternation over abortion. Many medical men believed that women doctors were the chief source of abortions. Storer, who chaired several panels on this topic, charged that the growth of abortions paralleled the expansion of women's hospitals, especially those allegedly for lying-in purposes. If women doctors, out of some misguided sympathy for their sisters, could participate in such crimes, what other damage would they do? What did women physicians mean when they declared that they would "open books that are sealed?" [92] Physicians, along with other nineteenth-

91. Horatio Storer, "The Causation, Course and Rational Treatment of Insanity in Women. A Gynaecist's Idea thereof," report to American Medical Association, as Chairman of its Standing Committee on Insanity, *Transactions of the American Medical Association* (1864).

92. Harriot Kezia Hunt, *Glances and Glimpses; or Fifty Years Social, Including Twenty Years Professional Life* (Boston, 1856; reprinted, 1970), p. 159. The charges about abortions being performed in female-operated lying-in hospitals were usually made, as Storer made them, by innuendo.

century men sought domestic tranquility. But, unlike most
other men, because of their special positions they found themselves charged with a major share of the responsibility of
maintaining the status quo.

The one serious charge against New England Hospital, in 1915, was
thoroughly investigated and the report indicates they were not guilty. See
folder "Abortion Controversy," New England Hospital Collections, SSC-SC.

5

A Break in the Barriers

Preserving the status quo in nineteenth-century Boston meant defending male dominance at Harvard Medical School, the Massachusetts Medical Society, and the major hospitals. These institutions, forming as they did a synergistic relationship, presented women with a formidable set of linked barriers. For example, graduates from Harvard Medical School were guaranteed admission to the Massachusetts Medical Society. Similarly, Massachusetts General Hospital, which had been founded by two Harvard professors, appointed only Harvard students to its internships. Harvard-educated physicians monopolized the staff appointments of all the major hospitals and many of the small hospitals founded by religious organizations. Thus, in the latter part of the nineteenth century, women hammered away at each institution in the hope that one victory would create a domino effect.

By ignoring the long years of planning, organizing, and sacrifice that went into this effort, historians have missed a significant chapter in nineteenth-century woman's struggle to gain equality. This failure is perhaps understandable since women physicians were forced to eschew the more dramatic tactics which have drawn attention to the suffragist movement. Seeking to be recognized as professionals, the women felt constrained to adopt a policy of proving their worth while working behind the scenes to develop support for their goals. Furthermore, the individualistic, free-enterprise concept of medicine in America precluded appeal to the legislative process. Finally, the complete masculine control of Boston's major medical institutions meant that the women had to attract and maintain friends at court. Male members would have to argue the women's case on the floor of the Massachusetts Medical Society; male trustees would have to vote on their pleas to enter Harvard: male physicians would have to admit them to the city's hospitals. Faced with a society which saw feminism and professionalism as mutually exclusive, the women physicians felt forced to carry on their battle in a carefully circumscribed arena.

Fortunately, however, there was some room for maneuvering. Although the medical establishment's counterattack achieved wide currency, the male medical world was not monolithic. A few physicians were persuaded that women had as much right as men to become doctors. Moreover, many male physicians, influenced in some measure by the success of their own rhetoric, became convinced that the number of women capable of becoming doctors was so small as to pose no threat to male domination of the profession. And although they rejected the Victorian argument that feminine modesty required women doctors, many male physicians had to admit that some women preferred doctors of their own sex. Moreover, a growing number of states were enacting legislation requiring the employment of female physicians in the treatment of women patients in state institutions, hospitals, and lunatic asylums. Thus, for good or evil, there appeared to be a market for the expected small number of women physicians who would practice. And once women physicians became a fact of medical life, the male medical establishment became vulnerable to a new line of attack. Indeed, if women, no matter how small a number, were practicing, did it not follow that they should be educated in sound medical schools and subject to the same certification process as men?

The women physicians were especially fortunate in attracting to their cause three of the most prominent physicians in Boston: Henry I. Bowditch, Samuel Cabot, and James Chadwick. As Martin Duberman has noted, we know far too little about why people do anything, let alone why they do something as specific as joining a reform movement.[1] These three

1. Martin Duberman, *The Uncompleted Past* (New York, 1969), p. 8. Evidence for the prominent role played by Bowditch, Cabot, and Chadwick

men differed in their areas of medical specialization and they ranged in age from Bowditch, who was seventy-one in 1879, to Chadwick who was thirty-five years younger. The one thing that all three seem to have shared was a combination of personal and public success which enabled them to bear the tension connected with supporting a highly unpopular cause. Each had personal friendships with women physicians, and each served as a consultant for a long period of time at New England Hospital: Bowditch for thirty years, Cabot for twenty-one years, and Chadwick for thirteen years. Each one appears to fit Gordon Allport's definition of the mature personality: the ability to get outside one's self-preoccupation and involve oneself in abstract ideals.[2]

Henry I. Bowditch, who championed the first female applicant to the Massachusetts Medical Society and whose motion thirty-two years later opened its doors to women, embodied these characteristics to the fullest. Bowditch served in several important positions in the Massachusetts Medical Society, held a professorship at Harvard, and became a leader in the public health movement. Having joined the abolitionist movement in its infancy in 1835, his threatened resignation from Massachusetts General Hospital in 1841 over a rule excluding Negroes as patients had forced the trustees to reconsider their position.[3] To Bowditch, the woman's struggle was an extension of the principles of the abolitionist movement. A letter to Zakrzewska recalling the early years of the fight to admit women to the Massachusetts Medical Society, illustrates the sense of security that enabled Bowditch to take part in more

is based on manuscripts in the Countway Library, HMS-A, as well as a variety of manuscripts preserved by the women physicians in several locations. These are listed in the back matter. See also Thomas W. Miller, "Male Attitudes toward Women's Rights as a Function of Their Level of Self-Esteem," Paper read at the Eightieth Annual Convention of the American Psychological Association, Division 9 Symposium: *Who Discriminates Against Women?*, Honolulu, Hawaii, September 4, 1972.

2. Gordon Allport, *Becoming: Basic Considerations for a Psychology of Personality* (New Haven, 1955), p. 45.

3. Vincent Y. Bowditch, *Life and Correspondence of Henry Ingersoll Bowditch*, vol. 1 (Boston, 1902), pp. 130–32.

than a half-century of reform: "At first I believed some of
the bigots thought I ought to be punished. But I cared not
for the dark hints of discipline impending, feeling sure as I
did that light would appear the next day and that with the
element of time and simple justice on my side, right would
certainly prevail." [4]

The women physicians of Boston attached special importance to membership in the Massachusetts Medical Society.
During the first half of the nineteenth century, that body
controlled medical licensing in the state. Although one could
practice without a license, the society's certification procedures were viewed as sifting out the regularly educated physicians from the sectarians and poorly educated practitioners.
Even after the state eliminated all licensing laws in 1859,
membership in the society was viewed as an important asset.
Not only did admission testify to one's ability, but it also
guaranteed cooperation and referrals of patients from other
physicians. Moreover, only society members were listed in
the official annual medical directory published by Francis
Brown. Although some of the society's members were willing
to consult with qualified women physicians not listed in the
official directory, such consultations were granted as a favor
and not as a matter of course, and most often with an air of
condescension which deterred many of the women from asking for one. Moreover, society membership was a prerequisite
for admission to the staffs of a number of hospitals and institutions. To be a member of a medical society in the nineteenth
century was the average physician's only hope for acquiring
comparative distinction among his or her peers.[5]

Because of the small number of qualified women physicians
at midcentury, the first attempts to crack the sexual barriers

4. Henry I. Bowditch to Marie Zakrzewska, June 15, 1884, reprinted in
Agnes Vietor, *A Woman's Quest: The Life of Marie E. Zakrzewska* (New
York, 1924), p. 391.
5. "Recollections of Dr. Emma Call," January 19, 1928, New England
Hospital Collection, SSC-SC; Rosemary Stevens, *American Medicine and
the Public Interest* (New Haven, 1971), p. 36.

were necessarily carried out on an individual basis. In 1852, two years after Harvard had rejected Harriot Hunt for the second time, Dr. Nancy Talbot Clark, a twenty-seven-year-old graduate of Western Reserve Medical College of Cleveland, became the first woman in the United States to seek certification from a state medical society. In her petition to the Massachusetts Medical Society, which was supported by Henry Bowditch, Clark stated that she was not asking for membership, but rather for an examination of her medical qualifications: "I ask this," she pleaded, "in order that, thereby, I may be publicly lifted from the rank of mere pretender to learning." [6]

Her personal appearance before the board of censors and her formal petition created such confusion among the five members who served as the society's application committee that the question was referred to the executive body of the society, the board of councilors. One of the censors, Dr. Edward H. Clarke, then only thirty-two years old, noted in his letter to the councilors that since the applicant had graduated from a reputable medical school and possessed the proper credentials, she appeared to meet all of the qualifications for membership, especially since the society's bylaws did not in any way bar women. Nevertheless, Clarke concluded his letter with the notation that the application was a "novel one." [7]

The censors did not automatically reject her application because a society bylaw required that every applicant who applied had to be examined. As a state licensing agency, the society was subject to a fine of up to $400 for each of the censors who failed to follow the law; moreover, the fine was payable to the applicant. After considering these issues, the councilors met in February 1853 and informed the censors that their obligation only applied to male applicants. More important, they also assured the censors that if their rejection

6. Henry I. Bowditch to Emma Call, December 25, 1884, New England Hospital Collection, SSC-SC.

7. Massachusetts Medical Society, Records of the Censors, February 1, 1853, HCL-A.

of Nancy Clark's application was challenged, the society would assume all costs of legally defending their action. Freed from all financial risks, the censors voted unanimously not to license Clark.[8]

The Nancy Talbot Clark decision, which must have appeared to the censors as an end to the matter, was merely the first exchange in a debate that spanned some thirty years.[9] In 1859, Marie Zakrzewska, newly arrived in Boston and still convinced of the city's liberality, informally approached the society and was informed that its policy remained unchanged. In 1864, having gained the friendship of a number of male physicians and no longer connected with Samuel Gregory, Zakrzewska again sounded out several members of the society. Encouraged at first by their response, she began studying for the examination, but after several months of discussion she was told that her application would not be considered. Angered by the decision, Zakrzewska promised herself that when the time came—and she was sure that it would come in her lifetime—the society would have to offer her an honorary membership to get her to join.[10]

Because of its influential position within the Boston medical network, the society's advice was often sought by other

8. Ibid., February 5, 1853.
9. There has been a recent effort to minimize the women's struggle, both in time and energy. See, for example, Everett R. Spender, Jr., "The Ten-Year Debate," *Massachusetts Physician* (July 1972), pp. 36–37, 42. Spencer argues incorrectly that Susan Dimock was the first applicant to the society whereas Nancy Clark had applied twenty years before Dimock.
10. Vietor, pp. 277–78, 395. Zakrzewska's anger may be better understood when viewed in the context of what the medical society required in an examination at this time and their policy in freely granting honorary memberships to males. An examination was not based on the kind of practical knowledge that Zakrzewska had built up in her medical practice but rather expertise in Greek, Latin, and subjects related to a liberal education. The exam changed in the years from 1860 to 1885. A list of the 152 male "honorary fellows" of the Massachusetts Medical Society is published in *A Catalogue of the Honorary and Past and Present Fellows 1781–1931* (Boston, 1931), pp. 3–6. Zakrzewska, needless to say, was never invited to membership.

medical institutions faced with the "woman question." For example, in 1867 Massachusetts General Hospital formally requested an opinion from the society on whether or not female students should be allowed to visit its wards. A few of the students of New England Hospital had been granted this privilege, but their presence in the wards of the hospital had resulted in a great deal of tension for certain male physicians on the staff. The inquiry in turn touched off a full-scale debate among the councilors who finally decided on a forty-nine to seven vote that it would be inexpedient to admit female students to hospitals and medical schools within the state.[11] "Inexpedience," that "little word," which had so angered Harriot Hunt when it was used by Harvard against her in 1850, was still deemed sufficient cause to block any further use of Massachusetts General Hospital by women medical students seventeen years later.

But, as the number of women physicians mounted, society members were increasingly called upon to explain and defend their position. The expanding female medical population also led to a shift in the arguments raised on behalf of the women doctors. Justice was the soundest reason for the admission of women into the Massachusetts Medical Society; however, there were only so many ways to state this proposition and, furthermore, many of the male physicians remained unmoved by this line of argument.

As early as Nancy Talbot Clark, women had also argued that certification by the society would help the public identify qualified women physicians. Convinced of its appeal to both the public and the society, the advocates of women's admission made this argument the central issue of their campaign. As a result, practicality replaced equity in the ensuing debates. Male physicians were informed that, like it or not, the question of women practitioners had already been decided; the only decision remaining was whether or not they would be screened and regulated on the same basis as men.

11. Massachusetts Medical Society, Records of the Council, June 4, 1867, HCL-A.

The question was one that was bound to appeal to a public increasingly baffled by the claims of a bewildering variety of practitioners. By the late 1870s a number of leading citizens advocated legislation to replace the licensing laws that had been eliminated in 1859. The Boston members of the medical society opposed any proposed legislation on the grounds that they would be forced to serve on the same licensing boards as the heretical homeopaths and eclectics. But, the more one argued that the regular practitioners should concentrate on regulating their own house, the more difficult it became to ignore the regular female physicians. As Dr. Robert Eddes reminded the members of the Dorchester Medical Society in 1878, "if membership is to be an honor, and non-membership disgrace, let no one be able to say that exclusion from the Massachusetts Medical Society is a mere matter of prejudice." Eddes pointed out that barriers must not only exclude the unworthy, but also include the worthy.[12] It took some time for this argument to sink in, but the growing number of women physicians in a period when the Massachusetts Medical Society faced the threat of having its preeminence eclipsed by a legislated certification board made it more palatable. Furthermore, some medical men began to recognize the paradox of rejecting applicants who were more qualified than many of the present society members.

The Massachusetts Medical Society was not the only group forced to confront the issue of medical women at this time. Dr. Alfred Stille's presidential address at the 1871 American Medical Association convention in San Francisco offered little

12. Robert T. Eddes, "What is the Object of the Massachusetts Medical Society, and How Can it Best be Fulfilled?" May 16, 1878, HCL-A; *Boston Daily Advertiser,* May 31, 1881; *Springfield Republican,* June 14, 1882; *Boston Herald,* June 14, 1882; *Boston Globe,* June 14, 1885; *Boston Transcript,* June 14, 1883. There were frequent articles in *BMSJ* responding to the public press but also acknowledging the existence of public concern and confusion. The best summary of the Boston medical establishment's objections to state licensing in Massachusetts is Reginald Fitz, "The Legislative Control of Medical Practice," *Medical Communications of the Massachusetts Medical Society* (1894), pp. 275–360.

encouragement to women physicians. "Certain women," he warned, "seek to rival men in manly sports . . . and the strong-minded ape them in all things, even in dress. In doing so, they may command a sort of admiration such as all monstrous productions inspire, especially when they tend toward a higher type than their own." Nevertheless, the question of women doctors surfaced indirectly in the form of a resolution acknowledging the right of its members to professionally consult with the graduates and teachers of the women's medical colleges. The debate quickly spilled over into the question of women physicians' membership in the association. Among the leaders of the opposition was Horatio Storer, who took the opportunity to expand at length on his favorite subject: "that uncertain equilibrium, that varying from month to month in each woman [which] unfits her from taking those responsibilities which are to control the question of life and death." When Dr. Gibbons of San Francisco retorted that a large majority of male practitioners fluctuated not once a month with the moon, but every day with the movement of the sun, because of the influence of alcohol, the convention dissolved into a shouting match. Cooler heads prevailed at the following session and, after apologies from both sides, the resolution was laid on the table without a vote. But the issue was not one that could be dismissed through parliamentary maneuvering, and in 1876 the association was presented with a fait accompli when Dr. Sarah Hackett Stevenson was sent by the Illinois State Medical Society as a delegate to the national convention.[13]

Equally encouraging were the actions of the state societies of Kansas, Michigan, and Rhode Island, all of which threw open

13. *BMSJ* 102 (1880), pp. 180–92; and Fitz, p. 142. See also references to women physicians in *Digest of Official Actions, American Medical Association* (1959) under "Consultations" (May 1871), pp. 41, 42; "Association in Medical Schools and Clinics" (May 1872), pp. 73, 74. That the acceptance of Dr. Stevenson did not entail the acceptance of women physicians as colleagues is evident from later official actions, see pp. 745–47 of the *Digest*. Morris Fishbein, *History of the American Medical Association 1847–1947* (Philadelphia, 1947), pp. 82–83.

their membership to women in 1877. Rhode Island not only voted to accept women, but also called attention to Massachusetts' backwardness: "Ever since Roger Williams found the breezes of the Narragansett so much more favorable to free thought, . . . we have had a certain advantage in being more guided by individual reason than in the old Bay State." [14] Encouraged by the other states and convinced that the threat of state regulation would force the Massachusetts society to reconsider its position, the medical women decided to stake their fortunes on the application of Dr. Susan Dimock. Her candidacy confronted the society with a real dilemma. Dimock, at this time a resident physician at New England Hospital, had graduated with high honors from the University of Zurich and had obtained an additional year of graduate medical training in Vienna and Paris. She carried out an extensive reorganization of the hospital's training school for nurses. She also earned a reputation among both male and female doctors as one of the most skilled surgeons in Boston. And, belying the popular stereotype of the unsexed woman physician, Mary Putnam Jacobi, a close friend, described Dimock as being "as fresh and girlish as if such qualities had never been pronounced by competent authorities to be incompatible with medical attainments. She had, indeed, a certain flower-like beauty, a softness and elegance of appearance and manner such as is abundantly lacking in the women most eager to denounce surgical accomplishments as outrageously unfeminine." [15]

The obvious qualifications again forced the censors to seek the advice of the councilors, who in turn formed a five-man investigation committee. In February 1873, four of the doctors signed a report recommending that since the bylaws made no distinction with regard to sex or color, a woman could be admitted to the society. Dr. Samuel Cabot appears to have been the prime mover advocating the acceptance of women, while Dr. W. W. Wellington alone filed a minority report which ad-

14. *BMSJ* 108 (1878), pp. 724–28. Chadwick's scrapbooks (HCL-A) include his correspondence with various state medical societies at this time.
15. *Medical Record* (1875), p. 357.

vised that legal counsel be consulted to learn "the rights of the society." A majority of the councilors sided with Wellington, however, and two lawyers were employed to study the issue. They reported that, although the bylaws did not in fact limit membership to males, the society could reject women if they thought sex a disqualification for medical and surgical practice. On June 3, buttressed by the legal opinion, the councilors voted forty-eight to thirty-two to instruct the application committee to reject the application.[16]

Once again the conservative forces had been able to hold the line, but it had been a close fight. The situation appeared to take a dramatic turn when Dimock died in a shipwreck off the English coast on May 7, 1875. Tributes to Dimock poured in from a number of medical men, and all eight of her pallbearers at the Boston funeral services a few weeks later were influential members of the Massachusetts Medical Society. Four days after the services, two consulting physicians at the New England Hospital, Henry Bowditch and Samuel Cabot, recommended that henceforth the society examine female as well as male applicants. Once again an investigating committee was formed, a majority of which recommended the admission of women. But the several intervening months served to undermine some of the impact of Dimock's death and on October 6, the councilors overturned the recommendation. Nevertheless, the thirty-six to twenty-seven vote was the closest to date, an encouraging sign to the women.[17]

The next attack came from an unexpected source—within —in the form of a petition on June 11, 1878, from the Middlesex South District, which declared that the time had come to admit women to the state society. The Middlesex chapter also furnished the council with the results of a statewide poll it had taken on its own initiative concerning the attitude of the society's members toward women physicians. A questionnaire had been sent to each member asking whether they were in

16. Massachusetts Medical Society, Records of the Council, February 5, 1873; March 11, 1873; June 3, 1873.
17. Ibid., June 8, 1875; October 6, 1875.

favor of admitting qualified women to the society or whether they favored certifying them without membership status, thus making them eligible for consultation with the society members along with other rights the society might grant them from time to time. Of the 60 percent who replied, 58 percent were in favor of the admission of qualified women to full membership, 13 percent were in favor of a certifying exam, and 28 percent were opposed to any recognition of female practitioners by the society.[18]

With 71 percent of the respondents in favor of some sort of recognition, the council appointed another five-man committee to consider the Middlesex resolution. The committee finally reported back at a meeting on October 1, 1879. Three members recommended a rejection of the resolution on the grounds that the society was established to include only males and, since the practice of medicine by women was still in the "experimental stage," there was no reason to reconsider the society's original objection. The minority report argued that the society's founders did not think to include women as none were then engaged in medical practice, but since a sizable number of women were presently practicing and the charter did not expressly exclude them, they should be admitted into the society. In a surprising move, the councilors adopted the minority report by a forty to thirty-two vote.[19]

Opposition within the society to the vote quickly surfaced. Pointing out that the bylaws describing membership used the pronoun *he,* it was charged that the councilors had exceeded their powers by changing the charter without a concurrent vote of the membership.[20] The charges of illegality were persuasive enough to change the position of a number of councilors, and the vote to admit women was rescinded the following February.[21]

18. Records of Massachusetts Medical Society, HCL-A; R. F. D. Adams to James Chadwick, January 28, 1879, Chadwick Scrapbook, HCL-A.
19. Records of Massachusetts Medical Society.
20. *BMSJ* 101 (1879), pp. 709, 851, 679, 527–28.
21. Records of Massachusetts Medical Society; *BMSJ* 102 (1880), pp. 160, 358–59, 501.

Although the revote was a setback, the advocates of female membership could derive some satisfaction from the fact that the opponents had been put on the defensive. Although they continued to cite the impropriety and impracticality of women as physicians, they had been forced to retreat to legalistic grounds in order to block the women. This shift dictated the next move of the women supporters: to build up support for a change in the bylaws which would enable women to enter the society.

Dr. James Chadwick, who by this point was in constant communication with the women physicians, readily responded to the need for more accurate factual information on the advancement of women outside Massachusetts. A few years earlier he had begun sending questionnaires inquiring about the status of women doctors to each state medical society in the United States and several foreign countries. In his published study, documenting the antiquated position of Massachusetts, he noted that seventeen state societies accepted women as members. The fact that 115 women had been so recognized, Chadwick concluded, meant that the time had come for the Massachusetts Medical Society to use its powers to protect the public by distinguishing between qualified and unqualified women physicians.[22]

Horticultural Hall's upper assembly room was filled to capacity for the 101st annual meeting of the Massachusetts Medical Society in 1882. When the woman issue came up, a motion was made to amend the bylaws so that women as well as men might become candidates for admission. The motion was followed by heated debate and parliamentary maneuvering on both sides. Dr. Wakefield of Leicester, "a venerable man with white hair and a beard," declared that thirty years ago he had been opposed to the idea of women physicians, but the world had moved ahead since then, and he had made up his mind to go with it in what little time he had left. Educated and uneducated women were practicing medicine in the state. "We want to sift them out," he cried, "so we will know who is

22. James Chadwick, "The Admission of Women to the Massachusetts Medical Society," *BMSJ* 105 (1881; reprinted in pamphlet form), p. 10.

educated and who is not. Those who are fit we want in the Society." [23]

The members voted that a change in the bylaws would have to originate in the council, but went on record as favoring the admission of qualified women. At the evening meeting of the council, Dr. Morrill Wyman of Cambridge, submitted a petition signed by 350 women citing the need for competent women physicians. "Now, these women might be all wrong," Wyman conceded, "but so long as they desired female advice, it is the duty of the society to examine practitioners." [24] Fighting desperately to check the growing sentiment in favor of women, Dr. George Cheyne Shattuck of Boston, drew on every argument that had ever been raised against the women. Once again, the councilors were reminded that God's plans for the universe had not included women doctors. Shattuck warned that he, along with other men, would not attend medical meetings that tolerated the unseemly practice of discussing medical topics in mixed company. Furthermore, only an "inferior style" of woman would be attracted to medicine; they might be intellectual," he warned, but they would be "women, whom the members of the society could not respect and love as they did the others." Finally, he reminded the councilors that since Harvard had only recently decided against educating men and women together in its medical school, the society should hesitate before taking such a "radical" step. Shattuck's arguments were followed by loud applause. Then, the council, persuaded by his rhetoric, adopted his motion to refer the question to one more committee.[25]

Enraged by what they considered to be a reactionary decision of the councilors, the defeated doctors decided to poll

23. *Boston Advertiser,* June 14, 1882.

24. Ibid. The petition has not been preserved, although the entire historical collection of the records of the Massachusetts Medical Society have been deposited in HCL-A.

25. Ibid.; *Springfield Republican,* June 15, 1882; *Boston Advertiser,* June 13, 1882.

the society again. Dr. Samuel Cabot and fourteen other physicians sent a questionnaire to the members of the society asking them if they had or would consult with women physicians and if they favored their admission to the society. Cabot found that 336 members had consulted with women while 684 had not. But, more significantly, 931 stated that they did not object to consulting with a woman because of her sex, while only 146 would refuse. Finally, 709 favored the admission of women to the society and only 400 were opposed.[26]

Bowditch, Chadwick, Cabot, and their colleagues went to the 1883 convention with high hopes. The questionnaire had apparently demonstrated that a clear majority favored the admission of women. The appearance of a woman physician in the audience, Dr. Alice Bennett, a member of the Pennsylvania Medical Society, appeared to be a successful omen.[27] But, once again, enough conservative councilors responded to the old arguments and the motion to change the bylaws was defeated on a sixty-two to fifty-eight vote. The *Boston Transcript* likened the "old fogyism" of the councilors to the conservatism of the British House of Lords.[28] The *Boston Globe*, agreeing with this analysis, branded the "autocratic" decision as unjust to "the many highly educated, efficient, and honored women physicians" and "unfair to the people." [29]

The conservative forces made one last stand at the 1884 convention but it was a losing effort. As one medical writer sadly noted, the woman question "like Banquo's ghost . . . stalked into the meeting in all its hideousness and would not be banished." [30] The members of the society voted 209 to 123 to adopt Henry Bowditch's motion that candidates for admission into the society may be either male or female. This time

26. Tabulated responses to the survey were printed on a circular signed by S. Cabot and others, April 10, 1883, Chadwick Scrapbook.

27. *WJ*, June 16, 1883.

28. *Boston Transcript*, June 13, 1883; *BMSJ* 108 (1883), p. 587.

29. *Boston Globe*, June 14, 1883; *Boston Transcript*, June 14, 1883; *Boston Herald*, June 13, 1883.

30. *JAMA* 3 (1884).

the councilors, with an air of accepting the inevitable, sustained the vote of the convention.[31]

The future of the society appeared to have been the main topic of conversation at the annual banquet. One speaker, gazing at the all male medical club, noted sadly, that "perhaps in 30 years from today, instead of sitting around the table, we shall have a ballroom scene before us."[32] The remark gave the homeopaths one of their rare opportunities to be condescending: "If such despondent ones . . . will accept comfort from outcasts of Israel," no such "Gilbert and Sullivan opera has as yet saddened the American Institute of Homeopathy of which women have been recognized and useful members since 1869."[33]

But it was difficult to console Dr. George Brune Shattuck, editor of the *Boston Medical and Surgical Journal*. Noting resignedly that the admission question had been settled, Dr. Shattuck sought some solace in his declaration that the action of a medical society could not alter the male and female physiology. But, the thought apparently only afforded fleeting comfort, for he ended the article on a pessimistic note, claiming the society's decision was one more addition to the "foolish fads and fancies" afflicting the women in the community. Who needed additional women doctors, he asked, in an age of "too much bad piano playing and too little good cooking and sewing?"[34]

In September 1884 Dr. Emma Call of the New England Hospital staff became the first female member of the Massachusetts Medical Society. That year's annual report of the hospital glowed with the pride of Call's appointment and looked optimistically to the future. Announcing the fall of what it hoped would be the last barrier to the women, the report declared that the woman physician was no longer an anomaly.[35]

31. *BMSJ* 110 (1884), pp. 585–87.
32. *New England Medical Gazette*, July 1884, p. 199.
33. Ibid.
34. *BMSJ* 110 (1884), pp. 594–95.
35. AR-NEH (1884), p. 5.

Unfortunately, both George Shattuck's pessimism and New England Hospital's optimism were premature. Did the shift of a few councilors' votes herald the coming of age of Boston's women physicians? Although the women's eagnerness to interpret the decision as a victory for equality is understandable, it must be remembered that the membership issue had been fought largely on the grounds of better regulation of Massachusetts medicine. Marie Zakrzewska, wise in the ways of Boston medical politics, privately noted that "necessity, not the acknowledgement of the principle of the right of women to practice, had finally conquered." [36]

Representative of much of the male point of view was Dr. George Lyman's declaration that the society's vote in favor of women physicians could not be interpreted as any sign of approval, but rather as a means of distinguishing between the "few educated exceptions and the whole festering mess of swindlers and abortionists." Moreover, despite the victory over the Massachusetts Medical Society, significant barriers remained in the way of a woman's advancement into medicine. Even if qualified women were admitted to membership, their numbers would be severely limited so long as they received separate and unequal medical training. As one woman physician put it, women sought entrance into the men's colleges "not because they are colleges of men . . . but because this is still so largely a man's world, with men so often holding possession of the Best." [37] In nineteenth-century Boston, the women doctors considered Harvard to have the "best" in medical education and they therefore embarked on a carefully orchestrated campaign which plunged the medical school into a controversy that one observer later described as unparalleled in its vehemence and personal animosity.[38]

36. Vietor, p. 393.

37. George H. Lyman, "The Interests of the Public and the Medical Profession," *Medical Communications of the Massachusetts Medical Society* (1875), p. 35. Public opinion polls are, of course, nonexistent except for the actual votes by the Massachusetts Medical Society membership. Lyman's focus is also evident in the Dorchester Medical Society minutes for 1875. (See pp. 131–35, "Dorchester Minutes," HCL-A.)

38. Vietor, p. 400; Thomas Francis Harrington, M.D., *The Harvard*

During the 1850s, Harvard, with a superior faculty and clinical facilities at Massachusetts General Hospital offered far more advantages than the women's medical colleges.[39] But Harvard's real claim to medical leadership came two decades later, when Charles Eliot's reforms brought the school into the national limelight. Eliot, who became president in 1869, transformed the curriculum by replacing the old system of two courses of four months each with a three-year and, ultimately, a four-year program. Furthermore, students were now required to pass each subject, whereas they previously were required to pass only five of nine courses. A building program was also launched to remedy the school's inadequate facilities. As Eliot noted in his annual report of 1871–72, a "revolution" had begun in the medical school and "a liberal endowment of the school would insure the complete success of the undertaking." [40]

Although it had been difficult for the women to penetrate the Massachusetts Medical Society, the struggle to gain admission to Harvard Medical School proved to be even more formidable. Here, too, cries for justice fell on deaf ears and the women again were forced to develop a strategy that would break through another barrier. But the task was complicated by the fact that Harvard lacked the society's quasi-legal role as medical watchdog. Appeals to a public responsibility which had influenced members of the medical society appeared to hold little relevancy for a private corporation such as Harvard. The women's task, therefore, was to find some means of connecting the issue of medical education of women to Harvard's self-interest.

After the final rejection of Harriot Hunt in 1850, no woman

Medical School: A History, Narrative and Documentary, 1782–1905 (New York, 1905), p. 1217.

39. Harrington, pp. 489–505; Martin Kaufman, *American Medical Education: The Formative Years, 1765–1910* (Westport, Conn., 1976), pp. 93–130.

40. Annual Report of the President and Treasurer of Harvard College, (1871–1872), p. 36.

had attempted to enter Harvard again until 1866 when two recognized women physicians in the city, Dr. Lucy Sewall and Dr. Anita Tyng of the New England Hospital staff, applied for admission. Sewall had graduated from New England Female Medical College and then spent an additional year of study in the hospitals of London and Paris, while Tyng, a graduate of Philadelphia woman's medical college, had served as Horatio Storer's surgical assistant, and then as a surgeon at New England Hospital. Despite their qualifications, both women found themselves victimized by the traditional prejudice that they were automatically less qualified because they were females. They therefore pointed out in their letter of application: "Finding, however, that our diplomas though legally sufficient, are not always considered satisfactory by male physicians, we are anxious to put our qualifications beyond dispute." In pleading their case as prospective students, they stated their willingness to accept whatever conditions, whether of study or examination, that Harvard could choose to impose. Their letter ended, as had Harriot Hunt's letter before them, by appealing to Harvard's "interest in justice and medical science." [41]

Dean Shattuck acknowledged the applications and informed the women that the matter would have to be decided on by the Harvard Corporation. Sewall quickly responded that since the school catalogue only referred to "graduates" rather than "male graduates," there appeared to be no obstacle to their acceptance. Moreover, her tactic now was one of assertiveness and confidence. Noting that their interpretation of the catalogue had been confirmed by "legal counsel," Sewall did not want to delay the matter. She wrote to Dean Shattuck informing him that the only matter which remained to be resolved was where and when they should report as students of the college.[42] But the matter was clearly not to be decided by

41. Lucy Sewall and Anita Tyng to Dean of Faculty of Medicine at Harvard Medical School, January 22, 1866, HCL-A.

42. Sewall's 1866 request referred to regulations published in the catalogue: "A graduate of another medical school of recognized standing may

either legal counsel or the confident manner of the applicants. Like Harriot Hunt, sixteen years earlier, Sewall and Tyng were politely informed that no provision had been made for the education of women in any department of the university.[43]

The following year another approach was made to Harvard, this time by two students at New England Hospital. The hospital women had obviously decided on a course of action designed to whittle away opposition, despite discouragement, polite or otherwise. The 1867 applicants were Susan Dimock and Sophia Jex-Blake and they concluded their letter of application by noting their agreement with a recent speech given by a Harvard spokesman: "American colleges are not cloisters for the education of a few persons, but seats of learning whose hospitable doors should be always open to every seeker after knowledge." But again Harvard made it clear that only males were to enjoy its hospitality.[44]

Unwilling to accept Harvard's rejection, Sophia Jex-Blake immediately began interviewing members of the medical school faculty on their attitude toward the admission of women. Armed with expressions of support from four faculty members (including Dr. Oliver Wendell Holmes), Jex-Blake and Dimock arranged a meeting with Dean Shattuck. But

obtain the degree of M.D. at this University after a year's study in the undergraduate course, passing all examinations required in the full undergraduate course and fulfilling all requirements for admission. These examinations may be taken only at the times set for regular examinations in September, February (mid-year examinations), and June" p. 3 of *Report of the Committee on Entrance Requirements for 1866,* cited by Lucy Sewall to George G. Shattuck, January 29, 1866, Harvard Medical School Dean's Records, HCL-A.

43. Harvard Corporation Records, Correspondence for 1866, HWL-A.

44. Harvard Corporation Records, March 11, 1867. President Thomas Hill's letter to Jex-Blake appears in Margaret Todd, M.D., *The Life of Sophia Jex-Blake* (London, 1918), pp. 190–91; the women's letter to Harvard appears in full in *Boston Daily Advertiser,* April 16, 1867. *The Advocate,* April 1867, contains the comment: "prominent Alumni of Boston are already taking measures for the prolonged agitation of the question."

those who were willing to admit women had warned them that they would only do so if the rest of the faculty was not opposed, and even this support melted quickly before the opposition at a faculty meeting in November 1867. Only one vote was cast against Dr. Edward Clarke's motion that the faculty did not approve the admission of any female to the lectures of any professor.[45]

Dimock and Jex-Blake reapplied to Harvard in January 1868. During the several months between their first and second application letters, the women had been able to gain a limited amount of clinical training at Massachusetts General Hospital. Declaring their willingness to submit to any examination and to abide by any regulation or restriction, the two women asked only to be granted "at least some of the advantages which are not denied any man." Still hoping to build on their four faculty friends, the two women suggested that in those cases where faculty members were unwilling to instruct females, substitute courses could be arranged with private physicians approved by the faculty.[46]

Although the applicants tried to achieve an optimistic tone in their letter, Jex-Blake's personal diary reveals the mounting frustration that accompanied the women's struggles. "Fighting on for Harvard with a sort of dull persistency," she recorded in March 1868. And, on another page, in a moment of despair at having achieved so little at her age, "A nice result at near 28 —Chaos!" [47] Nevertheless. Jex-Blake managed to get three women medical students to join her in attending the lectures of Dr. Hasket Derby at the medical school. Alarmed by what must have appeared to be creeping feminism, the medical faculty voted that the president be informed that they did not

45. Harvard Medical School Faculty Minutes, November 2, 1867, HCL-A. Todd, pp. 191–92.

46. Harvard Corporation Records, January 25, 1868. This time Matilda Towsley and Martha E. Hutchings also signed the letter. Neither of these names reappear in Todd's biography or other sources on Boston women physicians.

47. Todd, p. 196.

wish to have females attending any lectures or receiving any kind of instruction at the medical school.[48]

Thus, within a year, women felt the full power of the Boston medical establishment. As noted earlier in this chapter, Massachusetts General Hospital had, on the advice of the Massachusetts Medical Society, blocked female efforts to obtain practical training. Now Harvard had rejected the women's attempts to acquire the necessary theoretical preparation.

For the next four years, the women physicians confined their efforts to ironing out the tactical details and even arguing with more outspoken feminist allies about strategy.[49] It was not until 1872 that the women's hopes were even temporarily raised during the abortive merger discussions between the university and the New England Female Medical College. Although the negotiations were eventually broken off and Zakrzewska herself testified against a merger without sufficient guarantees by Harvard, the negotiations revealed a new possibility in the line of approach: Harvard's need for funds and better medical buildings.[50]

With Charles Eliot's plans for expansion of the medical school in the 1870s, the women felt an opportunity had emerged for them to begin bargaining on their own. The concept of women buying their way into medical school was not new. As early as 1865 a group of women in Boston and New

48. Harvard Medical School Faculty Minutes, May 20, 1868, HCL-A; Harvard Corporation Records, May 21, 1868.

49. Caroline Dall appears to have been the most outspoken of the feminist allies. See correspondence between Dall and Marie Zakrzewska, October 26, 1869 (*Caroline Dall Collection, MHS*) which discusses the strategy to be used with Harvard Medical School and advises Dall: "I don't doubt your honesty nor your desire to serve us medical women, and yes, I wish you would let them do their own business. I hope this letter will clear up a little your views on the subject and allow us to get on in our own way."

50. Vietor, p. 381. Although Zakrzewska testified before the legislature, her statements were not recorded and only briefly summarized in the newspaper as opposed to a merger. See the *Boston Daily Advertiser*, February 12, 1874.

York had raised $50,000 to endow a number of women's scholarships in some of the leading medical colleges in the country. But none of the schools were tempted and the fund was finally used to add a medical college to the Blackwell sisters' New York Infirmary.[51]

Several years later, a more attractive offer of a new building and also a $25,000 endowment did open Cornell's Ithaca campus to undergraduate women.[52] Jacobi cited the Cornell example, but also drew on personal experience in making some predictions at the first meeting of the Association for the Advancement of Women in 1873. While a student in Paris, Jacobi had managed—like most other American women students—to purchase a number of concessions in gaining access to facilities ordinarily open only to male students. More than once, her ready flashing of a "chez mon banquier" had opened doors more speedily at the Ecole de Medicine.[53] Now, a confident young physician, Jacobi dryly remarked to the women at the meeting that admission to medical schools in America could be similarly purchased. "It is astonishing," she asserted, "how many invincible objections on the score of feasibility, modesty, propriety, and prejudice will melt away before the charmed touch of a few thousand dollars." [54]

On March 21, 1878, Harvard Medical School was offered more than a few thousand dollars—$10,000 to be exact—by Marion Hovey of Boston, trustee of her late father's estate. There was, of course, the proviso that the money was to be used to educate women on equal terms with men at the medical school. In her letter, Hovey called Harvard's attention to the growing number of Boston women physicians, many of

51. Vietor, pp. 374–75.
52. Thomas Woody, *A History of Women's Education in the United States*, vol. 2 (New York, 1929; reprinted 1966), p. 248.
53. Rhoda Truax, *The Doctors Jacobi* (Boston, 1952), p. 84.
54. Dr. Mary E. Putnam Jacobi, "Social Aspects of the Readmission of Women into the Medical Profession," *Papers and Letters Presented at the First Woman's Congress of the Association for the Advancement of Woman, October, 1873* (New York, 1874), p. 177.

whom, to the consternation of the public, were poorly prepared. A good deal of this, she concluded, could be remedied
if Harvard would simply agree to admit women to its medical
college.[55]

As in previous cases involving the woman question, the matter was referred to the board of overseers. Only this time there
was no quick rejection; instead, a five-man committee consist-
ing of Alexander Agassiz, Morris Wyman, J. Elliott Cabot,
LeBaron Russell, and President Eliot, was appointed to study
the question. Harvard's willingness to consider the proposal
stemmed from a recognition that Victorian morality led some
women to insist that they be treated by physicians of their own
sex. Significantly, both the advocates and opponents of the admission of women to Harvard Medical School recognized this
expanding market for women physicians. By the last quarter
of the nineteenth century, the question for a growing number
of male physicians was no longer whether some women were
capable of becoming physicians. Convinced that the number
of women physicians would remain small, the issue became
how and where these women would receive their training.

The seriousness with which the Harvard committee approached its task was illustrated by its decision to poll the
membership of the Massachusetts Medical Society as to their
views on admitting women to Harvard Medical School. During
the previous year, 71 percent of the responding members of
the society had indicated their willingness to admit women.
This time, with a similar number of members responding, 51
percent favored the medical education of women at Harvard.[56]

Although the medical society members had divided almost
evenly on the question, four of the five committee members
voted in favor of accepting women. Only LeBaron Russell
opposed their admission. The majority report included a
lengthy survey of the medical education of women in both

55. Marion Hovey to Harvard Medical School, March 21, 1878, Harvard
Medical School Dean's Records.
56. Harvard Medical School, "The Majority Report," May 3, 1879, copy
in HCL-A.

Europe and the United States. Although they stated that it was too early to draw any positive conclusions from the European experience, they did note that in the country which had social conditions similar to America's—namely, Switzerland—female medical education had proven practical, had led to no evil results, and had not deterred the enrollment of male medical students. Pointing to the increased demand for the employment of women physicians in the treatment of their own sex and of children, the majority asserted that what was needed was not one more inadequate women's medical college, but the opportunity for women to receive a quality medical education. "Under these circumstances," the report concluded, "it is desirable that the experiment of admitting women to the medical school be tried." More specifically, the majority report recommended the acceptance of the Hovey fund and the raising of an additional sum of between $50,000 and $65,000 to cover the costs of a ten-year program.[57]

The minority report was written by Dr. LeBaron Russell of the Harvard medical faculty. He began by cautioning against dangerous and unnecessary ventures during a period when the medical school was still adjusting to the revolutionary changes instituted by Eliot. Furthermore, he continued, one innovation, the emphasis on practical work, made coeducation even more objectionable than it had been in the past when instruction was given almost entirely in the comparative safety of the lecture halls. Russell went on to point out that even the majority members had only recommended an experiment, indicating that they too harbored reservations about the decision.

Who could guarantee that the experiment would not lead to disaster? As Russell noted, a past president of the Massachusetts Medical Society who believed Harvard to be the most complete medical school in the United States had stated that he would not have sent his ward there, or, for that matter, would not have attended Harvard himself had women been

57. Ibid.

admitted to the school. It was clear, Russell concluded, that the advantages accruing to Harvard under the "experiment" were so few or nonexistent and the dangers so great that the Hovey offer should be rejected. But even Russell conceded the existence of "a legitimate demand for, and an important place to be filled by, well educated women as physicians." He recommended that the Hovey fund be pooled with other donations to form an independent woman's medical college in the city. In due time, if the school flourished, the women could then possibly bring it into the university as a separate college.[58]

Shortly after the two reports were filled, a special meeting of the medical faculty took place on May 24, 1879. After debating the issue at great length, the members voted thirteen to five against admitting women. Their vote hinged on the argument that all of the faculty's efforts should be reserved to ensure the success of the reform of the medical school. Fourteen of the faculty also signed a resolution stating that if the majority report was adopted, Harvard should demand no less than a $200,000 endowment.[59]

Three days later the board of overseers voted not to accept the Hovey offer. At the end of the meeting, Eliot, in an attempt to salvage something from the defeated majority report was able to secure the overseers' approval of his motion that under suitable restrictions the medical education of women at Harvard could be undertaken.[60] Eliot's profeminist parliamentary maneuvering did not go unnoticed. The *Boston Medical and Surgical Journal* lashed out at him in an editorial on "Harvard University and Female Physicians": "When the managers of political meetings secure the passage of pet resolutions in this manner, they are said to 'spring' them upon their victims . . . we have good reasons for supposing that several members of the board of overseers did not at the moment

58. Ibid.
59. Harvard Medical School Faculty Minutes, May 24, 1879.
60. Annual Report of the President and Treasurer of Harvard College (1878–1879), p. 31.

appreciate the inconsistent or hostile attitude of this eleventh hour resolution, and we believe they did not anticipate the use to be made of it." [61]

Eliot's "use" of the approved motion came swiftly—too swiftly as the medical journal pointed out. Eliot reviewed in detail the movement for admission of women to the medical school in his 1878–79 annual report. Advocates of coeducation probably were quite surprised by the fervor Eliot exhibited in championing women's medical education and certainly consoled by his claim that the joint position of the faculty and overseers was a temporary one, dictated by the ongoing innovations at the medical school. The admission of women, which had long been labeled inexpedient, now appeared to be merely inopportune. It was a small but encouraging step forward. Furthermore, the overseers' recognition of the need for women's medical education appeared to indicate that the door had not been completely closed.[62]

But it appeared equally clear that the next time the women appeared at the Harvard door they should be bearing gifts greater than $10,000. In the summer of 1880, a group of women including Marie Zakrzewska and Mary Putnam Jacobi began to discuss raising an endowment which could be used to "purchase direct partnership rights" into one of the larger medical colleges in the country. Although Harvard was the most desirable target (a reflection of its status in the medical world), the women agreed that all sectional jealousy must be laid aside: "Neither Boston, nor New York, nor Philadelphia must insist upon being the seat of the medical school." [63]

Despite the 1879 decision, Harvard still appeared to be the logical choice, primarily because of its expansion program and its sympathetic president. For example, in 1874 the medical school had launched a drive to secure $200,000 for a new building, but only half of the money had been raised by

61. BMSJ 102 (1880), p. 88.
62. Ibid.; Annual Report of the President and Treasurer of Harvard College (1878–1879), pp. 29–32.
63. Vietor, p. 379.

1880.[64] In May of that year, Eliot wrote to Dr. James Chadwick: "This is just the time to offer a round sum of money to
the university in order to procure the admission of women to
the medical school." Eliot estimated that $100,000 would be
a "good sum," which would be used for female classrooms and
additional faculty. Then, perhaps sensing that the amount of
money involved was considerable, he added: "If the sum
appeared large, it should be remembered that a separate
woman's school of equal quality would cost at least five times
as much." [65]

Moving quickly, the New England Hospital Society formed
a committee headed by Dr. Emma Call to spearhead the drive
for the necessary funds. Although the woman's medical college
in Philadelphia refused to participate, $50,000 in pledges was
raised in Boston and New York within a year. Eager to capitalize on the school's financial difficulties, a letter signed by
ten women physicians including Zakrzewska, Emily Blackwell,
and Mary Putnam Jacobi was sent to Harvard in September
1881 with the recommendation that the money be held in
trust until the income of the fund was large enough to cover
whatever additional costs would be incurred in the medical
education of women. If arrangements for this purpose could
not be made by 1891, the fund was to be returned to the
donors.[66]

Once again, the question followed the familiar route to the
board of overseers and on to majority and minority committee
reports which were presented at a meeting on January 11,
1882. Three members recommended the rejection of the offer,
while two advised its acceptance. Surprisingly, the overseers
voted eleven to six to accept the minority report. But the

64. Annual Report of the President and Treasurer of Harvard College
(1879–1880), p. 37.
65. Charles Eliot to James Chadwick, May 18, 1880, Chadwick Scrapbook. This letter has, before my discovery of it, been unavailable to
scholars. It was hidden away in the scrapbook.
66. Annual Report of the President and Treasurer of Harvard College,
(1881–1882), appendix I, p. 133.

losing side was able to delay the final decision until an overseers' meeting in March. Meanwhile, a group of enraged medical faculty members called a meeting to block the decision.
Threats of resignation punctuated the discussion and on a
fourteen to five vote, the faculty decided to officially protest
the January decision.[67]
The faculty hinted that if the overseers continued their
present course, they would risk seeing the experiment sabo-
taged from within. This threat combined with the rumor of a
mass faculty resignation caused a number of overseers to re-
evaluate their vote. Consequently, on April 24, 1882, in a
thirteen to twelve decision, the overseers voted not to accept
the women's proposal. What was even more discouraging was
their declaration that they could not "give any assurances or
hold out any encouragement that it would undertake the
medical education of women at Harvard." A final desperate
effort was made the following year. The faculty was approached with a plan to use the recently vacated old medical
building as a separate women's medical college. Women would
be instructed by either Harvard Medical School faculty or by
a separate faculty that would provide an identical education.
In either case, women would be awarded a Harvard medical
degree upon the completion of their work. This time there
was no need for prolonged discussion, and the medical faculty,
followed by the corporation, quickly rejected the proposal.[68]

The 1883 decision marked the end of the nineteenth-century
debate over women's admission to Harvard's medical college.
Frustrated by Harvard's intransigence, the women decided
there was nothing to be gained by prolonging the struggle.
Their decision was no doubt reinforced by President Eliot's
withdrawal from the alliance. Although President M. Carey
Thomas of Bryn Mawr later labeled his view on women's education as the "dark spot of medievalism" in his "otherwise

67. Ibid. pp. 32–36; *BMSJ* 106 (1882), p. 400.
68. Henry I. Bowditch to Harvard Medical Faculty, November 24, 1883,
HCL-A; Harvard Corporation Records, December 10, 1883.

luminous intelligence,"[69] Eliot had played an important behind-the-scenes role in the women's campaign. It was Eliot who first indicated in 1880 that Harvard might be willing to admit women in return for a sizable endowment, and he had also kept feminist hopes alive by gaining a favorable trustee vote on women's right to a medical education after Harvard had rejected the Hovey offer.[70] But Eliot was forced to chart a more careful political course after 1882. In 1883, for example, the overseers overturned and severely criticized Eliot's attempt to grant an honorary degree to Governor Benjamin Butler of Massachusetts.[71] By 1885 Eliot was in serious difficulty and one false step could have ended his administration at Harvard. The corporation was rumored, at one point, to have been ready to ask for his resignation if either of two fellows could have been persuaded to take on the presidency. Intent on protecting his own position, Eliot jettisoned the unpopular woman's issue.

Thus, in the late 1880s, when a group of women revived the plan to purchase admission to a medical college, Harvard was excluded from consideration. In 1889 an organized campaign was launched to endow Johns Hopkins University's long delayed medical school on the condition that women be admitted on the same terms as men. Funds were raised in several cities with Boston providing the second largest amount.[72] Mary Elizabeth Garrett, daughter of a trustee of Johns Hopkins and

69. M. Carey Thomas, "Notes for the opening address at Bryn Mawr College, 1899" (Bryn Mawr College Archives), abridged in Barbara M. Cross (ed.), *The Educated Woman in America* (New York, 1965), p. 142.

70. *BMSJ* 102 (1880), p. 88.

71. Hugh Hawkins, *Between Harvard and America: The Educational Leadership of Charles W. Eliot* (New York, 1972), p. 160.

72. "General Circular [for Women's Committee for Johns Hopkins University Medical School]," separate editions, c. Spring and Fall of 1890, SSC-SC; *Johns Hopkins University Circular, Catalogue and Announcement for 1910–1911 of Medical Department, 1910,* pp. 174–80; Alan M. Chesney, *The Johns Hopkins University School of Medicine: A Chronicle,* vols. I and II (1943–58); *WJ,* August 16, 1890, p. 260; *Retrospect of Twenty Years of Johns Hopkins Medical School, 1876–1896* (Baltimore, 1896), p. 38.

a resident of Baltimore, gave the largest individual donation, and finally offered to pay an additional $306,977 to complete the $500,000 endowment. With this sum the financially beleaguered Johns Hopkins surrendered to the women's terms. Still, some of the faculty refused to capitulate. Dr. William T. Councilman, for example, a distinguished pathologist and a vigorous opponent of coeducation, immediately resigned from Johns Hopkins and took a post at Harvard. As Sir William Osler wryly put it: "Johns Hopkins took the money, Harvard took the man; Johns Hopkins had coeducation without Councilman and Harvard had Councilman without coeducation." [73]

But the real question was what did the women have? The battle to gain access to a topflight medical school had been waged in Boston but was won in Baltimore. Was this the harbinger of a total victory or merely one more skirmish in an endless war?

73. *Bulletin of the Harvard Medical Alumni Association,* no. 7 (1894), pp. 41–42, reporting on the June 26, 1894, meeting. See also Dorothy Mendenhall's memoirs during the time she was a student at Johns Hopkins Medical School, 1896–1900, box 1, folder E, SSC-SC.

6

Moving Backward

The victory at Johns Hopkins touched off a wave of optimism among those who had fought for greater opportunities for women in medicine. To many it was the long-awaited break-through that would open the prestigious medical schools to women. What difference did it matter where the first triumph took place? The Baltimore capitulation would lead to other concessions across the land until every barrier was removed. The *Nation* echoed these hopes when it enthusiastically reported that Johns Hopkins could be the turning point for the fate of women as physicians.[1] *Century* magazine marked the decision by publishing a series of letters of approbation from a diverse group of public figures, including M. Carey Thomas, Dr. Mary Putnam Jacobi, Josephine Lowell, and Cardinal Gibbons. What is remarkable, the *Nation* noted, is that not a single one of these writers had "a word to say on the question of whether the quirls of a woman's brain have any peculiarities which necessarily unfit her from profiting from the most advanced medical instruction."[2] The only question that appeared to remain, the writer concluded, was whether similar groups of women would have to raise large sums of money in order to purchase their way into the other great universities or whether they would surrender peacefully.[3]

Thus, as the nineteenth century drew to a close, the opponents of women physicians appeared to be retreating on all fronts. Seemingly assured of ultimate success, many women

1. *Nation* (February 12, 1891), p. 131.
2. *Century* (May 1891), pp. 632–36.
3. *Nation* (February 12, 1891), p. 131.

physicians and their supporters began to abandon some of the
weapons they had employed in the battle. Thus, in 1893, when
the first class of men and women entered Johns Hopkins, the
Association for the Advancement of Women, which had championed the cause of women in medicine, embarked on a period
of decline that led to complete dissolution only six years
later.[4] Of even greater significance was the general conclusion
that separate medical colleges for women had outlived their
usefulness. By 1903 fourteen of the seventeen women's medical
colleges had either closed or merged with a coeducational university (see table 2).[5]

There were, of course, a few women like the president of the
Woman's Medical College of Pennsylvania who expressed
alarm at the trend, pointing out that since women would
always be a small minority in coeducational institutions, it
would be unreasonable to expect that their "peculiar requirements" or their individual interests would be protected.[6] But
such warnings were few and, considering the source, suspect.
The Board of Trustees of New York Infirmary clearly expressed the euphoria that swept through the ranks of medical
women. Announcing their decision to close the medical college
in 1899, the trustees declared: "It has now fulfilled its purpose,
and medical education may hereafter be obtained by women
in New York in the same classes, under the same faculty, with
the same clinical opportunities as men." Dr. Emily Blackwell,
cofounder with her sister Elizabeth of the infirmary school,
which in thirty-one years had graduated 364 women doctors,
summed up the efforts of the early female medical colleges:

4. See Edward James (ed.), *Notable American Women: 1607–1950* (Cambridge, Mass., 1971), vol. 1, p. 326 ("Ednah Dow Littlehale Cheney") and
vol. 2, p. 228 ("Julia Ward Howe").

5. The last survivor of the women's medical colleges, the Woman's
Medical College of Pennsylvania, became coeducational in 1969. See the
Newcomen Society of North America, *Pioneer-Pacesetter-Innovator: The
Story of the Medical College of Pennsylvania* (New York, 1971).

6. G. A. Walker, "The Woman's Medical College of Pennsylvania,"
WMJ 26 (1916), p. 44.

"We had held open the doors for women until broader gates had swung wide for their admission."[7]

Table 2   Decline of the Woman's Medical Colleges

College	Founding date	Enrollment 1893–94	Enrollment 1907–08
New England Female Medical College, Boston, Mass.	1848	merged 1873	—
Woman's Medical College of Pennsylvania, Philadelphia, Pa. (Female Medical College of Pennsylvania)	1850	192	138
New York Woman's Medical College, New York, N.Y. (homeopathic)	1863	43	20
Homeopathic Medical College for Women, Cleveland, Ohio	1868	merged 1870	—
Woman's Medical College of the New York Infirmary for Women and Children, New York, N.Y.	1868	82	extinct 1899
Woman's Hospital Medical College, Chicago, Ill.	1870	merged 1892	—
New York Free Medical College for Women, New York, N.Y.	1871	extinct 1876	—
Woman's Medical College, Baltimore, Md.	1882	28	28
Woman's Medical College, St. Louis, Mo. (homeopathic)	1883	extinct 1884	—
Woman's Medical College, Cincinnati, Ohio	1887	34	merged 1895
Woman's Medical College of Georgia and Training School for Nurses, Atlanta, Ga.	1889	extinct 1891	—
Woman's Medical College, St. Louis, Mo.	1891	extinct 1896	—
Presbyterian Hospital and Woman's Medical College, Cincinnati, Ohio	1891	not reported	merged 1895
Northwestern Woman's Medical College, Chicago, Ill.	1892	119	extinct 1902
St. Louis Woman's Medical College, St. Louis, Mo.	1894	43	extinct 1896
Woman's Medical College, Kansas City, Mo.	1895	—	extinct 1903
Laura Memorial Woman's Medical College, Cincinnati, Ohio	1895	—	extinct 1903
Total enrollment		541	186

Sources: Figures taken from *RCE* (1893–94), pp. 2045–50, and *JAMA* 51 (1908), pp. 586–87, 594–603.

Literary gates had also swung wide enough by the late nineteenth century to enable the woman doctor to enter a number of novels. William Dean Howells's *Dr. Breen's Practice* (1881), Sarah Orne Jewett's *A Country Doctor* (1884), Elizabeth Stuart Phelps's *Dr. Zay* (1883), and Annie Nathan Meyer's *Helen Brent, M.D.* (1891), all recognized this new phenomenon in American medicine. Even the male protagonist in Henry

7. *WMJ* 6 (1899), p. 249; Emily Blackwell, "The New York Infirmary and College," *Transactions of the Woman's Medical College of Pennsylvania* (1900), p. 80.

James's antifeminist novel, *The Bostonians* (1886), felt compelled to pay tribute to Dr. Prance, the female physician, when
he declared: "Whatever might become of the [woman's] movement at large, Doctor Prance's own little revolution was a
success." [8]

All signs pointed to the dawning of a new day in American
medicine, one that medical women could anticipate with hope.
Statistics indicated that the American woman doctor was far
in front of her European sisters. In 1900 there were 95 female
physicians in France, chiefly in Paris; there were 258 female
physicians in England; Germany, which opened its universities to female medical students in 1899, had only 406 women
enrolled; at the same time there were over 1,200 women enrolled in medical colleges in the United States and over 7,000
women physicians already in practice.[9]

In Boston the news of the Johns Hopkins registration of
women in its medical school in the fall of 1893 did much to
erase the mood of disappointment created by Harvard's rebuff
eleven years earlier. It was only reasonable to assume that
Harvard would soon follow the lead of its sister institution.
Meanwhile, a good deal of comfort could be derived from
other signs of progress. By 1890, for example, a half-century
after Harriot Hunt had first raised the banner of the women's
medical crusade, the number of women doctors in Boston had

8. *Boston Evening Transcript*, September 15, 1882; Henry James, *The
Bostonians* (New York, 1886; Penguin paper edition, 1966), p. 43.
9. *WMJ* 13 (1903), p. 116. The right of women to be physicians in the
respective countries was not recognized with graduation, however. For example, the debate in Germany continued until at least the year 1918
according to Mathilde Kelchner, *Die Frau and der weibliche Arzt* (Leipzig,
1934), p. 14, and Jill McIntyre, "Women and the Professions in Germany,
1930–1940," in Anthony Nicholls and Erich Matthias (eds.), *German
Democracy and the Triumph of Hitler* (London, 1971). For England, see
"Joan N. Burstyn, "Education and Sex: The Medical Case Against Higher
Education for Women in England, 1870–1900," *Proceedings of the American Philosophical Society* 117, no. 2 (April 1973), pp. 79–89; on France, see
Jeanne Chavvin, *Etude Historique Sur Les Professions Accessibles Aux
Femmes* (Paris, 1892).

expanded to 210, 18 percent of the physician population. Although a majority of these women doctors were the so-called irregular practitioners, the number of regular women physicians was expanding steadily, fueled by the women graduating from regular medical schools across the nation.

In 1893, three of Boston's four medical schools were open to women students: two regular medical schools, Tufts Medical School and the College of Physicians and Surgeons, and one homeopathic school, Boston University. Close to 25 percent of the classes at the two regular coeducational schools in Boston were female and 37 percent of Boston University's students were women. These numbers were expanding steadily, particularly at Tufts, where women accounted for 42 percent of the graduates by 1900. And this progress was not limited to Boston alone. Women made up 10 percent or more of the student enrollment at eighteen regular medical colleges across the nation. By 1893 women accounted for 19 percent of the University of Michigan Medical School, 20 percent of the University of Oregon Medical School and 31 percent of Kansas Medical College. These figures, of course, must be balanced against cities like New York, Philadelphia, and Chicago, where all of the regular medical schools were still sex segregated. In those cities all the women students were clustered in the women's medical colleges (see table 3).[10]

Evidence from the Boston sources suggests that many of the women graduates were experiencing financial as well as numerical progress. For instance, the *Boston Daily Advertiser* claimed that scores of women doctors, who counted among their patients the city's "most cultivated, influential, and high born women," had incomes of five figures. Another article in the *New York Herald Tribune* singled out the noteworthy success of Boston women physicians and called attention to the "surprising number of Back Bay offices luxuriant in appointment of tasteful furniture, paintings and bric-a-brac belonging to women who add M.D. to their names." The *Boston Post*

10. *RCE* (1893–94), pp. 2045–49.

singled out several newly graduated women physicians, "whose
practice is lucrative" and whose "professional services are in
demand in some of the best families of the city." [11]

Table 3   Percentage of Women Medical Students Enrolled
during Academic Year 1893–94 in U.S. Cities

Regular coeducational
medical schools

	No. women students	Women as % of total
Boston	52	23.7
Chicago	0	0.0
Los Angeles	6	15.4
Minneapolis	12	4.7
New York	0	0.0
Philadelphia	0	0.0
San Francisco	40	11.9

Source: All figures taken from RCE (1893–94),
pp. 2045–49.

Although the majority of women doctors may not have
carried on the fashionable practices described in the Boston
press, these women were confounding those critics who had
argued that women would not use their education. Two national surveys published in 1881 provided further hard data
to rebut the skeptics. Statistics were collected, for example, to
show that almost 90 percent of the women doctors who had
graduated from medical school were professionally active. The
incomes of women doctors were also subjected to careful scrutiny. In one of the studies that collected data on this topic, the

11. *Boston Daily Advertiser,* March 17, 1894; Ella M. S. Marble,
"Women's Contributions to Medical Literature," *WMJ* 5 (1896), p. 63;
New York Herald Tribune, November 7, 1886. See also *WJ,* August 16,
1890. The *Boston Post* article appeared in 1881 and was reprinted in the
Boston University yearbook, *The Imhotepian* (Boston, 1931), pp. 169–71.
See also M. L. Rayne, *What Can a Woman Do?* (Petersburgh, N.Y., 1893),
especially pp. 69–71.

average income of the seventy-six women reporting earnings was $2,907.30. Almost three-quarters of the women had incomes from $1,000 to $4,000 a year. This means that the average income of a woman doctor reporting was roughly three times that of a male white-collar worker of the same era.[12]

Perhaps economic motivation was an important part of some women's decisions to enter medicine in the first place. It is interesting that the decision to embark on a medical career came at a fairly mature age for most of the women. The average age upon entering medical school was 27; they began to practice at approximately the age of 31. The late entry age may be linked to the small but expanding opportunities for women in medicine in the 1870s. It is very likely that many women were interested in a medical career in the early periods but they had no hope that any opportunity for training or a career would materialize. Such women may have been encouraged by the success of others and may have made a delayed decision to enter medicine (close to 50 percent of the 1881 group had begun their careers in the five years preceeding the study). The women physicians also* married in greater numbers than did college-educated women of their same generation. Forty-one percent of the respondents had married, a figure higher than that for college-educated women as a whole.[13]

12. Emily F. Pope, Emma L. Call, and C. Augusta Pope, *The Practice of Medicine by Women in the United States* (Boston, 1881); Rachel L. Bodley, *Valedictory Address to the Twenty-Ninth Graduating Class of the Women's Medical College of Pennsylvania* (Philadelphia, 1881), p. 7; William G. Rothstein, *American Physicians in the Nineteenth Century: From Sects to Science* (Baltimore, 1972), p. 119; Rosemary Stevens, *American Medicine and the Public Interest* (New Haven, 1971), pp. 47–48; Stephen Thernstrom, *The Other Bostonians: Poverty and Progress in the American Metropolis, 1880–1970* (Cambridge, Mass., 1973), p. 298.

13. Pope et al., pp. 7–8; statistics on other college-educated women are cited by William H. Chafe, *The American Women* (New York, 1972), p. 100; Mary P. Ryan, *Womanhood in America* (New York, 1975), p. 236; Peter Gabriel Filene, *Him, Her, Self* (New York, 1974), p. 27. See also, Roberta Wein, "Women's Colleges and Domesticity, 1875–1918," *History of Education Quarterly* (Spring 1974), pp. 44–45.

Married or single, the woman doctor clearly had a preference for the city as a place in which to build her medical practice. During this period, Boston led the nation in the percentage of its physicians who were female. But, unbeknownst to women physicians in Boston and elsewhere, their "golden age" in medicine was already beginning to slip away by the turn of the century. The list of 300 women physicians in the 1900 Boston census, for example, accounting for 18.2 percent of the city's doctors, was destined to be the highwater mark for women.

Boston's experience was soon duplicated in other cities and the percent of women physicians nationally peaked in 1910 at 6 percent. The total number of women doctors in Boston began to decrease after 1900 and on a national level after 1910. As late as 1940, the 7,708 women physicians in the nation was actually a smaller *numerical* total than it was some thirty years earlier. And seventy-six years and two women's liberation movements after 1900, women still have not been able to match the earlier percentages (see tables 4 and 5).

Table 4   Percentage of Women Physicians in U.S. Cities

	1880	*1890*	*1900*	*1910*	*1920*	*1930*
Boston	14.9	18.0	18.2	13.7	9.7	8.7
Chicago	7.6	7.8	13.0	11.6	8.9	7.5
Los Angeles	—	7.4	14.9	17.9	13.3	9.5
Minneapolis	6.6	12.3	19.3	12.6	8.4	7.0
New York	5.0	4.9	7.2	6.6	5.3	5.5
Philadelphia	3.9	4.7	8.7	9.1	7.7	6.8
San Francisco	3.4	14.0	13.8	13.5	13.0	12.7
National average	2.8	4.4	5.6	6.0	5.0	4.4

Sources: Percentages based on figures from the U.S. Census, except for the 1880 figures for Boston and the 1890 figures for Philadelphia and New York which were handcounted from *Boston Directory* (Boston 1880) and *Polk's Directory* (Detroit and Chicago, 1890).

Thus, just as Boston had anticipated many of the steps that marked women's nineteenth-century struggles in medicine—a

separate women's medical college, the development of a
women's hospital, the fight for membership in the state medical

Table 5   Boston and the U.S.: Historical Patterns
of Women Physicians

	Boston			United States		
	Women physicians	Total physicians	% women	Women physicians	Total physicians	% women
1850	6	268	2.2	—	40,755	—
1860	31	351	8.8	200 *	55,055	0.4
1870	74	468	15.8	544	64,414	0.8
1880	132	882	14.9	2,432	85,671	2.8
1890	210	1,164	18.0	4,557	104,805	4.4
1900	330	1,816	18.2	7,387	132,002	5.6
1910	258	1,878	13.7	9,015	151,132	6.0
1920	166	1,717	9.7	7,219	144,977	5.0
1930	140	1,603	8.7	6,825	153,803	4.4
1940	142	1,569	9.0	7,708	165,989	4.6
1950	140	1,694	8.3	11,823	191,947	6.1
1960	200	3,447	5.8	15,672	260,484	6.0
1970	325	3,641	8.9	24,088	334,023	7.2
1973	527	4,478	11.8	30,568	366,379	8.3
1976	550	4,679	11.7	30,793	357,762	8.6

* Estimated.

Sources: Boston figures were handcounted from Boston City Directory
listings for 1850–80 and 1973; other years are from census data. National
figures are drawn from: Virginia Penny, The Employment of Women: A
Cyclopedia of Woman's Work (Boston, 1863), p. 25; J. M. Hooks, Women's
Occupations Through Seven Decades, Women's Bureau, Department of
Labor (Washington, 1947); U.S. Bureau of the Census, Census of the
Population, 1950, vol. 2 (Characteristics of the Population), part 1, U.S.
Summary, table 124, pp. 1–261; Health Resources Statistics, National
Center for Health Statistics, Washington, D.C. All figures for 1976 are
from James Battalino at Fisher-Stevens, Inc., Clifton, N.J.

society, entrance into coeducational medical schools, and the
battles for access to the city's hospitals—it also foreshadowed
much of the twentieth-century decline. Instead of victories, a
series of reversals almost erased the progress of the previous

century. There was no longer any illusion that the problems of women in medicine could be solved, or even viewed, from a strictly local perspective. Women would continue to push against local barriers, but they gradually came to realize that solutions called for action on a national level. And, as that realization gained momentum, the history of the barriers to women's entrance into medicine in Boston became more and more intimately connected with events in other cities.

Boston medical women suffered their first reversal in the area of medical education. The liberal currents that were expected to flow out of the Johns Hopkins victory never materialized. Instead of coeducational Boston University and Tufts engulfing Harvard, the two medical schools moved toward the entrenched position of their sister or, more appropriately, brother institution. In both cases, this reversal was tied to a conscious decision by the two schools rather than to some failure of female will.

The Boston situation was linked to the controversies that still swirled around the question of coeducation. On the one hand, Edward H. Clarke's warnings appeared to have proven groundless. More and more women were going to coeducational institutions and there was no evidence that their health had suffered or that they could not compete with men. In fact, the fear developed in some quarters that the women would outdo their male classmates. Male supremacists must have been at least momentarily shaken by the 1897 report of the commissioner of education which indicated that women were proportionately capturing a greater percentage of academic honors than men. Equally disquieting was the fear that the presence of these successful women might entice some men to abandon their "manly" ways in order to compete in the classroom. Thus, in the coeducation section of the 1905 report on education, a Professor Armstrong voiced his concern over the dangerous trend: "To put the matter in very simple terms . . . the boy in America is not being brought up to punch another boy's head, or to stand having his own punched in a healthy and proper manner: that there is a strange and indefinable air coming over the men; a tendency toward a common . . . sex-less tone of thought.[14]

Historians of education have by and large neglected the topic of coeducation. Some, like Lawrence Vesey in his history of the American university, touch lightly on the process, noting that during the progressive period, the university "peacefully accepted sexual diversity." The few like Thomas Woody who deal with the issue at length have taken the position that coeducation was a liberating experience for women and that access to professional education automatically placed the two sexes on an equal footing.[15]

Vesey is correct only in the literal sense, that the battle of the sexes did not break into open warfare. In fact, in almost every instance coeducation met with real resistance from both male students and the almost entirely male faculties. Many schools were, of course, forced to accept some women because of financial exigencies. Those schools who were in a better fiscal position either entered into coordinate arrangements such as that between Columbia and Barnard or rejected co-education entirely as did Yale.

A hierarchy soon emerged in the twentieth century which clearly equated prestige with, among other things, sexual seg-

14. *RCE* (1897–98), pp. 631–32; ibid. (1905), p. 7.
15. Lawrence Vesey, *The Emergence of the American University,* (Chicago, 1965), p. 333. A notable exception to the pattern of excluding women from the history of higher education is Patricia Albjerg Graham, *Community and Class in American Education, 1865–1918* (New York, 1974). Thomas Woody, *A History of Women's Education in the United States* (New York, 1929), vol. 1, pp. 329 ff., and vol. 2, pp. 224 ff. Sources that refute the description of sexual equality in coeducation include Helen R. Olin, *The Women of a State University: An Illustration of the Working of Coeducation in the Middle West* (New York, 1909), and issues of the *Association of Collegiate Alumnae Journal,* particularly those in the first decades of the twentieth century where the association's efforts to place women on par with men are described. Most accounts, even the most recent on professional education, continue to ignore women—see, for example, William R. Johnson, "Education and Professional Life Styles: Law and Medicine in the Nineteenth Century," *History of Education Quarterly* (Summer 1974), pp. 185–207.

regation. As late as 1962, Frederick Rudolph, a historian, could comment that coeducation helped to divide the subjects of the curriculum "into those which were useful, full-blooded, and manly, and those which were ornamental, dilettantish, and feminine." And, as he further argued, only a few of the men's liberal arts colleges were saved in the process: colleges like Yale, Princeton, and Amherst and coordinate institutions like Harvard and Columbia "preserved the liberal inheritance of Western Civilization in the United States by protecting it from the debilitating, femininizing, corrupting influences which shaped its career where coeducation prevailed." [16]

By the second decade of the twentieth century, the tensions surrounding coeducation had largely disappeared, but at the price of the liberating experience which Woody had so glibly described. Historians are just beginning to study the educational reform movements that may have affected the career opportunities of women at the turn of the century. One of these movements, the drive to legitimize home economics as a college curriculum exclusively for women, may have had a particularly critical impact. Even women who had pioneered in opening fields that had previously been exclusively male championed the cause of home management education.[17]

Ellen Richards, for example, had, in 1870, been the first woman student admitted to the chemistry department at the Massachusetts Institute of Technology. However, by the 1890s she had abandoned any pretense of furthering her career in chemistry as she channeled most of her energy into advancing the cause of home economics: "to study the economic and social problems of the home and the problems of right living." The small cadre of highly educated women who joined Richards no doubt felt they were responding to a social need—educating women to be better wives and mothers. It just hap-

16. Frederick Rudolph, *The American College and University: A History* (New York, 1962), p. 324.
17. Barbara Ehrenreich and Deirdre English, "The Manufacture of Housework," *Socialist Revolution* 5, no. 4 (October–December 1975), pp. 5–40, is a stimulating introduction to this topic.

pened, however, that the home economics movement meshed in many ways with the ideology of antifeminists who argued that motherhood and housewifery alone should be the careers women should follow. For example, in 1895 the American Medical Association came out in favor of the movement in the hope that it would extinguish a number of evils including "competition of labor between the sexes." [18]

By 1927, 240 colleges had established degree programs in domestic science or home economics; 243 other colleges and 168 normal schools offered it as an elective. Although home economics failed to make headway at most of the better women's colleges, they too seemed to be affected by the mood which legitimized it. Even Bryn Mawr, where President M. Carey Thomas had successfully championed equal opportunity for women, witnessed a new attitude on the part of its graduates as more married and fewer went to graduate school after 1910.[19]

With the fires of this hotbed of collegiate feminism reduced, it is not surprising that Arthur Calhoun could write in 1919 that a half century of coeducation, far from blurring sex roles, had strengthened women's "sense of maternal and connubial responsibility." He concluded that "college women make cheery, efficient homes." But domestic perfection came at the partial expense of career preparation as evidenced by the high rates of unemployed and underemployed female college graduates surveyed by the Collegiate Alumnae Association during the period. The net result was to make it clear that coeducational undergraduate schools posed no threat to home and family.[20]

18. Cited by ibid.; Editorial, "Public School Instruction in Cooking," *JAMA* 32 (1899), p. 1183.

19. Roberta Wein, "Women's Colleges and Domesticity, 1875–1918," *History of Education Quarterly* (Spring 1974), pp. 31–47.

20. Arthur W. Calhoun, *A Social History of the American Family* (New York, 1919), vol. 3, p. 95; Woody, vol. 2, pp. 296–303; The Association of Collegiate Alumnae journals and meeting reports provide ample documentation that women college graduates had a chronic employment problem. See particularly *Association of Collegiate Alumnae Journal* 3

Professional education, on the other hand, in a competitive occupation like medicine, presented a distinct and more dangerous situation. There, women were obviously preparing for careers that put them on a collision course with men. Women had been steering this course for some time, but in large part they had been doing so in isolated women's medical colleges. The nineteenth-century Wellesley College and Smith College graduates demonstrated the trend among the most highly qualified group of female medical students.

Of the thirty-eight Wellesley and Smith women who entered medical school after graduation in the 1880s, all entered a women's medical college. In the next two decades, this trend was completely reversed and more than 70 percent chose a coeducational medical school. By the end of the nineteeth century, women began increasingly to compete with men for admission to male-dominated schools. Moreover, the additional number of female physicians challenged the assumption held by some male physicians that only a few women would seek professional careers in medicine. As Gordon Allport has noted, fear of a particular group is in large part a function of its size and density.[21]

With practically one of five Boston physicians a woman, the period of salutary neglect for women physicians came to an

-----

(April 1910), pp. 61–74; Kate Holladay Clagborn, "Occupation for the College Graduate," ibid. 3 (February 1900), pp. 62–66; Elizabeth Kemper Adams, "The Vocational Opportunities of the College of Liberal Arts," ibid. 5 (April 1912), pp. 256–65; and especially the entire issue entitled "The Vocational Number," ibid. 6 (April 1913).

21. Wellesley statistics are based on lists of graduates in Alice Ames Kavanagh, Edith Midwood Perrin, and Jean Watt Gorely, "Wellesley in Medicine," *Wellesley Magazine* (March 1939), pp. 284–90; and, Jean Watt Gorely, "Comments on Wellesley in Medicine," ibid., pp. 506–07. The Smith statistics are compilations done by Myra Melissa Sampson and they appear on several lists in folder 42 of Sampson, Smith College Archives. Radcliffe College did not offer adequate premedical laboratory courses at this time according to Dorothy Mendenhall, who became a student at Massachusetts Institute of Technology in 1895 after investigating the Radcliffe situation first. The Gordon Allport reference is taken from *The Nature of Prejudice* (New York, 1954), pp. 220–22.

abrupt close. But the virtual disappearance of the women's medical colleges by 1903 did not mean that the women medical students also needed to disappear. Coeducational institutions, such as the ones that accepted Smith and Wellesley graduates, could have filled the educational void by becoming coeducational, in fact as well as name. That this trend did not develop is one of the major reasons why women fared so poorly in the medical profession in the twentieth century (see table 6).

Women, of course, were not the only group to experience restrictive admissions policies after the 1890s. The decline in the number of medical schools from 162 in 1906 to 69 in 1944 led to increased competition for medical school openings and increased limitations on opportunities for blacks and Jews in the professions. During this period, the number of black medical colleges dropped from seven to two, and although the proportion of black physicians climbed sharply from 1900 to 1910 (from 1.3 to 2.0 percent), thereafter only marginal gains were made up to the early 1960s. The well-known limitation of Jewish medical students became especially oppressive during the Depression when many medical schools adopted an unofficial quota of 10 percent.[22]

22. Researchers have generally ignored the problem of women as minority group members and the subject is just now being systematically investigated. Cynthia Epstein and Helen Mayer Hacker have excellent theoretical discussions of this subject. See especially, Helen Mayer Hacker, "Women as a Minority Group," *Social Forces* 30 (October 1951), pp. 60–69; and "Women as a Minority Group—Twenty Years Later," Paper delivered at the American Sociological Association Meeting, 1972 (reprinted by Know, Inc., No. 1974). Both the Jewish and black studies on the medical profession ignore the problems of female members of their respective groups. On Jews, see Reuben A. Kessell, "The A.M.A. and the Supply of Physicians," *Law and Contemporary Problems* 35 (Spring 1970), pp. 267–83; Jacob A. Goldberg, "Jews in the Medical Profession—A National Survey," *Jewish Social Studies* (1939), pp. 327–36, esp., p. 332; James Burrow, *AMA: Voice of American Medicine* (Baltimore, 1963), p. 187; Seymour M. Lipset and Everett Carll Ladd, Jr., "Jewish Academics in the United States: Their Achievements, Culture and Politics," *American Jewish Year Book* 72 (1971), p. 95; Ernest Van den Haag, *The Jewish*

Table 6 The Coeducational Retrenchment: 1894–1908
(regular medical schools with female enrollment of 10 percent or more in 1893–94)

College and location	1893–94		1907–08	
	Total enrollment	% women	Total enrollment	% women
University of Southern California	39	15.38	89	10.11
Cooper Medical College (Calif.)	228	12.28	97	3.09
University of California	109	11.01	36	13.89
Medical Department, University of Colorado	42	19.05	52	11.54
Denver Medical College (Colo.)	36	25.00	79 *	5.06 *
Gross Medical College (Colo.)	72	26.38	79 *	5.06 *
National University (George Washington), D.C.	88	12.50	198	1.51
Council Bluffs Medical College (Iowa)	12	25.00	extinct 1895	
Kansas Medical College	45	31.11	69	4.35
College of Physicians and Surgeons (Mass.)	135	21.48	162	0.00
Tufts University (Mass.)	80	28.75	371	9.43
Johns Hopkins University (Md.)	83 †	15.66	281	6.76
University of Michigan	375	18.93	390	5.38
University of Buffalo (N.Y.)	186	11.83	176	5.68
Syracuse University (N.Y.)	56	12.50	150	5.33
National Normal University (Ohio)	30	13.33	extinct 1900	
Toledo Medical College (Ohio)	38	10.53	29	10.34
University of Oregon	29	17.24	88	6.82

* These schools merged in 1902.
† Includes graduate physicians enrolled in 1893–94. (The first-year class included in 1893–94 three women and fifteen men: 16.66 percent female enrollment.)
Sources: Figures taken from RCE (1893–94), pp. 2045–50, and JAMA 51 (1908), pp. 586–87, 594–603.

Any real comparison of the discrimination by the medical profession that women, blacks, and Jews have experienced must await further research on the experience of the latter two groups. However, certain broad parallels and contrasts are apparent. As three vulnerable groups, all suffered from the medical establishment's fear of overcrowding and were singled out for differential and unequal treatment. Still, each group seems to have experienced a leveling off or cutback during different periods: women in the decade before 1910, blacks in the 1910s, and Jews in the 1930s. When one uses the crude yardstick of percentage of total population, blacks and women appear to have experienced the greatest discrimination. Jews, on the other hand, have successfully overcome the quotas, as is indicated by a recent study that finds them overrepresented by 231 percent in the medical profession. Black doctors, averaging 2.5 percent of the total population of physicians in the twentieth century, are drawn from a group that has accounted for about 11 percent of the population; they are, therefore, underrepresented by a factor of 1 to 4. Women doctors, who have averaged about 6 percent of the total number of physicians for the century, are underrepresented in terms of their share of the total physician population by a factor of 1 to 7.[23]

Mystique (New York, 1969), p. 23; Marshall Sklare, The Jew in American Society (New York, 1974). On blacks, see Edward Henry Corwin and Gertrude E. Sturges, Opportunities for the Medical Education of Negroes (New York, 1936); W. Montague Cobb, Progress and Portents for the Negro in Medicine (New York, 1948); Dietrich C. Reitzer, Negroes and Medicine (Cambridge, Mass., 1958). Cobb, while ignoring the sex-specific problems of black women doctors, does contain listings of the graduates of Howard University Medical School and Meharry Medical School by sex from the 1870s to 1947. The percentage of women in these schools, 3.4 percent, is lower than the national average for women during this period. See also, James L. Curtis, Medical Schools and Society (Ann Arbor, 1971).

23. Curtis; Saul Jarcho, "Medical Education in the United States, 1910–1956," Journal of the Mount Sinai Hospital 26, no. 1 (1959), pp. 358–60; Oscar Handlin and Mary F. Handlin, "The Acquisition of Political and Social Rights by the Jews in the United States," American Jewish Year

Boston University represents an archetypal betrayal of the women's medical struggle. The school, which had taken over New England Female Medical College in 1873, was the first coeducational medical college in Massachusetts and one of the first in the United States. In its early years the school, led by Dean Israel Talbot, brother of Dr. Nancy Clark, took great pride in its commitment to women. But there were other and more crucial reasons why the school accepted so many women. Although Boston University did include "regular" courses such as anatomy and surgery in its curriculum, the school was committed to homeopathy, a system of medicine based on the idea of like curing like. Samuel Hahnemann, a German physician who founded this system, was a strong critic of regular medicine. He developed a method of treating disease that involved giving minute doses of drugs, which would produce in a healthy person symptoms similar to those of the disease. In transporting homeopathy to the United States, Hahnemann started a schism within the ranks of American medical practitioners. In Boston, a major purge of homeopaths from the Massachusetts Medical Society occurred one month after Boston University's takeover of the Female Medical College in 1873. Even more damaging were the bacteriological discoveries of the 1870s and 1880s which made it more and more difficult for such medical sects to justify their existence. The zenith of homeopathy occurred around 1880. Subsequently, increasing numbers of homeopaths began to abandon their dogmas and edge toward the mainstream of medicine.[24]

Book 56 (1955), p. 43. For the Jewish overrepresentation see Van den Haag, p. 23.

24. *New England Medical Gazette*, March 1875, p. 115, is but one example. See also an unpublished biography of Israel Talbot in BUMS-A. Rothstein, pp. 230–48, 278, contains detailed discussions of the rise and fall of homeopathy as does Martin Kaufman, *Homeopathy in America: The Rise and Fall of a Medical Heresy* (Baltimore, 1971), pp. 56–58, 77–86; and Harris L. Coulter, *Divided Legacy: A History of the Schism in Medical Thought* (Washington, 1973), vol. 3, pp. 328–508.

Thus, Boston University offered its students an education in a branch of medicine that was disappearing rapidly. The high percentage of women medical students in the school's early years must be viewed within this framework. As homeopathy came under increasing fire, the school experienced difficulty in attracting competent students. Women, who had few schools open to them, were a major source of qualified applicants. Thus, as the number of students leveled off and began to decline in the 1880s, the percentage of women increased. For example, the class of 1886, which had the smallest number of graduates in ten years, was 56 percent women. Because they had so few options in terms of medical schools, women were attracted to Boston University from a much wider geographic area than the male students. Consequently, 83 percent of the male members of the class of 1882 came from within Massachusetts while 75 percent of the women in that same class were drawn from outside the state. Women also seemed to outdistance the men academically. The Boston University Medical School did not regularly publish the honors rating of its graduates. When it did, as in 1905, though only four of the nineteen graduates were women, they walked off with the two highest academic positions. During Talbot's administration, he often pointed out that women regularly achieved the highest grades and did the best academic work.

Although the school boasted of its dedication to women's education, female students expressed doubts about the depth of this commitment. One of the woman editors of the school newspaper, *The Medical Student,* pointed out that when appeals for money are made to Boston's wealthy women, the school is "PRE-EMINENTLY" a "coeducational college," but "the *sentiment* of the school is not." The existence of two student medical societies, the male "Hahnemann Society" and, ironically, the female "Gregory Society," symbolized to the women their second-class status. Only the male students were allowed to send delegates to the state Hahnemann Society. Even more galling to the women students, the society provided sumptuous banquets for the male seniors of each graduating class in the 1880s while the female students were left to fend for themselves. When in 1889 the women requested admission to the Hahnemann Society, they were roundly rejected—a move that the women denounced as Boston University's "Dred Scott Decision." [25] A much more serious piece of discrimination during the school's early years resulted when only male students were allowed to witness operations in Boston City Hospital's amphitheatre. This restriction was especially disturbing to the women since the school's catalogue failed to mention it. At a time when women medical students throughout the country found it almost impossible to gain hospital experiences, many were attracted to Boston University by its announcement that since Boston City Hospital was in the "immediate proximity to the school, the lecture hours of the senior and middle classes are so arranged, that without loss of time, they can be present at all important operations.[26]

Protests by several of the more militant women prodded the administration into writing a polite letter requesting the hospital authorities to grant equal privileges to the women medical students. The hospital's unwillingness to change its policy forced the school to revise the next year's catalogue, substituting "male students" for "students" in the section that referred to the surgical privileges and clinical facilities of the school.[27]

However, the women were not interested in the administration's agreement to recognize the existence of injustice, but rather in its willingness to amend the situation. The prohibition against observing operations remained an issue and beginning in 1882 the Boston University women headed by a thirty-nine-year-old student, Martha Ripley, again took the initiative and petitioned Boston City Hospital to change its

25. *Medical Student* (January 1889), pp. 86–88; the women gained entrance to the society by 1896—*Medical Student* (November 1896), p. 9.

26. *Boston University Medical School Announcement*, 1877, p. 11; *BMSJ* 114 (1886), p. 452; *Boston Transcript* clippings in Warren Scrapbook, BU-A.

27. *Boston University Medical School Announcement*, 1879, p. 11.

rules. Although the trustees of the hospital tabled the request,[28] there is evidence that the hospital relaxed its enforcement and some women students were able to attend some of the operations. The horrified editor of the *Boston Medical and Surgical Journal*, commenting on the female infiltration, warned that the patients would refuse to be operated on if women continued their presence, especially, "When they are armed with opera glasses." [29]

Finally in 1886, after continued pressure from the women, the Boston University administration requested the hospital trustees to formally admit women to the operations. The trustees agreed to the request with the qualification that the attending surgeon (always a male at this time) could request either sex to leave if the case was improper to view on a coeducational basis.[30]

However, in the final analysis, these victories can be likened to securing better accommodations on a sinking ship. Boston University made every effort to keep the homeopathic vessel afloat, even to the point of distributing 3,000 copies of a "prize" essay, "Why Students of Medicine Should Select the Homeopathic School." [31] But pamphlets could not stem the trend that saw the number of homeopathic schools drop from twenty-two to nine and the number of students reduced by two-thirds between 1900 and 1917. Each year the decline became more precipitous. Thus, within a span of five years after 1913, the Boston University student body fell by 50 percent.[32]

Unwilling to continue on a course that was leading to oblivion, the administration, with overwhelming support from the faculty, students, and alumni, decided in 1918 to reorganize

28. Trustee Minutes, Boston City Hospital, February 21, 1882, BCH-A.

29. *BMSJ* 114 (1886), p. 452. G. H. M. Rowe, Superintendent of Boston City Hospital, to Dr. C. P. Worcester, Secretary of the Faculty, Harvard Medical School, June 18, 1892, HCL-A.

30. *Boston City Document*, vol. 97, p. 9, BCH-A.

31. *Report of the President of Boston University for 1903–04*, p. 45, BUMS-A.

32. *History of the Reorganization of the Boston University School of Medicine* (Boston, 1918), p. 4.

the medical curriculum along regular lines.[33] What is significant for the history of women in medicine is the effect of this reorganization on female enrollment. The school's transformation into a regular medical school meant that it would be able to attract a much larger pool of applicants. As the school found itself in a more selective position, it could ignore the women students that had once been a major source of strength. Whereas, during the twenty years leading up to the change-over, 29.5 percent of the senior class consisted of women, their proportion of the "regular" medical classes dwindled to 9.9 percent in the following twenty years and hit a low in 1939 when there were no women in the graduating class.

The experience of women at Tufts Medical School presents an even sharper example of the dashing of the early hopes of coeducational medical education. Tufts, which began in 1893, expanded rapidly so that thirteen years later it was the largest medical school in New England and the seventh largest in the country as measured by the number of annual graduates. Moreover, by 1906 it was so successful that it showed a profit for the year.[34] But, in its opening years, when the future was uncertain, the school had accepted a large number of women so that in 1900, 42 percent of the graduating class was female.

As in the case of Boston University, the women appear to have been academically more successful than the men, regularly accounting for a far higher percentage of honors than their numbers warranted. Thus, in 1902, although women were only 26 percent of that year's graduating class, they accounted for 60 percent of the honors.[35] However, rather than strengthening their position within the university, their success seems to have led to their undoing. As Mary Putnam Jacobi had noted several years earlier: "Opposition to women

33. *A Confidential Communication to the Alumnae of Boston University School of Medicine* (Boston, 1918), p. 12; *History of Reorganization*, pp. 1, 2. See also *BMSJ* 185 (1921), pp. 331–33.

34. *Tufts University Annual Report of the Medical School*, 1906, p. 5.

35. Computed from listings in the Tufts University Medical School Commencement Announcements in year by year tally.

physicians has rarely been based upon any sincere conviction that women could not be capable. Failure could be pardoned them, but—at least so it was felt in anticipation—success could not." [36] A Tufts Medical School trustee admitted that the objections to coeducation did not lie in any failure on the part of the women: "They have done their work well—too well if anything." Such an appraisal certainly holds true when the women graduates of Tufts are compared to a national sample. Five of the women in these early years later merited fellowship status in the American College of Surgeons when it was formed, giving Tufts the distinction of having the largest number of women fellows of any coeducational medical college in the nation. [37]

Although no records survive documenting a deliberate decision to cut the number of women medical students, we do know that such a decision was made at the undergraduate level. By 1900 a strong male reaction to coeducation had set in at Tufts. [38] The 1905 selection of a strong antifeminist president, Rev. Dr. Frederick W. Hamilton, only served to accelerate the trend and complete the movement toward a sex-segregated campus. Although the men argued that segregation would attract more male students, which would improve the reputation of the school, the underlying cause of their animosity stemmed from the academic success of the women. In 1906, for example, all five seniors elected to Phi Beta Kappa were women. [39] President Hamilton took up the cry that male under-achievement was due to the declining numbers of men en-

36. Mary Putnam Jacobi, "Women in Medicine," in Annie Nathan Meyer (ed.), *Woman's Work in America* (New York, 1891), p. 196.

37. *Hartford Courant*, quoted in *WJ*, October 26, 1907, p. 172; Ida Clyde Clarke (ed.) *Women of Today* (New York, 1925), pp. 126–28.

38. *Tufts Weekly*, March 28, 1900, p. 1.

39. *WJ*, July 30, 1910, p. 123. In 1910 there were sixteen women and fourteen men in the undergraduate graduating class, the top three ranking students were women. See also Russell E. Miller, *Light on the Hill* (Boston, 1966). Miller's historical account does not document the material on women and he draws different conclusions from this data. His focus is on the undergraduate, not the medical education of women.

rolled at the school, down to 30 percent of the 1907 freshman class. Hamilton argued that men were intimidated by the women in their classes: "I have known men to say that they often hesitate to recite or to enter into discussion in mixed classes for fear of making themselves ridiculous before the women." [40] M. Carey Thomas visited Tufts the following year and confirmed Hamilton: "I saw about twenty girls and five or six boys. The boys were huddled together in a corner just as we women used to huddle together in the old days of co-education at Cornell." It is interesting to note that during the Tufts controversy, Dr. Charles M. Green of Harvard Medical School, argued that the chief disadvantage of coeducation was the nervous strain which women experienced when they competed for class honors.[41] Green appears to have been right about the existence of nervous strain; his error was to associate it with the wrong sex.

Similarly, the *Boston Transcript* seems to have confused heroines and villains. Likening the controversy to an academic variation of Gresham's Law, the paper argued that just as "cheap money drives dear money out of circulation . . . the weaker sex drives out the stronger." Neither the president nor the men were willing to be driven out. On the undergraduate level, the answer was simple. In 1910, after three years of planning and promotion, a separate college for women, Jackson College, was established. The announcement of the decision touched off a joyful celebration among the men. Bonfires were lit, horns blew, and the women were forced to run a gauntlet of insulting men.[42]

A separate medical school for women, however, would have been too expensive a proposition. Tufts seems to have modified the pattern Western Reserve University used to exclude

40. *Tufts University Presidential Report*, 1906–07, p. 21; *New England Journal of Education* 66 (1907), pp. 485–86.

41. M. Carey Thomas, "Present Tendencies in Women's College and University Education," *Association of Collegiate Alumnae Journal* 3 (February 1908), pp. 53–54. *WJ*, April 23, 1910, p. 67.

42. *WJ*, January 1, 1910, pp. 2–3 (reprint of *Boston Transcript* article).

women a few years earlier. Western Reserve was a pioneer in educating the early women doctors and two of the prominent physicians in Boston, Nancy Clark and Marie Zakrzewska both received their degrees in the 1850s. Several decades later, the Ohio school debated coeducation for its undergraduate college, decided against it, and then without any formal action to bar women students in its medical school, simply stopped enrolling them. Likewise, the sharp decline in the percentage of women in Tufts Medical School followed closely the controversy in the undergraduate school.[43]

It appears to be more than a coincidence that in 1904 and 1905, the first years when official statistics were published in the American Medical Association journal, Tufts did not report its numbers of female students. More significantly, during this same period the medical school deleted the boldface phrase acknowledging coeducation on its catalogue cover. Where formerly "For Men and Women" appeared to welcome prospective female students, the 1906 catalogue showed no outward evidence of coeducation. The results of these actions were quickly apparent. Only 7.6 percent of the 1910 medical school graduating class consisted of women, far from the record of 42 percent ten years earlier. But the end was not yet in sight. In 1919 the long decline bottomed out as the two female seniors accounted for only two percent of the graduates.[44]

43. The Western Reserve solution is described by Frederick C. Waite, "The Medical Education of Women in Cleveland, 1850–1930," *Western Reserve University Bulletin*, no. 16 (September 15, 1930), pp. 1–29. Waite's account omits mention of the pamphlet by Carroll Cutler, "Shall women now be excluded from Adelbert College of Western Reserve University? an argument presented to board of trustees Nov. 7, 1884."

See also Frederick C. Waite, *Centennial History of the Western Reserve School of Medicine* (Cleveland, 1946), pp. 125–28. Tufts Medical School sources for the coeducation controversy included Tufts Medical School Faculty Minutes and all internal correspondence of the medical school which have been preserved in the Tufts Archives and published reports.

44. All statistics are based on *JAMA* education issues beginning with the first one in 1904. Before this date, statistics are based on college cata-

The College of Physicians and Surgeons in Boston moved just as quickly to close its doors to women students. Founded in 1880, the school had no university affiliation and therefore always remained on the periphery of medical education in the city, its students barred from the hospital and clinical facilities controlled by the larger institutions. As early as 1881, the college catalogue actively solicited women students and dismissed Victorian charges that it was immodest for women to attend classes along with men: "there can be no more impropriety in instructing women in the knowledge of the practice of medicine than in training her for the office of a nurse." A year later the faculty went on record as favoring the idea that women "with the same mental vigor, with greater enthusiasm and ambition than the opposite sex" should become physicians.

But the college, caught up in the antifeminism that was sweeping the nation's medical schools, reversed its position in the twentieth century. The first ominous note was struck in 1900 when the college catalogue contained a new paragraph warning women that they would meet the "same obstacles" in their medical studies as would men. In 1908 the college invited one of the nation's leading antifeminist speakers, G. Stanley Hall, to address its graduating class. Hall's speech was unequivocally hostile to the aspiring woman doctor as he reiterated the old stereotypes of feminine hysteria and menstrual disability. Significantly, Hall's appearance occurred during the first year that the college did not report its female enrollment to the American Medical Association journal. By 1912 only 2.3 percent of the student body were women, down from a high of 21.4 percent in 1894.[45]

logues, commencement lists, or published figures in the *RCE*. The statistics on Tufts graduating female seniors appear to be affected by both world wars because of the school's policy of accepting female transfer students in large numbers. Aside from these periods, the female percentages remain fairly stable, averaging 4.3 percent from 1924–39 when the graduating class was about 100 seniors annually. Before this period the size of the class was smaller. As the school grew, the numbers of women diminished.

45. Internal files of the College of Physicians and Surgeons in Boston are housed in the Rare Book Room of Countway Library, HMS, but will

Elsewhere in the nation, the pattern of declining female enrollment in medical schools was repeated, sometimes even
more abruptly than in Boston. No better illustration of how
women were forced out of medicine exists than the case of
the Medical College of Chicago. Founded in 1870, the college
had graduated 350 women doctors by 1892 when it became
part of Northwestern Medical School. The women's division
continued to function within the university as a separate unit
with its own faculty, which included Dr. Alice Hamilton, professor of pathology, and Dr. Bertha Van Hoosen, a leading
surgeon.

In 1902, without warning, the university decided to close
the women's division. As Van Hoosen later recalled, she first
learned of the decision one morning when, while eating break-
fast before an eight o'clock clinic, she read the *Chicago Daily
Tribune* headline: "Northwestern University Woman's Medical School Closed."

> It was very definite, and absolutely final. I never knew
> the reason for this action, or the suddenness of it—two
> months before the end of the school year. No disposition
> had been made for the students, teachers, or teaching
> material. As an earthquake, the earth had opened and the

---

not be open to scholars until 1980. The information about the college and
statistics were taken from *RCE*, the *JAMA* education issues, the Flexner
Report (1910), and publications of the college. Quotations are from the
Annual Announcement of the College of Physicians and Surgeons (1881–
1882), pp. 6–7; ibid. (Summer 1900), p. 7; ibid. (December, February, 1909);
circular entitled "Value in Mind Cures, G. Stanley Hall Discusses the
Subject at Commencement Exercises of College of Physicians and Surgeons,
June 10, 1908," HCL-A. For further validation of G. Stanley Hall's stature
as an antifeminist, see Thomas, p. 46; G. Stanley Hall ("Coeducation,"
American Academy of Medicine [June 4, 1906], p. 654) argues that the
study of biology and laboratory work "either confuses or strains the girl"
making her education in this area an impossibility. For a detailed study of
Hall, see Dorothy Ross, *G. Stanley Hall: The Psychologist as Prophet*
(Chicago, 1972). Hall's antifeminism is not dealt with in this account.

Northwestern University Woman's Medical School had disappeared.[46]

It was not until 1926 that women were again allowed to enter Northwestern Medical School, and then only because of Mrs. Montgomery Ward's casual inquiry about coeducation after her gift to the school's endowment fund. Unwilling to take any chances on Mrs. Ward's possible feminist sympathies, the university quickly decided to admit women and was rewarded handsomely when she doubled the original gift. From the start, the representation of women in each class was set at four, the number necessary for a complete dissecting team, and with the exception of a few World War II classes, this figure varied only slightly until the 1960s.[47]

In medical schools that remained coeducational during the period from the late nineteenth century to the 1920s, the percentage of women students dropped sharply. At Johns Hopkins, the decline was from 33 percent in 1896 to 10 percent in 1916. At the University of Michigan, the percentage fell from 25 percent in 1890 to 3.1 percent in 1910. Between 1916 and 1926 only 6 percent of Michigan's medical school graduates were women, a situation which can be attributed neither to

46. Esther Pohl Lovejoy, *Women Doctors of the World* (New York, 1957), p. 94; Bertha Van Hoosen, *Petticoat Surgeon* (Chicago, 1950), pp. 137–38; Leslie B. Arey, *Northwestern University Medical School 1859–1959: A Pioneer in Educational Reform* (Chicago, 1959), pp. 120–22, 214, 441–42. See also Helga M. Ruud, M.D., "The Women's Medical College of Chicago," *MWJ* 49 (1956), pp. 41–46, 64. I am indebted to William K. Beatty for copies of letters surrounding the 1902 closing of the Woman's Medical College of Northwestern University, NWUMS-A.

47. Arey, pp. 214–15; see AMA statistics for each year. Internal records for the Northwestern University Woman's Medical College appear to have been lost, but investigation of the resources in the Northwestern University Medical School Library did turn up an interesting source of primary data: *Woman's Medical School, Northwestern University (Woman's Medical College of Chicago); The Institution and Its Founders* (Chicago, 1896). Several other Chicago medical histories give cursory attention to the college.

their lack of premedical qualifications nor their performance once they entered medical school. In fact, the women who were allowed to enter Michigan were clearly superior to the men as a result of higher entrance requirements for women. During the years 1923 to 1926, 84.8 percent of all graduating female students and only 44.1 percent of all male graduates had bachelor's degrees before beginning medical studies. Moreover, women had a better scholastic record during the same period with a grade point average of 3.87 compared to the men's 3.46. Although the author of the article reporting these statistics applauded Michigan's liberal attitude toward women in medicine, clearly his claim that Michigan required "only that women meet the same scholastic requirements for entrance as do men, and maintain a passing grade" was patently false.[48]

The net effect of this retrenchment was the dissolution of the optimism created by the Johns Hopkins victory. Although medical coeducation had not been abolished, it had only survived in token form. Nor could there be any turning back. Except for the homeopathic New York Woman's Medical College, which dissolved in 1918, Woman's Medical College of Pennsylvania was the only college of its type in existence after 1910; separate women's medical colleges were no longer a viable alternative. The only option was for women to fight a holding battle in the hope that new opportunities would somehow materialize.

48. Arthur C. Curtis, M.D., "The Woman as a Student of Medicine," *Bulletin of the Association of American Medical Colleges* 2, no. 1 (January 1927), pp. 140–48.

7

Lonely Battles

To a number of medical women viewing the gloomy prospect of narrowing opportunities, the only possible solution to their plight was some form of organized action. But their relatively small numbers limited their potential for saving the situation or for influencing the course of American medicine. Although a woman's medical association could serve as a gadfly, reminding the medical world of the condition of women physicians, some outside force was needed to serve as a catalyst for progress. The nineteenth-century experience had shown that neither the desire of women for change nor an appeal for simple justice had been enough. Each step forward had resulted from the ability of women to take advantage of problems within the medical world. The medical establishment's war with the irregulars had helped open the medical societies to those women who had attended regular medical schools while the financial needs of schools like Johns Hopkins had improved their chance to obtain a first-rate medical education.

The outbreak of World War I provided twentieth-century medical women with an opportunity to recoup, but the short duration of the war precluded any meaningful advance. It was not until World War II that a scarcity of male medical students and physicians caused serious reconsideration of women as a source of medical practitioners. Between the wars, aspiring female physicians were forced to confront a new barrier in the form of internship appointments.

At the same time, old barriers remained firmly in place. Not surprisingly, in a period of widespread retrenchment in co-educational medical schools, Harvard had experienced little

difficulty in defending its exclusionary policy. This had not
been due to a lack of effort on the part of the women, who
were, no doubt, encouraged by what they may have viewed as
a trend toward "creeping coeducation" at Harvard. In 1894,
the university had made its own accommodation to the pressures of coeducation and incorporated Radcliffe College as an
independent undergraduate college within the university. The
new woman's college was permitted to grant degrees which
were then countersigned by the president of Harvard and
embossed with Harvard's seal. Over the next several years, the
Radcliffe women made every effort to achieve a closer relationship with the university. Radcliffe students were allowed
to take courses at Harvard, but only as a result of individual
negotiations by the students involved. After Harvard refused
for several years to grant women a Harvard Ph.D., Radcliffe
granted its own doctorate in 1902.[1]

Three years later, eight women physicians, all members of
the Massachusetts Medical Society and affiliated in some way
with New England Hospital, petitioned Harvard to accept
women medical students. Their arguments—that there was
now a need for trained women physicians, that women had
proven themselves in the profession, and that qualified women
medical students would not lower the school's standards—had
all been raised before. In fact three of the signers—Emily
Pope, Augusta Pope, Emma Call—had been petitioning for
some thirty years.[2]

Harvard, of course, had even greater experience in rejecting such petitions and dismissed the latest one with no difficulty. Despite the existence of Radcliffe, little had changed
in the thinking of Harvard about the role of women. For that

1. The complex history of the Radcliffe doctorate is detailed in Mary
Roth Walsh, "Women and the Harvard Ph.D. 1879–1902," unpublished
manuscript. See also *Graduate Education for Women: The Radcliffe Ph.D.
A Report by a Faculty-Trustee Committee* (Cambridge, Mass., 1956).

2. "Petition for the Admission of Women to the Harvard Medical
School," October 30, 1905, HCL-A; Harvard Medical School Faculty
Minutes, December 2, 1905, and January 6, 1906, HCL-A.

matter, Radcliffe was saddled with a male president, Le Baron Russell Briggs (1903-23), who believed that if women's colleges "teach women to compete with men, they will fail." To Briggs, a woman's best chance for wealth and success was through marriage rather than a career.[3]

What over fifty years of efforts to gain Harvard medical degrees proved was that petitions and negotiations were in vain unless Harvard could derive some benefit from coeducation. The women petitioners had come close to victory in the 1880s when for a time it appeared that the only question was how much it would cost the women to purchase their way into Harvard. However, the university's gradually improving financial situation seemed to preclude a similar opportunity from emerging in the twentieth century, and there appeared little likelihood of any other opening until World War I created a momentary crisis in American medical education.

The war was a two-edged sword for the medical schools; not only did it create a new demand for doctors in the military, it also cut the supply of medical school applicants as many college graduates entered military duty instead of continuing their studies. These pressures led thirteen medical schools, including Columbia and Yale to break with their all-male tradition and admit women for the first time. After much discussion, the Harvard administration finally decided in August 1917 that it too would train a small number of women at its medical school.[4]

Fragmentary evidence makes it difficult to piece together the complete story of the events that transpired in the months following this decision. One thing is clear: Harvard made the original decision grudgingly, pushed by the belief that it should make some contribution to the war effort and by its concern over the possibility of a dip in qualified male appli-

3. Rollo Walter Brown, *Dean Briggs* (New York, 1926), pp. 217-18; L. B. R. Briggs, *Girls and Education* (Boston, 1911), p. 4.

4. The official Administrative Board action took place on September 7, 1917 (cited in C. Sidney Burwell memo, October 17, 1942, Harvard Medical School Dean's Records, HCL-A).

cants. As late as August 28, 1917, the administration was still mulling over the best method of how to admit the women or, more accurately, how to keep them at arm's length. It finally decided that though the women were to be trained at Harvard Medical School, they would not be awarded the esteemed Harvard degree. After discussing various alternatives which included the possibility of a Wellesley or Simmons College medical degree, it was finally decided that Radcliffe would grant the degree. Internal correspondence indicates that the proposed Radcliffe M.D., like its Ph.D., was not to be considered the equivalent of the Harvard degree—at least by Harvard officials.[5]

Even though the women were to be taught separately, the idea was too much for a number of male students who drew up a petition against the women's admission, arguing that "whenever a woman proved herself capable of intellectual achievement, the area in question ceased to constitute an honor to the men who had previously prized it." [6] Luckily for the men, there were only a few weeks between Harvard's announcement and the opening of the fall semester. Consequently, only twenty women applied, sixteen of whom were judged to be unqualified. Three of the remaining four had already been accepted by other medical schools. Although the three women apparently would have preferred Harvard, they were not given a choice. The administration quickly announced that it was abandoning the plan to admit women

5. These points are documented in the A. Lawrence Lowell correspondence of this period (folder 1459, Lowell Papers, HWL-A), which includes the following letters for 1917 to: Dean Bradford, August 11; Dean Briggs, August 24; Dean Bradford, August 25; Otto Folin, August 26; Dean Briggs, August 28; Dean Bradford, September 18; Yale University and Columbia University (seeking statistics on women medical students), September 21; Mrs. Thayer, September 25; Miss Ellen F. Pendleton, September 17; Miss Ellen F. Pendleton, September 29. See also *Harvard Crimson*, October 9, 1917; Harvard Medical School Faculty Minutes, October 5, 1917, HCL-A.

6. Student petitions are not preserved for this period in HCA. The direct quotation of the content of the petition is in *Woman Citizen*, October 30, 1920, p. 600.

because of insufficient numbers—despite the fact that they had
only contemplated accepting five women per year in the first
place!

Nevertheless, President A. Lawrence Lowell insisted that
the women had been given a "fair chance." In a letter to
President Ellen Pendleton of Wellesley College, Lowell wrote
that he was very glad to have made the offer because it showed
that there were few women in the New England area with the
necessary preparation for entering the school. Several months
later, Pendleton along with the presidents of Massachusetts
Institute of Technology, Smith, Vassar, Bryn Mawr, Mount
Holyoke, and thirty other prominent individuals signed a
petition to Harvard urging Lowell to reconsider his decision.
The petition was promptly rejected, although Lowell did declare that if the war continued for any length of time, Harvard
would be "forced" to train women physicians. Fortunately, the
war ended quickly, and not only was the world made safe
for democracy, but Harvard Medical School was kept safe
for men.[7]

The appointment of Dr. Alice Hamilton as an assistant professor at the medical school one year after this episode was,
not surprisingly, viewed by some as a feminist victory. But far
from any signal that Harvard had reconsidered its position
on coeducation, Hamilton's appointment was one more example that the university would only accept women when it derived some benefit from the action. Hamilton's stature as an
expert on industrial diseases was unexcelled in the United
States at this point. She had few illusions about the reason
for her selection, and she wrote in her autobiography: "In-

7. A. Lawrence Lowell to Miss Ellen Pendleton, Wellesley College,
September 29, 1917, Lowell Papers, HWL-A. "Petition to the President and
Fellows of Harvard University, June, 1918," HCA. The petition begins:
"We, the undersigned, wish to express to the President and Fellows of
Harvard University our sincere appreciation of their recent offer to open
the courses of the Medical School to women as a war measure and our
regret that the time was too short to bring forth an adequate response."
See also Annual Report of the President and Trustees of Harvard College
(1918), p. 144.

dustrial medicine had become a much more important branch during the war years, but it still had not attracted men, and I was really about the only candidate available." [8]

Nevertheless, at the time of her appointment Hamilton expressed the hope that the next step by Harvard would be the admission of women as medical students. College women were quick to respond to this cue. The announcement of Hamilton's appointment stimulated another round of petitions, this time from a number of Wellesley students and a group of Boston women physicians. Harvard's prompt rejection of the petition plus Hamilton's initial experiences at the school must have quickly disabused her of such ideas. President Lowell, in fact, carefully stipulated that her appointment was not to be construed as a precedent for admitting women students into the medical school. To drive this point home, Lowell demanded that Hamilton accept three limitations: she was not allowed into the faculty club, she was not to participate in the academic processions at commencement, and she was not eligible for faculty tickets to the football games. Beyond her original appointment, Harvard also was wary of giving Hamilton any further recognition as a leading international scientist. When she retired fifteen years later, she still held her original faculty rank—the only assistant professor emeritus at the medical school. The crowning insult, however, came after her death when Harvard President Nathan Pusey, in a remarkable display of hubris, stated that her unique position at the school had given her "extraordinary visibility," implying that Harvard had given more to Hamilton than she had given to it. [9]

8. *Boston Globe,* February 25, 1959; Alice Hamilton, *Exploring the Dangerous Trades* (Boston, 1943), pp. 252–53.

9. *Boston Herald,* March 25, 1919; ibid., April 7, 1919. Lowell to Wolcott, December 21, 1918, folder 311, Lowell Papers. See also Jean Alonzo Curran, *Founders of the Harvard School of Public Health with Biographical Notes* (New York, 1970) pp. 17–19, 157–59. *Official Registrar of Harvard University* 68 (August 12, 1971), p. 29; p. 37. Harriet L. Hardy, *Announcement of the School of Public Health,* Harvard (1934). "Dr. Alice: First Lady of Harvard," *Harvard Medical Alumni Bulletin* 43 (Spring

While hopes for greater opportunities stemming from co-education were dashed by the retrenchment during the first three decades of the twentieth century, a similar fate befell those who anticipated a larger role for women in the national and state medical societies. Dr. Bertha Van Hoosen attended an American Medical Association meeting in 1904 and was disappointed at the small number of individually isolated and ineffectual women doctors present: "A generation 'earlier, women doctors were on the outside standing together. Now they were on the inside sitting alone. Their influence was nil." This was also true in the various state organizations. In 1917, for example, a little over thirty years after the admission of Emma Call to the Massachusetts Medical Society, there were only 179 female members in an organization of 3,616. Such a small number of women precluded any political leverage within the state societies as witnessed by the fact that in some years as few as two state societies in the nation had a woman on their program of speakers.[10]

Furthermore, whether intentional or not the male doctors appear to have formed a second line of defense in the form of new special interest or local medical societies. One historian views the rush to form medical societies after 1890 as a consequence of scientific advances in medicine during the previous two decades. This is undoubtedly true, but to the women doctors of the period these new organizations must have often appeared to be a further extension of the old boy network. In greater Boston alone, 87 of the 121 existing medical societies in 1910 had been formed since 1890. A comparison of the organizations to which the Boston women doctors belonged

---

1969), pp. 4–5. Hamilton gives only a passing description of her Harvard experience in her autobiography; her personal letters, which may provide more detail, are not yet open to researchers at the SA.

10. Esther Pohl Lovejoy, *Women Doctors of the World* (New York, 1957), p. 97; Bertha Van Hoosen, *Petticoat Surgeon* (Chicago, 1950), p. 201. Women were first admitted to the AMA in 1876 as delegates (described more fully in chapter 5). *WMJ* 27 (1917), pp. 52–53; *WMJ* 35 (1928), p. 198; *WMJ* 36 (1929), p. 217.

and a list of the new societies indicates that practically all were exclusively male.[11]

Ironically, the women doctors in Boston and the nation began to lose ground during the same period when the suffrage drive was reaching its triumphant conclusion. The explanation for this apparent contradiction may be found in the feminists' decision to channel their efforts into winning the vote— the most respectable, but at the same time, most limited of their demands. Beatrice Hall, writing in 1914, complained that the struggle for the ballot had become so dominant "that it overshadowed all others [demands], and the public is apt to regard the woman's movement as synonymous with the suffrage cause." [12]

Once the decision had been made to concentrate on the suffrage, the feminist focus shifted away from the professional woman. This was, no doubt, practical politics. The professional woman had already been converted to the cause; it was the woman in industry and the home who had to be won over. Women physicians (along with other professionals) did not quarrel with this tactic and, in fact, supported it enthusiastically. In one statistical sample, 43 percent of the women physicians were suffrage leaders.[13]

Dr. Anna Howard Shaw, a Boston University Medical School

11. Robert Wiebe, *The Search for Order: 1877–1920* (New York, 1967), p. 114. A complete breakdown of societies and membership was done for the *Medical Directory of Greater Boston* 1910 (2nd edition) but comparative profiles for the 1915 directory were also obtained. Whenever possible, actual membership lists were consulted in published organization directories or in manuscript.

12. Beatrice Forbes-Robertson Hale, *What Women Want: An Interpretation of the Feminist Movement* (New York, 1914), p. 86. Recent research on the nineteenth- and early twentieth-century movements provides additional evidence for this point of view. See Sharon Hartman Strom, "Leadership and Tactics in the American Woman Suffrage Movement: A New Perspective from Massachusetts," *Journal of American History* 62, no. 2 (September 1975), pp. 296–315.

13. Richard Jensen, "Family, Career, and Reform: Women Leaders of the Progressive Era," in Michael Gordon (ed.), *The American Family in Social-Historical Perspective* (New York, 1973), p. 273.

graduate and vice-president or president of the National Woman Suffrage Association from 1892 until 1913, spoke for many professional women when she declared that medicine had its limitations in aiding the vast majority of women. She asserted that feminism's efforts "must begin at the very foundation of the social structure, laws for [women] must be made and enforced and some of those laws could only be made and enforced by women." The net result was that the women physicians were left to fend for themselves. In Boston, for example, the *Woman's Journal,* which had done so much to champion the women doctors in earlier years, all but ignored their plight in the twentieth century.[14]

Finding themselves outside both the mainstream of male medical societies and the current feminist focus, some women physicians decided to form their own organizations. In the 1890s, a group of Boston women doctors formed the Twentieth-Century Club in order to gain experience in conducting meetings and in delivering professional papers, opportunities that were unavailable to them in the state and local societies. Unable to attract a large enough membership, the club disbanded in a few years. Another group of women physicians, all members of the Massachusetts Medical Society, organized the Woman's State Medical Society of Massachusetts in 1908. One of their explicit goals was to "encourage social and harmonious relations within the profession." The group met during the week of the annual session of the Massachusetts

14. Anna Howard Shaw, *The Story of a Pioneer* (New York, 1915), pp. 141–42. By the 1890s almost all the leading women physicians began to support the suffrage to the detriment of their own professional concerns because they felt the suffrage was a critical battle. Mary Putnam Jacobi, for example, published *"Common Sense" Applied to Woman Suffrage* in 1894, but long before this she had begun to move away from strictly medical concerns and toward the woman's movement and reform. Lovejoy describes the support women doctors gave to the suffrage in *Woman Doctors of the World,* p. 109. The conclusion on *WJ* is both a quantitative and qualitative one based on systematic counting of articles and analysis of the contents of each issue beginning in 1870 to the time when it was replaced by the *Woman Citizen.*

Medical Society in June, but by 1915 they had also dissolved, presumably because of a lack of sustained membership.[15]

The only group of women physicians in Massachusetts able to survive the first flush of organizing enthusiasm proved to be the New England Hospital Alumnae Society, no doubt aided by the fact that they had an institutional base. In 1910 the society, then more than thirty years old, changed its name to the New England Women's Medical Society in an effort to broaden its membership appeal. But even this society had difficulty; seven years later it had been able to attract only sixty members, although there were approximately four times that many eligible women doctors in the Boston area alone.[16]

The first call for a national organization of women doctors went out as early as 1867 when Boston feminist Caroline Dall declared that women doctors should organize now that they had achieved success on an individual basis. An abortive attempt to form a separate women's medical organization took place in Washington, D.C., in 1888. Five years later, a group of women doctors in Toledo launched the *Women's Medical Journal,* a monthly magazine devoted to instilling a sense of group consciousness in its readers.[17] All of these efforts to develop a stronger voice for women physicians were capped off in 1915 by the formation of a group known as the National Women's Medical Association, shortly thereafter (in 1919) renamed the American Medical Women's Association (AMWA). The appearance of this national organization touched off a panic among some male physicians and caused a number of

15. *Medical Directory of Greater Boston,* 1910, p. 163; and ibid., 1915–1916, p. 171.

16. Margaret Noyes Kleinert, "Medical Women in New England: History of the New England Women's Medical Society," *JAMWA* 11 (1956), pp. 63, 64, 67. This historical account is taken verbatim from the 1908 booklet of the society, SSC-SC.

17. Caroline Dall, *The College, the Market, and the Court; or Women's Relation to Education, Labor and Law* (Boston, 1867), pp. 22, 432–33; Van Hoosen, pp. 200–01; *WJ,* October 27, 1888, p. 342; "Organizations of Medical Women," *WMJ* 13 (1903) is one report on organizing efforts. These reports begin with the first issue in 1893, however. See *WMJ,* passim.

women physicians to circulate petitions condemning the group. Although the association was able to survive this initial hurdle and go on to be a reasonably effective lobbyist for women doctors, its membership never exceeded one-third of the women physicians in the country. As the official publication of the association complained: "But all our Big Women have not come in. They know that this National Society is a factor in the life and progress of Women in the profession, but for one reason or another they withhold cooperation." [18]

The membership figures reflect the dilemma that confronts every minority group: integration versus separation. The victories of the nineteenth century meant that women would be allowed into medicine, but only at the periphery. On the other hand, after having struggled so long to be accepted, many women viewed any step which identified them with a separate woman's movement as a move away from whatever chance they had for advancement into the medical mainstream. As Dr. Kate Hurd-Mead, the regional director for the association in New England and New York reported, it seemed impossible to get women doctors to "pay any more attention to us [AMWA] than an advertisement of Lydia Pinkham." [19]

Aware of these fears, the American Medical Women's Association required that all of its members simultaneously join the American Medical Association and purposely held its meetings at the same time and place as those of the AMA. De-

18. *Bulletin of the Medical Womens National Association,* no. 12 (April 1926), p. 10; Lovejoy, p. 302; Sophonisba P. Breckinridge, *Women in the Twentieth Century: A Study of the Political, Social and Economic Activities* (New York, 1933), pp. 27, 62–63; Rosalie Slaughter Morton, *A Woman Surgeon: The Life and Work of Rosalie Slaughter Morton* (New York, 1937), pp. 167–74; Van Hoosen, *Petticoat Surgeon,* pp. 200–02. My generalizations about AMWA are based on reading of all the minutes, bulletins, and journal issues as well as manuscript material in AMWA archives.

19. Minutes of the American Medical Women's Association, June 10–11, 1921, p. 4, box 7; ibid., June 8–10, 1924, box 7; Kate Hurd-Mead to President Taylor-Jones, March 24, 1930, box 17; see also her letter to Taylor-Jones, September 27, 1930, box 17, in which she reports that her people in New England were "stone-cold," AMWA Collection, CUA.

spite its minority position, the AMWA represented the only voice of women doctors and defended women's interests on a variety of fronts. One of their first campaigns (and perhaps what saved the group from dissolution by providing it with a rallying point) was the effort to have women doctors commissioned on the same basis as men during World War I. Dr. Bertha Van Hoosen, who helped form the association, waited with apprehension when she heard that women doctors were circulating another petition in 1917. But when the petition arrived, it was not directed at the association but "against the class and sex discrimination made by the Surgeon-General." With that petition, declared Van Hoosen, "the AMWA's future existence was assured." [20]

Numerous women doctors had already applied to the military at this point but they had been rejected because of their sex—army officials stipulated that the word "person" meant men, not women. In June 1917 women doctors enthusiastically endorsed a resolution demanding that women be given "the same rank, title and pay given to men." In the end, patriotism won out, and just as black doctors supported the war effort despite the government's segregationist policies, the American Medical Women's Association urged women doctors to contribute their services in any manner acceptable to the government.[21]

The net result was that their direct contribution to the war effort was limited to the establishment of a number of hospitals in Europe and the use of some fifty-five women doctors as contract surgeons. These women performed surgery in military hospitals without any military status or benefits such as pen-

20. Lovejoy, p. 302. Van Hoosen, *Petticoat Surgeon*, p. 202. On the founding of the Medical Women's National Association see specifically, Minutes of the American Medical Women's Association, June 10–11, 1921, p. 4, and Ibid, June 8–10, 1921, box 7, AMWA Collection, CUA; and reports in the *WMJ* and *MWJ* beginning with vol. 16, (1916), p. 245.

21. "Medical Women's National Association, Report of the Second Annual Meeting, New York City, June 5–6, 1917," *WMU* 27 (1917), p. 141; "Medical Women Ready to Serve Their Country," ibid., p. 149; ibid., p. 184.

sions or military bonuses. As one contract surgeon later recalled, "The only reward we can receive is . . . to be buried
in Arlington Cemetery." [22]

Although important, the issue of military commissions for
women doctors faded in comparison to the association's major
concern: the decreasing number of women doctors. In addition
to calling upon the medical colleges to accept more women
students, the association sought to reverse the decline in a
number of other ways. One approach was an attempt to interest young women in the medical profession through a speaker's program and by supplying financial aid to prospective,
needy female medical students. Constant appeals were also
sent to members urging support for the Woman's Medical College of Pennsylvania, the last of the female medical schools.[23]

But it was the issue of internships that increasingly occupied
the association in the years between the wars. Thus, while the
medical women were fighting educational battles they thought
they had already won, they were confronted with the additional challenge provided by the growing emphasis on postdoctoral medical training. Internships had not been a significant part of nineteenth-century medical education, but by 1904
when the American Medical Association's Council on Medical
Education first investigated the question, it estimated that 50
percent of medical school graduates went on to hospital training. Nine years later the figures had shot up to between 70 and
80 percent and as high as 90 percent at some of the better
medical schools such as Harvard and Johns Hopkins. In the
late 1920s, at least one expert claimed that for successful medical practice, the internship was mandatory. By 1932, seventeen

22. Lovejoy, pp. 301–02; Dr. Ollie Baird-Bennett, in *Hearings Before
Subcommittee No. 3 of the Committee on Military Affairs, House of
Representatives*, 78th Congress, First Session on H.R. 824, March 10, 11, 18,
1943 (Washington, 1943), p. 87.

23. *WMJ* 25 (1915), pp. 97, 107; "Report of the Committee on Medical
Opportunities for Women, American Medical Women's Association, 1929,"
box 17, and Minutes of the American Medical Women's Association,
May 23, 1923, box 7, AMWA Collection, CUA.

state boards had made the internship a requirement for licensing. Moreover, internship barriers—formidable in themselves —threatened women with a "systems effect." Women's inability to gain internships could be (and often was) used as a reason for not admitting them to medical schools. Opponents argued: what profit was there in educating women doctors if they could not continue on to critical postgraduate training? [24]

Long before the question of internships had reached such crucial proportions, however, women had begun their struggle to gain postmedical school training. In Boston, as in the other medical centers of the country, these efforts had been marked by continuous frustration. As early as 1857, Dr. Sarah W. Salisbury, a graduate of the New England Female Medical College and later a member of its faculty, unsuccessfully petitioned the trustees of Massachusetts General Hospital to be admitted to its wards for postgraduate training. Salisbury was so desperate for clinical training that she wrote again to the trustees, declaring that she was even willing to be admitted as a patient if that were the only way she would be allowed into the wards. But the trustees were unmoved by Salisbury's rather creative offer and informed her that they saw no reason to change their views.[25]

Throughout the remainder of the nineteenth century, with the exception of New England Hospital, women physicians found themselves barred from internships at any of Boston's regular hospitals, though sometimes more or less welcome at the city's homeopathic hospital. Consequently, when Boston City Hospital adopted a policy of competitive exams for their coveted internships, the trustees saw no contradiction in their

24. Rosemary Stevens, *American Medicine and the Public Interest* (New Haven, 1972), pp. 116–18; *Science* 37 (October 1913).

25. Trustees Minutes, Massachusetts General Hospital, November 22, 1857, p. 316, and June 11, 1858, p. 368, Massachusetts General Hospital Archives. Frederic A. Washburn, *The Massachusetts General Hospital: Its Development 1900–1935* (Boston, 1939), p. 170; this tactic was also tried unsuccessfully by Mrs. Batchelder in 1866 at Boston City Hospital. See Committee of the Hospital Staff, *A History of the Boston City Hospital from Its Foundation until 1904* (Boston, 1906), p. 217.

announcement that the posts would then go "impartially to the best men." [26]

The situation was, if anything, worse in the rest of the country. In the 1890s there were only six American hospitals in addition to New England Hospital that regularly accepted women: Woman's Hospital of Philadelphia, West Philadelphia Hospital for Women, Woman's Hospital and Foundling Home in Detroit, Women's and Children's Hospital in Chicago, Women's and Children's Home in San Francisco, and the New York Infirmary for Women and Children.[27]

It was World War I, with the resultant decrease in male interns, that provided women doctors with their first breakthrough. A number of hospitals that had responded negatively in 1917 to a questionnaire sent out by the American Medical Women's Association asking if they accepted women applicants, wrote to the organization the following year requesting names of interested women. The case of Massachusetts General Hospital illustrates the pressures that led to the appointment of its first woman intern in 1919. With the United States at war, male interns were interested only in general medical or surgical training, as a valuable preparation for military service. So the head of the pediatrics division, who was unable to fill the internship in his department with a male, petitioned the board of trustees to allow the appointment of a woman. The board rejected the request twice, but finally relented when the only male interested in pediatrics resigned in June 1918 to enter the service. The choice of a substitute lay between one of two "undesirable male Hebrews" and a woman. The result was the grudging appointment of Dr. Mary Wright, who was somewhat overqualified insofar as she had interned the previous year at Peter Bent Brigham Hospital in Boston.[28]

26. *A History of the Boston City Hospital until 1904,* p. 291.

27. Helen MacMurchy, "Hospital Appointments: Are They Open to Women?" *New York Medical Journal* (April 27, 1901), is a national and international survey listing opportunities by hospital and by city.

28. Dr. Fritz Talbot to Dr. Joseph Howland, August 15, 1917 and June 25, 1918, Massachusetts General Hospital Letters, HCL-A.

Not surprisingly, most hospitals ceased appointing women interns as soon as the war was over. Institutions owned and operated by women (such as New England Hospital), which had been shorthanded due to the lack of intern applications, were again inundated with more applications than they could accommodate after 1919. Similarly, Peter Bent Brigham, one of the newest major Boston hospitals (opened in 1913), was adamant about excluding women interns in 1916, but reversed its position as the military call went out in April 1917. Martha Eliot, then a student at Johns Hopkins, commented in a letter to her mother on Peter Bent Brigham's intern shortage, noting that a friend of hers, a senior at Johns Hopkins, Mary Wright, had been "invited" to apply for a medical internship at the hospital. By the fall, Eliot felt confident enough about the intern shortage and the receptiveness of both Massachusetts General and Peter Bent Brigham to send for internship applications. Both Eliot and another female graduate of Johns Hopkins interned at Peter Bent Brigham in 1918–19 and the chief resident, perhaps as a patriotic gesture, gave up his room to the two women; but once the war was over, the hospital refused to accept another woman intern for the next thirty years! Similarly, after the appointment of Mary Wright at Massachusetts General in 1918, only six other women were appointed to internships before World War II—three in pediatrics and one each year between 1938 and 1940 in the new medical specialty of anesthesiology.[29]

Some hospitals did not even have to break with their all-male traditions during World War I. Even with appeals to the mayor of Boston to intercede on behalf of the women doctors,

29. AR-NEH (1919); Martha Eliot to her mother, February 14, 1916; ibid., April 29, 1917; ibid., September 4, 1917; ibid., October 15, 1917; ibid., February 11, 1918; personal communication from Martha Eliot to Mary Roth Walsh, March 1, 1974. I also utilized the oral history transcripts for Martha Eliot which, with the letters cited above, are in SA. Statistics on the individual hospitals cited were obtained from systematic checking of names listed in hospital annual reports for each year.

Boston City Hospital, a major teaching hospital, did not yield until 1931 when Dr. Madelaine Ray Brown, who had already completed one internship at the University of Michigan Hospital, was appointed. Boston Lying-In Hospital, a logical place for the training of women physicians, did not admit women into its internship program. By 1922 this maternity hospital had trained 299 interns, all men. In contrast to the Boston Lying-In, New England Hospital, highlighting its role as a fortress for women physicians, had trained 400 women interns in approximately the same number of years. As late as 1941, 11 of the city's 13 women interns were at New England Hospital.[30]

When approached by the American Medical Women's Association, spokesmen for the segregated hospitals, which found no difficulty in housing nurses, matrons, and female patients, defended their policy by arguing that they could not find rooms for women interns. The result was a situation where most men were able to intern in the geographical area where they had gone to medical school and where they would more than likely establish their practice. Women, on the other hand, were forced to seek internships in the few cities where they were available to them. Thus, for women interns at least, the "new freedom" of women in the 1920s simply meant the freedom to travel for internship training. In 1925, for example,

30. *Boston Transcript*, February 8, 1923. Hospital scrapbooks were also checked along with archives at the Lying-In Hospital. Trustee records were consulted for the Boston hospitals whenever they were available. The 1920s were a period of growing staff and intern shortages at Boston City Hospital and it is likely that the "breakthrough" in 1931 was actually a response to this, rather than a victory for the women on other grounds. See Trustee Minutes Boston City Hospital, May 22, 1931; November 23, 1923; August 1, 1924; and August 15, 1924, BCH-A. See also "Records of the Medical Staff," Boston City Hospital, February 1, 1927, vol. 2, for a discussion of the small number of applications to the medical staff. Trustee Minutes, Boston City Hospital, June 13, 1919, shows that Dr. Mabel Ordway was appointed as Second Assistant Visiting Physician for six months beginning July 1, 1919. On November 17, 1919, she was reappointed. This was an obvious response to the World War I shortage. *MWJ* 48 (1941), p. 142.

50 percent of all women interns trained in nine widely separated hospitals, one of which was in the Philippines! [31]

According to statistics published in the American Medical Association Directory for 1921, out of 482 general hospitals approved for intern service, only 40 admitted women interns; in other words, 92 percent of the hospitals did not train women doctors, however excellent the woman's medical school record. As late as the mid-1930s, twelve states (one of which required the internship before licensing) had no hospitals available for women interns. In twelve other states, women medical graduates had only one hospital available to them. New York City has often been cited as more hospitable to women doctors; yet, in 1940 only 42 of 1,190 internships there were held by women.

At the outbreak of World War II, only 105 of 712 American Medical Association-approved internship hospitals accepted applications from women. As late as the 1930s, an average of 250 women medical graduates faced what was described as the "heart-rending task" of competing for 185 internships "open to women." Meanwhile, the 4,844 male medical graduates could choose from among 6,154 internship opportunities available to them.[32]

By the end of the 1930s the mood of women physicians stood in sharp contrast to the optimism with which they had welcomed the new century. The hopes for genuine coeducational medical schools had long since faded in the face of a quota system that grudgingly rationed a few places in each class. Between the two world wars, quotas for women medical students averaged 5 percent. The existence of a few women in most medical classes was used to demonstrate the absence of sexual

31. See also Bertha Van Hoosen, "Opportunities for Medical Women Interns," *MWJ* 33 (1926), pp. 102–05, 194–96. She found that many hospitals listed in the AMA directory as accepting women interns had no accommodations for women and had never appointed any women (Annual Report, May 9, 1932, box 17, AMWA Collection, CUA).

32. *MWJ* 48 (1941), p. 142; *MWJ* 47 (1940), p. 260; *MWJ* 45 (1938), p. 309; boxes 7 and 17, AMWA Collection, CUA.

discrimination, while at the same time the small number of women meant that their existence could be ignored as medical professors addressed their classes as "gentlemen only." The situation of women in medicine during this period is well illustrated by Dr. Herman Weiskotten's 1928 study of the graduates of fifty-two medical schools. The author originally intended to devote a special section of his report to the subject of women's medical careers, but he quickly deleted that section when he found "the number of women graduates included was too small to warrant any conclusions." The token participation of women in the medical profession had thus eliminated any serious consideration of their separate career patterns and problems. A decade later when Weiskotten published a new and painstaking survey of the nation's seventy-seven medical schools, he did not repeat his original "error," but simply treated all medical students as if they were male. Women students, as far as the medical establishment was concerned, were no longer worthy of notice.[33]

Still, despite the obstacles, college women continued to batter away at the gates of medical schools. In 1933, 507 women filled out 833 applications to medical schools across the country; eight years later, 636 women sent out 2,283 applications in an effort to take advantage of any opportunity which might develop.[34]

Once again, war provided women with a new set of opportunities. With the onset of World War II, American medical women for the first time found themselves treated as a valu-

33. H. G. Weiskotten, "A Study of Present Tendencies in Medical Practice," *Bulletin of the Association of American Medical Colleges* 3 (1928), p. 132; Herman G. Weiskotten, Alphonse M. Schwitalla, William D. Cutter, and Hamilton H. Anderson, *Medical Education in the United States, 1934–1939*, Commission on Medical Education (Chicago, 1940).

34. Reported in Fred C. Zapffe, *Journal of the Association of American Medical Colleges* 14 and 17 (1939 and 1942) and summarized by the Harvard Medical School Report on the Admission of Women, table 2, 1943, HCL-A.

able national asset. Nothing better illustrates the fallacy of the
argument that women were not interested in careers as physicians than the experience during the war years. As the barriers
were grudgingly lowered, the number of women who entered
medical training increased; when they were raised again at the
end of the war, the number began to drop.

Symbolic of medical women's progress in World War II was
their successful campaign to be commissioned in the military
medical corps. During World War I, Surgeon General Gorgas
had agreed with the American Medical Women's Association that justice demanded equal opportunity for women
doctors, but he argued that time could not be spared from the
war effort to pass the necessary legislation. He had, however,
promised that in any future wars women physicians would be
commissioned on an equal basis with men.[35]

A few of the members of the association were angered by the
fact that nurses were commissioned in 1920, but since World
War I had been fought "to end all wars" most women doctors
lost interest in the subject during the interwar years. The beginning of the war in Europe in 1939 immediately revived the
issue. In the spring of the following year, the American Medical Women's Association appointed a committee on emergency
service registration and mailed out questionnaires to nearly
8,000 women physicians in the United States. Some 2,000 responded, half of whom offered their services wherever needed,
in this country or abroad. In June the faculty of the Woman's
Medical College of Pennsylvania unanimously expressed a desire and willingness to serve in the armed forces. And only one
day before Pearl Harbor, the Board of Directors of the American Medical Women's Association forwarded to President
Roosevelt a set of resolutions requesting commissions for wo-

35. Dr. Sophia Kleegman, "Appointment of Female Physicians and
Surgeons in the Medical Corps of the Army and Navy," *Hearings Before
Subcommittee No. 3 of the Committee on Military Affairs, House of
Representatives,* 78th Congress, First Session, on H.R. 824 and H.R. 1857,
March 10, 11, and 18, 1943 (Washington, 1943), p. 67.

men doctors in the Medical Reserve Corps of the U.S. Army and Navy.[36]

These and a number of individual requests were immediately rejected by the government. It expressed the hope that the additional physicians required for complete mobilization would be drawn from the available supply of male physicians. Women doctors were informed that if, by chance, certain women specialists were needed, they would be employed on a contract basis as in World War I.[37]

Even after the United States entered the war, there was no immediate change in the government's stand. A few women doctors such as Dr. Margaret Janeway accepted positions as contract surgeons, but filed protests with the War Department stating that they hoped this would lead to a regular commission. Some women doctors were not even accepted on a contract status. One physician had her M.D. status ignored while her employer, an army camp, classified her as a special technician. Along with the demotion, they refused to grant the living expense allocation paid to doctors, forcing her to pay this out of a salary of $150 a month.[38]

Another option was open to women physicians; beginning in 1942, they could serve as physicians in the Women's Army Auxiliary Corps (WAACS). But both contract surgeon status and medical duty in the WAACS were rejected by the American Medical Women's Association as representing an inferior form

36. Helen E. Marshall, *Mary Adelaide Nutting: Pioneer of Modern Nursing* (Baltimore, 1972), pp. 260–61; National Committee to Secure Rank for Nurses, "Victory," bulletin no. 15, August 18, 1920, Department of Nursing Education Archives, Teachers' College, Columbia University; Mrs. Frank Vanderlip, *Hearings, 1943*, p. 53. Women's Bureau, United States Department of Labor, *Women Physicians*, bulletin 203, no. 7 (Washington, 1945), p. 5. Dean Martha Tracy to Maj. Gen. McGee, Surgeon General, June 25, 1945, box 17, AMWA Collection, CUA; AMWA Minutes for Board of Directors, December 6, 1941, box 17, AMWA Collection, CUA.

37. Maj. Gen. McGee, Surgeon General, to Martha Tracy, July 2, 1940, box 17, AMWA Collection, CUA.

38. Dr. Emily Barringer, *Hearings, 1943*, pp. 17–18.

of medical service: contract surgeons, because of the low salary, low status, and lack of both uniform and promotion; the WAACS, because women would be prohibited from the combat zone and grouped with a military unit whose primary purpose was to fill jobs such as clerks, stenographers, and telephone operators—thus freeing men for a more direct role in the war. Running through the association's objections to both positions was a conviction that women doctors should not be forced to serve their country in a second-class capacity. Eager to serve, yet unwilling to accept lower status, nine women doctors (including Barbara Stimson, niece of the secretary of war) had joined the British Medical Corps by 1942.[39]

Of even greater importance was the fear that medical schools, charged with supplying the military with doctors, might cut back on the already limited quotas of women medical students. The dean of the University of Arkansas Medical School, citing patriotic motives, announced in the fall of 1942 that the university would accept no women for the duration of the war. Although protests by the American Medical Women's Association and other women's organizations forced the dean to rescind his order, the idea posed a real threat to the future supply of women doctors. By 1942 women college students across the nation were complaining that other medical schools were rejecting women for similar reasons.[40]

The passage of Public Law 252 on September 22, 1941, authorizing the president to make temporary appointments of "qualified persons" as officers in the U.S. Army, had initially appeared to be an answer to the women's problems. But when women applied for appointments as officers under the terms of the law, the War Department, on the advice of the comptroller general, in effect informed them that nothing had changed since World War I—where the words *person* or *persons* were used in the law, only a man or men were intended.[41]

39. June 1940, box 17, AMWA Collection, CUA; *Hearings, 1943*, p. 9.
40. Emanuel Celler, *Hearings, 1943*, p. 3; ibid., pp. 18, 19; Military Commissions folder, box 16, AMWA Collection, CUA; *New York Times Magazine*, August 30, 1942, p. 10.
41. *Hearings, 1943*, p. 2.

At this point, the American Medical Women's Association launched a major campaign to overturn this ruling. Individual women doctors were advised to write to Mrs. Roosevelt and sympathetic congresswomen such as Edith Norse Rogers, sponsor of the WAACS bill. The board of directors of the association established a special committee to direct the fight; the committee appointed Judge Dorothy Kenyon of New York as legal advisor and Miss Pauline Mandigo, a well-known public relations expert, as publicity director. Resolutions of support were gathered from such diverse groups as the International Ladies Garment Workers Union, the Ladies Catholic Charities of New York, and the National Women's Party. There was even a letter of encouragement from eighty-three-year-old suffragist leader, Carrie Chapman Catt: "If there was anything I could do to help, I would gladly do it, but I am an old lady now and not able to do very active work; however, I still see the wrong and the need of action." Women doctors were able to gather resolutions of support from some of the eastern state medical societies, only to see them defeated three times in a row when they were brought to the floor of the American Medical Association annual meetings. Spokesmen for the association made it clear that women's place, if not in the home, was, at best, on the homefront.[42]

However, the American Medical Women's Association campaign in combination with the growing needs of the military, led Congressmen Emanuel Celler of New York and John Sparkman of Alabama to file separate bills allowing women to serve in the medical corps of the army and navy. As Celler pointed out, the War Department's ruling that women were not "persons" was at best "mid-Victorian." Dr. Emily Barringer, chairperson of the association committee to secure military commissions, demonstrated at the congressional hearings on the Celler and Sparkman Bills that the military was not making the best use of American doctors. Noting that the army

42. Ibid., pp. 2, 15, 17–18, 59; Minutes of the Medical Women's National Association, 1942, p. 22, and Military Commissioner's folder, box 16, AMWA Collection, CUA; *Washington Evening Star*, March 13, 1943; *New York Times*, March 23, 1941.

had taken some of the most skillful male obstetricians abroad and left at home some of the best female plastic surgeons, Barringer dryly added that if there was one type of operation that soldiers did not need, it was a Caesarean section. Finally on April 16, 1943, President Roosevelt signed into law the Sparkman-Johnson Bill enabling women to enter the Army and Navy Medical Corps.[43]

By the middle of the war the growing demand for doctors led many medical schools to accept more women applicants. But women, despite the passage of the Sparkman-Johnson Bill, were forced to pay for these new opportunities. While up to 80 percent of the male medical students in some war years had their expenses entirely financed by the government through such plans as the Navy's V-12 program, women received no such incentives. Nevertheless, the portion of medical students who were women increased steadily from 5.4 percent in 1941 to 8.0 percent in 1945. Moreover, women accounted for 14.4 percent of the medical school class that began its studies in the last year of the war. A glance at table 7 demonstrates how each suc-

Table 7   U.S. Medical Student Breakdown by Class, 1945–46

	Year entered medical school	No. of women	Total enrollment	Women as % of total
Freshman	1945	875	6,060	14.4
Sophomore	1944	416	5,750	7.2
Junior	1943	318	5,751	5.5
Senior	1942	259	5,655	4.5

Sources: Education issues of the JAMA for respective years.

ceeding medical school class in the war included more women students.

Boston's two coeducational medical schools experienced a similar increase in women medical students. Between 1942 and

43. Hearings, 1943, pp. 2, 20. Congressional Record 89, no. 61, p. 2962.

1945 the percentage of females in the entering medical school classes at Boston University and Tufts rose from 1 percent to 19 percent and from 4 percent to 15 percent respectively.[44]

The pressures which had led other institutions to revise their policies finally forced Harvard to reverse its nearly 200-year exclusion of women. During the 1930s the medical school had regularly received application letters from women, often supported by letters of recommendation from male relatives who had graduated from Harvard and by an occasional endorsement written on congressional stationery or the stationery of a foreign embassy. This was all to no avail. The only accommodation made by Harvard was to devise a form rejection, known as the "letter to ladies." [45]

By 1943, however, the medical school was no longer in a "buyer's market." Applications were down sharply, and the quality of those applying left much to be desired. After what was described as a "heated debate" at the January meeting of the medical school faculty, a committee was appointed to investigate the question of whether women should be admitted to Harvard Medical School. On March 16, the committee unanimously recommended that the school break with its all-male tradition and thereby replace the available pool of "mediocre men" with a group of "very superior women." The result was a meeting filled with "scenes of disorder and confusion." [46]

Those faculty advocating the admission of women were surprisingly far ahead of their own generation of male medical colleagues. Outlining the advantages of coeducation, the Harvard professors wrote: "part of the education of a young man for the modern world is that he learn to recognize the capacity

44. Hulda E. Thelander, "Opportunities for Medical Women," *JAMWA* 1 (1946), p. 326. Computations are based on the published lists in the two medical school catalogues for the years involved.

45. Harvard Medical School Dean's Records, HCL-A.

46. Harvard Medical Faculty Minutes, April 2, 1943, HCL-A; ibid., May 22, 1943, vote of fifty-six to three. Dr. Robert Morrison to Dean Sidney Burwell, March 17, 1943; Dr. John Williams to Dean Sidney Burwell, March 17, 1943, Harvard Medical School Dean's Records.

of women to take an equal part in the duties and responsibilities of life." The absence of such an experience at the all-male medical school, the report concluded, led to a situation where Harvard graduates saw women in the medical world "only in subordinate, almost menial capacities, and are, therefore, subtly imbued with the point of view that women as a group are incapable of reaching a professional level similar to that attained by men." Harvard Medical School, according to the committee, owed its male students the opportunity to make up their own minds on the capabilities of women doctors "unweighted by artificial impediments." [47]

If those faculty members in favor of women's admission were ahead of their time, the opponents appeared to be moored to the nineteenth century. They argued that the committee's recommendation was unpersuasive, and at least one faculty member (shades of Edward H. Clarke) asserted that the "pro-feminists" had overlooked "the fundamental biological law that the primary function of women is to bear and raise children." Nevertheless, a large majority of the faculty, mindful of the decreasing quality of the student body and another law, that of self-preservation, voted to accept women into the medical school. [48]

Despite the favorable vote, the governing board of the university decided to hold out and rejected the faculty recommendation. But the increasing gravity of the manpower shortage forced its hand in 1944. An administrative subcommittee reported that there was no lack of interested women and pointed out that the mere rumor of coeducation in 1943 had resulted in 153 applications. More important was the committee's conclusion that the question was no longer one of merely improving the medical school, but of preventing it from falling both in numbers and quality to a "dangerously low level." The subcommittee reminded the administration that in the previous two years the admissions committee had

47. "Committee Report, Harvard Medical School," 1944, p. 2, Harvard Medical School Dean's Records.
48. Ibid.

been forced to accept males who at the time of their application were less than seventeen years old and in their first year of college. Female applicants were all graduates of four-year schools and their scores on the medical school aptitude test were significantly higher. In addition, prospects for the immediate future appeared to be even more dismal. In the spring of 1944, the army announced that it was releasing 2,800 of the 6,500 places it had reserved for the following year's entering class of medical students. The curtailment of the army's medical education program would mean more medical school places thrown open to civilians—either women or those men rejected from military service. Finally, unable to delay any longer, the Harvard Corporation voted on June 5, 1944, to admit women into the medical school's 1945 freshman class. The twelve women who graduated four years later had begun medical school at ages ranging from twenty-one to twenty-seven and had graduated from college in the years between 1940 and 1945; one had begun her M.D. study with a master's degree in public health. They were a far cry from the teenage college boys who had entered Harvard Medical School during the war.[49]

Advances were also made in the area of internships during the war years. The *New York Times* declared in 1942: "Hospitals are hanging out the welcome signs to women physicians these days. Fledgling women doctors, once excluded . . . are now being snapped up as fast as the ink dries on their diplomas." The *Medical Woman's Journal* joyously informed its readers that the unprecedented demand for women had forced almost all hospitals in the country to open their doors and to beg women to enter. Although both the *Times* and *Journal* articles exaggerated the amount of real progress, the figures on women's internships were impressive. In one year alone, the number of hospitals accepting women doctors increased by 400 percent—from 105 in 1941 to 463 at the end of 1942—although

49. Based on biographical data in *The First Decade of Women in Harvard Medical School, 1949–1959,* Harvard Medical Alumni Association Publication (Boston, 1949).

the latter figure still accounted for less than half the hospitals
approved for internship by the American Medical Association.
The reason for the shift was, of course, because of the rapidly
dwindling supply of male interns. By January 1943 there were
2,392 unfilled intern slots in the civilian hospitals across the
nation.[50] Massachusetts General Hospital opened its first internship in general medicine to a woman in 1943; by the end
of the war, women were eligible for training in all areas except
surgery. During the war years, 1942–45, Massachusetts General
Hospital appointed nine women interns—more than it had in
all its previous history.[51]

As the United States emerged from the war, women physicians naturally hoped that their recent gains would be preserved and expanded. As Dr. Elizabeth H. Hewkin wrote in
the *New York Times* after the war: "The girls who riveted and
welded . . . have returned to their peacetime pursuits, but
women doctors . . . who took the place of men and worked
long hours . . . have come into their own. They have arrived,
they are wanted, and their position is at last secure." Similarly the *Journal of the American Medical Women's Association* noted that the women physicians' wartime record would
ensure other women "for all time an undeniable right to consideration for entrance into the country's finest medical schools
and acceptance for training . . . in the foremost hospitals
throughout the land." [52]

But once again, as fifty years before, optimism quickly dissolved in the face of reality. Within a year after World War II,
the medical establishment moved swiftly to reverse the feminist

50. *MWJ* 49 (1942); *New York Times,* June 21, 1942. *Women Physicians,*
p. 8.

51. Nathaniel Wales Faxon, *The Massachusetts General Hospital* (Cambridge, Mass., 1959), pp. 255–56. Published records of Massachusetts
General Hospital, the annual reports for those years. Seven women had
been admitted in all the years through 1941.

52. *New York Times Magazine,* November 10, 1946, p. 10. *JAMWA* 1
(1946), p. 149. See also R. R. Spencer, "Opportunities for Women in War
Medicine," *The Diplomate* 15 (January 1943), pp. 24–25; *Women Physicians,* p. 19.

gains. A number of women doctors were removed from hospital staff and clinical positions in order to make room for returning veterans. Other women were switched to routine jobs that any well-trained nurse could perform. As one writer summed up the medical events in postwar America: "Hospitals have pitched women off their staffs as promptly as many shipyards told Rosie the Riveter to go home and peel potatoes." By the fall of 1946 a full-page advertisement with protests from leading women doctors appeared in the *New York Herald Tribune* under the caption: "DOCTORS WANTED: NO WOMEN NEED APPLY." [53]

53. *New York Herald Tribune,* October 27, 1946 (supplement, advertising section); H. Whitman, "M.D. for Men Only?" *Woman's Home Companion* 73 (November 1946), p. 32.

8

What Went Wrong?

Why were women unable to capitalize on the victories of the past, not only those of the war years, but also those of the previous century? Any answer must take into account the historical and sociological forces that have affected women's role in American medicine. The story of women in medicine enables us to see how little has changed until recently.

Much of this history has long been unnoticed. Consequently, later generations of women interested in medical careers did not know that the late nineteenth century had been a truly progressive period. As recently as 1968, Dr. Charles Phelps wrote in the *Journal of Medical Education* to applaud the current percentage of women in medical school (7.7 percent); he noted that this "represents a rather remarkable change considering the fact that there were no women in medicine only 100 years ago." Similarly, in 1972 the Boston University Medical School handbook welcomed that year's entering class with the news that their class (21 percent women) had the largest proportion of women in the medical school's history, forgetting the fact that almost a century earlier women regularly exceeded the 30 percent mark and, for several years running, passed 50 percent.[1]

The past few years have witnessed a dramatic increase in the number of women medical students and a rebirth of the optimism that marked the late nineteenth century. But failure to understand the forces that blocked the earlier advances

1. *Boston University Freshman Facts* (Boston, 1972), p. 8; Charles Phelps, "Women in American Education," *J. Med. Ed.* 43 (1968), pp. 916–24.

could condemn the current movement to a similar fate. One might argue—as do many current feminists—that the past is irrelevant and that we are in a new age where women for the first time have a chance for success. But those women who confidently entered the twentieth century had similar views. Certainly, everything seemed to point to enlarged opportunities for medical women. The rapidly growing population demanded more medical care as a result of the scientific advances of the previous quarter century. Women were gaining entrance to a number of occupations, and women doctors, although not accepted as the equals of men, were no longer regarded as eccentrics. When all of this was combined with the recent inroads into education and medical societies, there seemed every reason for optimism.

The question of why the twentieth century became an era of stagnation and even regression for women in medicine has been almost completely ignored by historians. Scholars who have directed attention to the issue have divided along two lines: those who believe that women were the victims of a professionalization process in medicine, marked by licensing laws and the reforms stemming from the 1910 Flexner report, and those who adopt a "blaming the victim" approach which makes the women responsible for their own demise.[2]

As noted in chapter 1, the argument that women physicians were "driven out" of medicine in the early nineteenth century by licensing laws and educational requirements is unsubstantiated by the historical evidence. Nor do the events connected with the passage of the Massachusetts Licensing Act of 1895 explain the twentieth-century downturn. First, the 1895 act was a liberal piece of legislation with a grandfather (and grand-

2. Andrew Sinclair, *The Emancipation of the American Woman* (New York, 1965), pp. 147, 149; Barbara Ehrenreich and Deidre England, *Witches, Midwives, and Nurses: A History of Women Healers* (Oyster Bay, N.Y., 1972), p. 30; Richard Shryock, "Women in American Medicine," *JAMWA* 5 (1950), pp. 371, 377; Reuben A. Kessell, "The A.M.A. and the Supply of Physicians," *Law and Contemporary Problems* 35 (Spring 1970), p. 270.

mother) clause that automatically licensed graduates of legally chartered medical colleges who were practicing in the state as of July 1894, those who had practiced medicine in the state for a period of three years prior to June 1894, and graduates of medical colleges legally chartered by the commonwealth. Those who were not covered by these categories were eligible for written examinations which by 1898 were taken under a numbering system that made it almost impossible for the graders to identify the candidates. Moreover, as late as the 1920s Massachusetts was considered to have one of the most lenient licensing laws in the country. The fact that between 1890 and 1900 the number of women physicians in Boston increased almost 60 percent indicates that the new law did little to check the flow. Perhaps the most significant fact of all is that there is no evidence that any of Boston's women physicians or their organizations ever attacked the licensing requirement.[3]

On the contrary, women physicians regularly boasted of how well they did on licensing examinations. Official records of these examination results categorized by sex do not exist, but women physicians occasionally compiled their own statistics. One study published in the *Transactions of the Woman's Medical College of Pennsylvania,* for example, shows that only 4.9 percent of the graduates of the three remaining women's medical colleges (the Pennsylvania, Baltimore, and New York [homeopathic] schools) failed between 1901 and 1903. During the same period, 16.3 percent of the total number of graduates

3. The developments in medical licensing in Massachusetts are documented in the public documents of the Board of Registration beginning with the first annual report in Jan. 1895 and continuing to 1912. Medical journals regularly published lists of the pass-fail rates of graduates of the various medical schools on the state licensing examinations. See also Lawrence M. Friedman, "Freedom of Contract and Occupational Licensing 1890–1910: A Legal and Social Study," *California Law Review* 53 (1965), pp. 487–534; Frederick C. Waite, "Recent Licensing of Graduates in Inefficient Medical Schools," *Federation Bulletin* (September 1926), p. 6; Frederick C. Waite, "Some Types of Fraudulent Medical Diplomas and the Uses Made of Them," *Journal of the Missouri State Medical Association* (April 1926), pp. 121–31.

of the other medical colleges in the country failed the examinations.[4]

Others, noting the national decline in the number of women physicians after the publication of Abraham Flexner's famous report in 1910, have assumed a cause-and-effect relationship.[5] Flexner's report, sponsored by the Carnegie Foundation, was a hardhitting attack on the low level of medical training in the United States. Long viewed by historians as a watershed in American medical education, the report has been depicted in more recent scholarship as a capstone at the end of a long crusade to reform and regularize medical training.[6] In fact, the pace and rate of consolidation to eliminate the proliferation of medical colleges was as rapid before the report as after. As the Boston and national figures demonstrate, the decline

4. See Clara Alexander, "A Forecast in Medical Education," *Transactions of the Woman's Medical College of Pennsylvania* (1905); Clara Marshall, "Fifty Years in Medicine," *Virginia Medical Semi-Monthly* (January 27, 1899).

5. Shryock, p. 377; in agreement with Shryock are Barbara Ehrenreich and Deidre English, "Witches, Midwives and Nurses," *Monthly Review* 25 (October 1973), pp. 36–37; Louise Tayler-Jones, "Medicine as a Field for Women . . . ," *Journal of the American Association of University Women* 31, no. 3 (April 1938), p. 153.

6. See particularly, Robert P. Hudson, "Abraham Flexner in Perspective: American Medical Education, 1865–1910," *Bulletin of the History of Medicine* 46 (September–October 1972), pp. 545–61. Also Carleton B. Chapman, "The Flexner Report by Abraham Flexner," *Daedalus* (Winter 1974), pp. 105–17; H. David Bants, "Medical Education, Abraham Flexner—A Reappraisal," *Social Science and Medicine* 5 (1971), pp. 655–61; J. Richard Woodworth, "Some Influences on the Reform of Schools of Law and Medicine, 1890–1930," *Sociological Quarterly* 14, (Autumn 1973), pp. 496–516; Kessell, pp. 267–83; Saul Jarcho, "Medical Education in the United States, 1910–1956," *Journal of the Mount Sinai Hospital* 26, no. 1 (1959), pp. 339–85; Stephen J. Kunitz, "Professionalism and Social Control in the Progressive Era: The Case of the Flexner Report," *Social Problems* (1975), pp. 16–27; Michael Schudson, "The Flexner Report and the Reed Report: Notes on the History of Professional Education in the United States," *Social Science Quarterly* 55, no. 2 (September 1974), pp. 347–61; Gerald E. Markowitz and David Karl Rosner, "Doctors in Crisis: A Study of the Use of Medical Education Reform to Establish Modern Professional Elitism in Medicine," *American Quarterly* 25 (March 1973), pp. 83–107.

in women medical students had begun a decade before the
Flexner study. The author himself noted in his report that
the total number of women medical students had dropped
some 19 percent in the previous six years (see table 8). Flexner

Table 8   Enrollment Figures for Women Medical Students,
1894–1909

	1894	*1904*	*1905*	*1906*	*1907*	*1908*	*1909*
Coed medical colleges *							
Number of colleges	72	97	96	90	86	88	91
Total women students:							
United States	878	946	852	706	718	649	752
Boston	101	82	93	85	73	63	79
Total women graduates:							
United States	—	198	165	200	172	139	129
Boston	22	16	15	21	18	12	11
Women's medical colleges							
Number of colleges	7	3	3	3	3	3	3
Total students	541	183	221	189	210	186	169
Total graduates	120	56	54	33	39	46	33
All medical colleges							
Number of colleges	152	160	158	162	159	151	140
Total women students	1,419	1,129	1,073	895	928	835	921
Total women graduates	—	254	219	233	211	185	162

* In the absence of an official "coed" designation in 1894, colleges were
designated as such if they had female students enrolled.
Sources: RCE (various years) and JAMA education issues. Boston figures computed from these and locally published lists.

became the first to conclude from the national figures that
women were showing a decreasing inclination to enter the
medical profession.[7]

One of the few historians to venture an interpretation on the
subject, Andrew Sinclair, has merely echoed Flexner's sugges-

7. Abraham, Flexner, *Medical Education in the United States and
Canada, A Report to the Carnegie Foundation for the Advancement of
Teaching* (New York, 1910), pp. 178–79.

tion that women themselves were to blame for their demise. According to Sinclair's view, female medical pioneers derived greater pleasure from the struggle to gain access to the profession than from the actual practice of medicine; once the barriers had been broken, succeeding generations had no real interest. Furthermore, he argued that those who did pursue medical careers were "few and often untalented." [8]

The story of women's efforts in the twentieth century to secure careers in medicine stands in sharp contrast to the simplistic views which place the burden of failure on the women's shoulders. Further, the decline of the irregular fields of medicine—the homeopaths, the eclectics, and the physiomedicals—does not explain the women's failure to maintain their nineteenth-century momentum. Although women physicians were more likely to be found among the irregulars, they were making substantial inroads into the ranks of the regulars. By 1894, 66.4 percent of women medical students were enrolled in regular schools. And, as one woman doctor of the period commented, there were "about as many women practicing 'regular' medicine as 'homeopathic' and 'eclectic' practitioners." Their success seemed to indicate that the gains of the nineteenth century would continue.[9]

But, as we have seen, the institutional barriers that appeared to have been overcome showed a remarkable resiliency in the twentieth century. The expectation that the gaps opened in the educational barriers of the nineteenth century would continue to widen until the walls fell from lack of support proved unfounded. In fact, the gaps were quickly filled so that eventually only the most persevering woman could be admitted. What is clear is that women were not blocked by their inability to meet the increasing admissions requirements, per se, but by those who controlled the system of medical education. Beachheads were effected in some medical schools and a few hospitals, but they remained just isolated outposts of women unable

8. Sinclair, p. 149.

9. RCE (1893–94), pp. 2045–50; Mary A. D. Jones, "Editorial," *American Journal of Surgery and Gynecology* (January 1899), p. 146.

to expand their position. On occasion, barriers were lowered to solve a problem extraneous to the needs of women—such as a war or a manpower shortage—but once the problem had been overcome, the barriers were again raised, if not to their original height, at least to a height great enough to remain an obstacle. Thus, medical schools would accept women when they themselves were stigmatized (such as Boston University during its homeopathic era), when a school desperately needed students in its early years (as in the case of Tufts), or because of wartime shortages of qualified students (as in the case of Harvard). But in none of these instances were women ever accepted as a result of any real commitment to their medical education.

The question of quotas for women and minorities is a sensitive issue which is often rejected out of hand by medical school spokesmen. Admissions decisions have always been closely guarded secrets and therefore difficult to assess. But the fact that the percentage of women entering medical school, compared to total enrollment, shifts with the needs of the institution and society seems to indicate that a woman's fate in the admissions committee rests on forces independent of her medical aptitude. Certainly a 1968 Women's Bureau report raises serious suspicion that admissions decisions are not sex blind. The study noted that the number of women applicants to medical school increased over 300 percent between 1930 and 1966 while the number of male applicants increased only 29 percent. Yet, the proportion of women accepted by medical schools during this period had decreased and that of the men had increased. Separate statistics were published, beginning in the late nineteenth century, which grouped medical students on the basis of gender. By 1970 this had led to what Dr. Frances Norris called the "equal rejection theory" in which medical schools grouped women apart from men and then rejected approximately half of the female applications solely on the basis of sex, regardless of qualifications.[10]

10. Dr. Frances Norris, *Hearings before the Special Subcommittee on Education of the Committee on Education and Labor, House of Repre-*

In the 1920s and 1930s, women applicants to medical school talked openly about the "places" allocated to female students. By 1950 this was referred to in sociological journals as the "traditional five per cent quota on women students." Even as recently as 1969–70, four medical schools (Albany Medical College, Yale Medical School, Emory University Medical School, and Loyola Medical School) openly expressed discriminatory policies toward women students in the handbook for prospective medical students, *Medical School Admission Requirements,* published by the Association of American Medical Colleges. Medical school spokesmen usually publicly deny the existence of sex discrimination, but the mathematical consistency of the number of women accepted indicates that an internal quota system existed for each school.[11]

When guaranteed anonymity, a number of medical school officials have admitted that quotas, in fact, exist. In 1946, for example, the dean of one large eastern medical school frankly admitted establishing a 6 percent quota for women and giving priority to men. In 1961 another dean admitted to a similar practice: "Hell, yes, we have a quota; yes, it's a small one. We do keep women out, when we can. We don't want them here—and they don't want them elsewhere, either, whether or not they'll admit it." Similar positions have been unconsciously revealed by representatives of other universities. A case in point is the medical school spokesman who felt that his school's policy was generous to a fault: "Yes, indeed, we take women, and we do not want the one woman we take to

---

sentatives, 91st Congress, 2nd Session on Section 805 of H.R. 16098, part 1 (Washington, 1970), pp. 512–13.

11. Interviews with practicing women physicians in New England in 1974 and 1975. See also published information on this in the women's medical journals. See especially, *MWJ* 22 (1929), p. 299, which described a doctoral dissertation by Mrs. Leslie Bartlett, "The Present Status of Medical Women," based on a questionnaire study done under the auspices of the Women's Bureau of the Department of Labor. Unfortunately, this study was never published in its entirety. See, for example, Josephine J. Williams. "The Woman Physician's Dilemma," *Journal of Social Issues* 6, no. 3 (1950), p. 43.

be lonesome, so we take two per class." All of these statements were corroborated by a Special Subcommittee on Education, Discrimination Against Women, of the Ninety-first Congress in 1970 which cited a survey of admissions officers in nineteen of twenty-five northeastern medical schools who admitted that they accepted men in preference to women unless the women applicants were demonstrably superior.[12]

Certainly, when one looks at postwar statistics, it is difficult not to conclude that a decision to limit female applications had been made. The figures in table 9 are based on the graduating classes from 1941–56. It must be remembered that there is a four-year lag between entrance into medical school and graduation. Thus, the class of 1949 represents decisions made in the spring of 1945, several months before the close of the war when qualified male medical applicants were still in short supply. The class of 1950 was accepted during the transitional year of 1946, and the class of 1951 reflects the first real postwar entering class. The peak year for women coincided with the year when the male student supply was at lowest ebb.[13]

The downward trend continued so that by 1955 the low point had been reached. At certain medical schools the percentage of women was much lower than the national average. In 1955, for example, only 1 percent of the graduates were female at Tufts Medical School. At nine other coeducational medical schools, there were no women graduates at all in 1956. One of these was the University of Michigan Medical School, which had pioneered in admitting women to its classes eighty-six years earlier.

The long tradition of hostility to women physicians by the male medical profession has succeeded in reinforcing the

12. Norris, *Hearings, 1970*, p. 518, referring to *Medical School Admission Requirements, U.S.A.*, 19th edition, 1968–69 and 20th edition, 1969–70 (Evanston, Ill.). Jacqueline Seaver, "Women Doctors in Spite of Everything," *New York Times Magazine*, March 31, 1961, p. 67; *Hearings, 1970*, pp. 521, 568.

13. Computations based on published lists in Tufts Medical School catalogues and the *Boston University School of Medicine Alumni Directory* for 1966 which contains corrected listings.

stereotype of medicine as a man's world. Although women physicians are no longer subject to the invidious attacks of the nineteenth century, there is no mistaking the animosity that remains. Foreign women who have studied in our medical

Table 9   Women Medical Students and Graduates, 1941–56

	Women students	Percentage of all students	Women graduates	Percentage of all graduates
1941	1,146	5.4	280	5.3
1942	1,164	5.3	279	5.4
1943	1,150	5.1	241	4.6
1944	1,176	5.0	239	4.7
1944 (2nd)	1,141	4.6	252	4.9
1945	1,352	5.6	262	5.1
1946	1,868	8.0	242	4.2
1947 *	2,183	9.1	342	5.4
1948	2,150	9.5	392	7.1
1949	2,100	8.9	612	12.1
1950	1,806	7.2	595	10.7
1951	1,564	5.9	468	7.6
1952	1,471	5.4	351	5.7
1953	1,463	5.3	363	5.5
1954	1,502	5.3	360	5.2
1955	1,537	5.4	345	4.9
1956	1,573	5.5	340	5.0

* Includes additional classes.
Source: Based on AMA statistics, JAMA 161 (1956), p. 1658.

schools have often commented on how hostile the environment is for women. A 1949 poll of 100 hospital chiefs of staff could include, among many other negative comments about women physicians: "Women doctors are emotionally unstable . . . they talk too much . . . they're always on the defensive . . . they get pregnant . . . if she is married and childless she is frustrated . . . or if she raises a family she is neglecting her practice." Dykman and Stalneker's 1957 questionnaire concerning the role of women in medicine elicited a number of similar responses from male physicians, for example, "Women were created to be wives" and "I dislike female doctors of either sex." One medical school dean even admitted that he preferred a third-rate man to a first-rate woman doctor.[14]

What effect the rapid development of nursing as a profession exclusively for women had on the supply of women doctors awaits further research. In 1890 there were 30 nursing schools in the nation, graduating 470 female nurses annually. By 1926 there were over 2,000 schools with a graduation figure of 17,500. Preliminary findings indicate that nurses were drawn from a different social class than women physicians. Consequently, it is doubtful that nursing diverted many women from pursing careers as doctors. Nevertheless, the existence of nursing clearly reinforced the notion that only men should become doctors. If women were interested in medicine, the argument went, nursing was the natural vehicle by which they could realize their objectives. The result was a neat division of responsibilities: men would cure the patients through surgery and medicine; women would provide care and maintenance—the traditional female "nurturing" role.[15]

Of course these stereotypes are not limited to the medical world, but are part of society at large. There is little wonder that so few young women are attracted to careers as doctors when all of society's cues are negative. In childhood, the girl is given a nurse's kit, while the boy receives "Dr. Dan—The

14. The hospital study is cited by Janet Travell, M.D., in *Office Hours: Day and Night* (New York, 1968), p. 246; the editorial was in *Westchester Medical Bulletin* (August 1949) under the title "Sex and Medicine"; see also Roscoe A. Dykman and John M. Stalnaker, "Survey of Women Physicians Graduating from Medical School, 1925–1940," *J. Med. Ed.* 32 (1957), p. 30; Charles Phelps, "Women in American Education," *J. Med. Ed.* 43 (1968), p. 916.

15. Olin Anderson, *The Uneasy Equilibrium* (New Haven, 1968), p. 39. Kessell, p. 269; Everett C. Hughes, *Education for the Professions of Medicine, Law, Theology, and Social Welfare* (New York, 1973), p. 28; Abraham Flexner, *Medical Education: A Comparative Study* (New York, 1925), pp. 137–38; Kathleen Cannings and William Lazonick, "The Development of the Nursing Labor Force in the United States: A Basic Analysis," *International Journal of Health Services* 5, no. 2 (1975), pp. 185–216.

Bandage Man." In high school, boys are encouraged to think of professional careers in science, while girls with scientific talents are directed toward teaching, nursing, and auxiliary jobs such as in medical technology. Not surprisingly, women students rejected by medical schools (even those with higher grade point averages than their male peers) are more apt to view their rejections as "just" and switch to careers with lower educational requirements. Unfortunately, there is more truth than humor in the cartoon in which a guidance counselor, having been informed of a young woman's interest in medicine tells her: "Yes, the medical profession can be a very rewarding career. Why not plan to *marry* a doctor?" A series of oral histories of women physicians conducted in 1974 and 1975 revealed that the women had been consistently discouraged by high school and college guidance counselors and other advisors. Such discouragement continues even if a woman is admitted to medical school and successfully graduates. For example, letters submitted to the intern selection committee at a California hospital included the following statements: "Patty is an attractive, mature, personable young lady who is a pleasure to have around and who has no 'hangups' sometimes associated with female physicians"; "Nancy proved to be a very pleasant and friendly individual who is delightfully feminine at all times"; and "Ms. ——— is intelligent, mature, pleasant, and dependable—she is also an excellent cook." [16]

Equally destructive to the motivation of women for professional careers in medicine is the position taken by those who

16. "Women M.D.'s Join the Fight," *Medical World News* 2, no. 43 (October 23, 1970), p. 27. Marshall H. Aecker, Marilyn E. Katatsky, and Henry M. Seidel, "A Follow-up Study of Unsuccessful Applicants to Medical Schools," *J. Med. Ed.* 48 (1973), pp. 991–1001; David M. Levine and Carol S. Weisman, *Career Patterns of Unaccepted Applicants to Medical School: A Case Study in Reactions to a Blocked Career Pathway,* Office of Health Manpower Studies, School of Health Services, The Johns Hopkins University (Baltimore, 1974). The intern letters are in Sonia Bauer, "Correspondence," *NEJM* 291, no. 21 (November 21, 1974), pp. 1141–42. The oral histories were collected by Mary Roth Walsh.

label themselves "friends" of women physicians and who write articles recruiting women to the profession. Dr. John Parrish, for example, in a recent article in *Woman Physician,* urges women to take advantage of paraprofessional opportunities in medicine. Although he recognizes the existence of highly talented women, he insists that the solution to finding employment for them lies in the creation of more "in-between" jobs. So restricted is his vision of female potential that he does not sense the contradiction when he happily concludes: ". . . it is within the realm of possibility that a decade hence the rest of the world will be studying this country, rather than the reverse, in the utilization of talented women in medicine." [17]

Only a few young women have been able to withstand these pressures. Thus, a recent survey of National Merit scholars shows that many women who were somehow able to nurture the idea of a career in medicine through high school discarded it in college. Although women made up one-third of the group which stated that they intended to become doctors, only 8 percent of the medical school applicants consisted of women three years later. A career orientation study at Cornell University showed that women undergraduates differ from their male classmates in ways which may be occupationally crippling. Despite higher academic distinctions, the women reported a lower estimate of their intelligence than men and tended to remain in disciplines traditionally attractive to women.[18]

The crippling effects of undergraduate education on women are further reflected by comparing women who enter a six-year medical school program directly out of high school with women who enter medical school at the usual age of twenty-two, after four years of college. At Boston University, where two separate medical school programs operate, the contrast in female enrollment is quite sharp. The four-year medical school program in 1974–75 had an average of 18.4 percent female enrollment in its four classes. In the six-year medical school program for the same year, the average female enrollment was

17. *WP* 26, no. 7 (July 1971), p. 357.
18. Phelps, p. 917; *Boston Sunday Globe,* October 13, 1974.

37.3 percent. The different female enrollment patterns may reflect the number of women who are discouraged by the socialization that occurs during the undergraduate years.[19]

An important by-product of male medical culture is the role conflict which it produces in women. As early as 1882, Mary Putnam Jacobi pointed out that the most serious obstacles are not always the most real. People do not ask if a woman physician is capable, but "will she upset our ideal of womanhood . . . and the social relations of the sexes? Can a woman physician be lovable; can she marry; can she have children; will she take care of them? If she cannot, what is she?" Although we have come a long way from the early twentieth century when it was popularly believed that women doctors could be recognized on the street by their masculine dress and bearing, there is still a conviction that a woman who becomes a physician will be defeminized. As Dr. Estelle Ramey, a noted endocrinologist, declared recently, the popular image of a woman doctor is still a "horse-faced, flat chested female in supphose who sublimates her sex starvation in a passionate embrace of the *New England Journal of Medicine.*" [20]

Any woman who hopes to succeed as a physician must be talented, productive, and ambitious, but these qualities, which are encouraged in men, are perceived in women as aggressive, mannish, and castrating. Women applicants to medical school have commented on the dilemma that this produces for them at the time of their interview. They must convince the admissions officer (usually a man) that they are feminine, but strong; dedicated, but healthy in their social needs; intelligent, but not domineering. In addition, feminists claim that "medical

19. Statistics are based on those for the academic year 1974–75. Enrollment in the six-year medical school program was 99 men and 37 women; enrollment in the four-year medical school program was 478 men and 88 women. Information obtained from Dean William McNery, October 1974.

20. Mary Putnam Jacobi, "Shall Women Practice Medicine?" *North American Review* (1882), p. 54. Dr. Estelle Ramey, "An Interview with Dr. Estelle Ramey," *Perspectives in Biological Medicine* 14 (Spring 1971), pp. 424–31.

admission committees don't like to admit 'uppity broads.' And
the medical school grind takes the fight out of even the
feistiest of students." This is particularly true of women students, who are apt to have more anxiety about their education
in the first place.[21]

This anxiety is especially well illustrated by Matina Horner's studies of female motivation. In one of the projective tests
that she has devised, a group of women college students are
asked to describe Anne, who finds herself after first term finals
at the top of her medical school class. Their responses were
filled with negative consequences for the student, reflecting
their belief that when a woman trains to become a doctor, the
results are a loss of femininity and social rejection. Anne is
pictured by many as unhappy, aggressive, unmarried, or as
someone who uses others in order to get ahead. Other respondents simply could not cope with feminine success and resolved their anxiety by rejecting the cue. Thus, in one
response, she becomes a nonexistent person created by a group
of male medical students who take turns writing exams for the
fictitious Anne.[22]

21. Judith Bardwick, "Women's Liberation: A Nice Idea, But It Won't
Be Easy," in Carol Tavris, *The Female Experience* (Del Mar, Calif., 1973),
p. 87; Joan Savitsky, "Getting into Medical School These Days is as
Difficult as Finding a Doctor Who'll Make a House Call on Wednesday,"
Boston Sunday Globe, January 23, 1972, pp. 8–9; Office of Career Services
and Off-Campus Learning, Harvard-Radcliffe College, *A Guide for Pre-
medical Students at Harvard and Radcliffe*, 1973–74, pp. 65, 57. See also
M. D. Howell, C. C. Tentindo, and J. B. Walter, "What If You Were
Married to a Cab Driver?: Medical-School Admissions Interviews with
Women Applicants," unpublished manuscript, Harvard Medical School,
1973; Chris Coste, "Women in Medicine: Progress and Prejudice," *New
Physician* 24, no. 11 (November 1975), p. 28.

22. Matina S. Horner and Mary R. Walsh, "Psychological Barriers to
Success in Women," in Ruth B. Kundsin (ed.), *Women and Success: The
Anatomy of Achievement* (New York, 1974), pp. 138–44; Matina S. Horner,
"Toward an Understanding of Achievement Related Conflicts in Women,"
Journal of Social Issues 28, no. 2 (1972), pp. 157–76. The concept of the
Motive to Avoid Success has been updated and clarified in Matina S.
Horner, David W. Tresner, Anne E. Berens, and Robert I. Watson, Jr.,

If women are able to overcome all other barriers, there are
still those problems created by the existence of patriarchy and
its accompanying expectations for the role of women in marriage and family life. In 1882 Jacobi outlined what she believed was a workable plan for aspiring women physicians.
The woman would begin her medical studies after her college
degree at twenty-two and would be ready to practice at twenty-
seven, marrying at that time or a year later. Her children
would be born during the first years of the marriage, a period
when her newly established practice made relatively few demands on her time. What must have been a little too neat
even for the 1880s is completely unrealistic in an age of internships and residency requirements which make heavy demands
on a doctor, usually up to the age of thirty-one or thirty-two.[23]

Today the great majority of women physicians do marry,
with 71 percent doing so before they complete postdoctoral
training. Since fathers seldom assume half the responsibility
for rearing children in our society and the coordination of
household tasks usually rests on women, there are difficulties
for women physicians at many stages of the family cycle. Not
the least of these is the fact that inflated notions of the effects
of marriage on the productivity of women physicians have
been consistently used to block many women from even entering medical school. As one medical school dean put it: "How
can you justify more of them? The girls are just looking for
something to do until they get married." As early as 1894 an
official at Johns Hopkins Medical School was quick to assess
coeducation as a failure on the strength of a 33.3 percent female attrition rate because of marriage. What he failed to

"Scoring Manual for an Empirically Derived Scoring System for Motive to
Avoid Success," preliminary draft, August 1973.

23. Dr. Alice Rossi, in her seminal 1964 essay, "Barriers to the Career
Choice of Engineering, Medicine, or Science Among American Women,"
reported that 80 percent of the 1961 female college graduates cited the
doctor's job as "too demanding to combine with family responsibilities."
See Jacquelyn A. Mattfeld and Carol G. Van Aken (eds), *Women and
the Scientific Professions* (Cambridge, Mass., 1965), pp. 51–127. I have
taken the Jacobi quote from Jacobi, p. 69.

mention was that there were only three women students in that particular class to begin with. Similarly, others have casually referred to a 50 percent dropout rate in a class of two women.[24]

In 1940 Dean Dwight O'Hara of Tufts Medical School paid homage to the myth by applauding the gallantry of medical schools to even accept women students "because they have to train two or three to get one who will practice medicine." Twenty years later, in a similar (albeit more subtle) vein, Dr. Alfred Ingegno, a columnist for *Medical Economics,* wrote that since male doctors were more productive, it would be "socially logical" to deny women even the 5 or 6 percent of the places that were then being allocated to them. Ingegno gallantly hastened to add that he was not suggesting such a move since women doctors were a luxury he thought we could afford: "Besides there's always the possibility of a medical shooting star in skirts." [25]

Especially disappointing is the willingness of medical sociologists to accept and reinforce the myth. In 1970, for example, a Carnegie Commission report on health careers contained a typographical error stating that only 45 percent of women were active in medical work (the statement should have read 91 percent).[26] Similarly Eliot Freidson, cited in 1972 by the American Sociological Association for "developing new perspectives on the medical profession," merely echoed an old perspective on a woman's role when he wrote that "only a modest proportion" of women physicians in the United States qualified to practice actually do so. But the study that Freidson cited in support of his argument actually showed that 87 percent of the women physicians in that sample were prac-

24. Seaver, p. 6; *Harvard Medical Alumni Bulletin* (1894).

25. Dwight O'Hara, *Medicine* (Boston, 1940); Alfred Ingegno, *Medical Economics* (December 1961, pp. 41–48).

26. Carnegie Commission on Higher Education, *Higher Education and the Nation's Health: Policies for Medical and Dental Education* (New York, 1970), p. 26. Dr. Leon Eisenberg, a Harvard Medical School professor, was quick to point this out in "Medical Womanpower: A Statistic Goes 'Astray,'" *American Journal of Orthopsychiatry* 41 (April 1971), p. 349.

ticing.[27] Similarly, Eli Ginzberg in *Men, Money, and Medicine* (the title alone is instructive) claimed, without supporting evidence, that the male physician worked during his career an average of one-third longer than the female.[28] The strength of the stereotype of the dilletante woman physician is evidenced by its persistence in the face of an exhaustive number of studies, dating back to one by a group of Boston women physicians in 1881, all of which reach the same general conclusion: between 84 and 93 percent of women practice medicine after graduation. The most recent research, available to both Freidson and Ginzberg, indicates that fewer than 7 percent of female physicians are not employed.[29]

27. See Eliot Freidson, *Profession of Medicine* (New York, 1973), p. 55, which cites the Dykman and Stalnaker study. See p. 33 of the study itself. This is Freidson's only citation for the topic of women doctors.

28. Eli Ginzberg, *Men, Money and Medicine* (New York, 1969), p. 144. Ginzberg has no footnote for the statement I have quoted here. His footnoting of the chapter in general indicates that he was familiar with a number of 1967–68 sources on women physicians, including Carol Lopate, *Women in Medicine* (Baltimore, 1968). Her book has much evidence, including preliminary reports of unpublished data, to refute such a generalization.

29. The research done on this subject agrees that between 84 and 91 percent of women physicians are professionally active, working either full or part-time. The controversy seems to revolve around the definition of full or part-time, not the fact that women are professionally active. Until relatively recently, investigators did not systematically record the actual number of hours physicians were working at their profession. In 1952 and again in 1965, when this variable of hours was included in research studies, the model numbers of hours of practice per week were 45 for women physicians and 50 for men physicians. On the point of hours, see Dykman and Stalnaker, pp. 3–38; and, I. Powers, R. D. Parmelle, and H. Wiesenfelder, "Practice Patterns of Women and Men Physicians," *J. Med. Ed.* 44 (1969), pp. 481–91. These two studies and the following all investigated the subject of percentages of professionally active women physicians, sometimes with male comparisons. See Emily F. Pope, Emma L. Call, and C. Augusta Pope, *The Practice of Medicine by Women in the United States* (Boston, 1881); Martha Tracy, "Women Graduates in Medicine," *Bulletin of the Association of American Medical Colleges* 2 (1926–27), pp. 21–28; Florence de L. Lowther and Helen R. Downes, "Women in Medicine," *JAMA* 129 (1945), pp. 512–14; Helen R. Downes and Florence

It is true that women "drop out" of active medical practice an average of 4.8 years, usually during the childbearing portion of their life cycles, compared to the male average of 2.1 years. However, men terminate their medical careers much earlier—84.6 percent having permanently retired by age sixty —while women are more apt to work longer at the other end of the life cycle—only 50 percent of women having retired by age sixty. Moreover, when we consider that the female life expectancy is seven years longer than that of the male, one might even argue that women physicians are the more productive of the two groups over their respective life cycles.[30]

This is not to say that the strain of marriage and family life has not taken its toll on women physicians. From 1949 to 1958 twice as many women as men dropped out of medical school (15 percent versus 8 percent). Although the dropout rate for academic reasons was about the same for both sexes, non-academic reasons accounted for 8 percent of the women's dropout rate and 3 percent of the men's dropout rate.[31]

---

de L. Lowther, "Group of Women Physicians," *MWJ* 53 (1946) pp. 39–49; Ruth Glick, "Practitioners and Non-Practitioners in a Group of Women Physicians," Ph.D. dissertation, Western Reserve University, 1965; Jane Gaudette Jones, "Career Patterns of Women Physicians," Ph.D. dissertation, Brandeis University, 1971; C. S. Shapiro, B. J. Stiber, A. A. Zerkovic and J. S. Mausner, "Careers of Women Physicians," *J. Med. Ed.* 43 (1968), pp. 1033–40; Phelps found that a large number of women worked fewer hours due to their work site, i.e., federal government fixed hours and salaried positions: "It would appear that it is the nature of the jobs women hold, rather than the nature of women themselves that tends to limit their hours of medical practice" (p. 921).

30. Dr. Francis Norris cites these facts in her testimony before Congress (*Hearings, 1970*, pp. 516–17). See also Margaret A. Campbell, M.D., *Why Would a Girl Go Into Medicine?* (New York, 1973), pp. 102–03.

31. G. O. Johnson and E. B. Hutchins, "Doctor or Dropout: A Study of Medical Student Attrition," *J. Med. Ed.* 41 (1966), pp. 1107–1204; Campbell cites an unpublished study that shows the positive impact of feminist support groups for women graduate students. See L. W. Sells, "Sex Differences in Graduate School Survival," paper presented at the annual meeting of the American Sociological Association, New York, August 28, 1973. More recent published research shows male and female students have the same

Since this data was collected in an era when there was a great deal of hostility to women's careers in medicine, it is likely that at least some of the dropouts of women students were due to sex-related factors. Shortly after World War II, for example, Cornell University Medical School required a woman student to leave medical school for a year after giving birth to a child. Other medical schools adopted a punitive attitude toward a woman student as soon as she became pregnant. One midwestern medical school, for example, required the woman to discontinue classes until the child was born.[32]

A recent study by Dr. Jane Gaudette Jones at Boston University, Tufts, and Harvard medical schools on *temporary* female dropouts—that is, those who eventually reentered medical school and graduated—suggests that sex-related reasons play an extremely important role. Jones found that 53 percent of those women who left medical school once, and 67 percent of those who left twice did so for marriage- and family-related reasons. In addition 21 percent of the first interruptions and 33 percent of the second interruptions were because of financial problems. When we consider that studies show that women have more difficulty in obtaining economic support from parents and that medical schools have had a firm policy of not providing *any* financial assistance to female first-year students as well as limiting aid to other women students, then prejudice against women becomes the overriding force behind female attrition. If we can include economics among the sex-related factors, then as high as 74 percent of the first group of temporary women dropouts and up to 100 percent of the

attrition rate—see Davis G. Johnson and William E. Sedlacek, "Retention by Sex and Race of 1968–1972 U.S. Medical School Entrants," *J. Med. Ed.* 50 (1975), p. 927. (This study is discussed in chapter 9.)

32. "The Intern and Resident Situation in the Voluntary Hospitals: A Panel Discussion," *JAMWA* 4 (1949), p. 373. Statement by Dr. Emerson Day. See also *Hearings, 1970*, vol. I, pp. 559–62, for a sampling of the extremes of medical schools on the question of pregnancy: either requiring the student to drop out or requiring her to conform to exactly the same timetable as nonchildbearing students.

second group are linked to the "disadvantage" of being a woman.[33]

Jones also found that nearly one-half of the married women students who do graduate, attempt to minimize their sex-role strain by choosing an area of medicine that will give them time to spend with their families. The difficulty of combining marriage and a medical career is illustrated by the case of one woman physician who reentered medicine after devoting fifteen years to raising a family. Even though her husband was also a physician, his opposition to her medical work caused her to sneak out to night calls as guiltily as if she were meeting a lover. Another woman doctor wrote angrily in the *New England Journal of Medicine* detailing the sex-role advantages married men have in their careers and concluded that "only when the institution of wifehood in its present form is either abolished or made available to doctors of both sexes will women physicians be able to do as much as their male colleagues." [34]

More than a century of charges that women physicians physically and/or emotionally cannot stand the strain of competing family demands has made it extremely difficult for women to discuss these and similar problems with their professional colleagues. Male physicians, having warned women against entering medicine in the first place, see no reason why any special accommodation should be made for them. The

33. Jones, p. 91, contains a chart of reasons for women dropping out of medical school. A 1973 study shows 82.5 percent of the men but only 58.6 of the women had parents who were willing to financially support their medical education: Marshall H. Becker et al., *Hearings, 1970* p. 997, provides information on federal funding of medical schools and Lopate, pp. 74–80, cites several research reports on this subject. Since only 17 percent of medical students in one study (compared to 81 percent of life science graduate students) received financial support, the financial problem for women is considerable. See also Campbell, pp. 11–12, who also calls for new research on female attrition.

34. Jones, p. 102; Betty Friedan, *The Feminine Mystique* (New York, 1964, Dell Paperback edition), p. 340; letter to the editor, *NEJM* 285, no. 5 (July 29, 1971), p. 304.

result is that during their pregnancies many women medical students and interns work dangerously close to delivery out of the feeling that they must hold up their end of the bargain. If women delay their childbearing until they become residents, they may be able to locate a part-time residency.[35] But even when such schedules are available, deepseated feelings among women that they must prove themselves force many to view such adjustments with suspicion. Several years ago, Dr. H. S. Kaplan became convinced that prejudice against women doctors manifested itself in the unwillingness of medical schools and hospitals to make adequate provisions for women students and interns in cases of childbirth and childcare. Consequently, Kaplan, with the aid of a federal grant, developed a more flexible training program in psychiatry for married women with families. In seven years it trained sixty-four physician-mothers, not one of whom had to terminate her training because of pregnancy or family problems.[36] Nevertheless, Kaplan's study touched off a flood of critical letters to the *Journal of the American Medical Women's Association,* the thrust of which was that women did not want any special favors, nor did they intend to become second-class medical citizens by pursuing part-time training.[37]

Although many of the responses were reflex reactions to anything that might compartmentalize women's medical training and isolate it from the medical mainstream, the writers had hit upon a real weakness in Kaplan's program. Any medical training program that grants women what appear to be special favors (although they are in fact concessions to the extra family burdens women bear), invokes anger from the men who feel that they are being exploited. The women, in turn, feel guilty for having the extra time off. Whether recent fed-

35. Harold Kaplan, "Women Physicians," *New Physician* 20, no. 1 (January 1971), pp. 11–19; Harold Kaplan, "Part-Time Residency Training: An Approach to the Graduate Training for Some Women Physicians," *JAMWA* 27 (1972), p. 648; *Hearings, 1970,* pp. 560–62.

36. Kaplan, "Women Physicians," pp. 11–12.

37. *JAMWA* 30 (1965), pp. 876–78.

eral legislation requiring hospitals to offer part-time programs to men as well as women will aid women by reducing their guilt remains to be proven.[38]

It is not surprising that many women, after weighing the cost in time, personal stress, and money, decide that a career in medicine is not worth the effort. Dr. Barbara Kehler's 1974 study shows that female doctors annually earn only 57 percent as much as do their male counterparts. One reason for the disparity in both annual and hourly earnings is the assumption in our society that a woman should receive a lower salary than a man. Practically every woman doctor, at one time or another, has been told by a patient who has just learned of the fee, "Why, I might have had a man doctor for that." It is equally important that women have been tracked into the less remunerative branches of medicine. The importance of patronage or sponsorship in professional careers, the "old boy" network of contacts, probably plays an even greater role in medicine than in any of the other professions. The result is that women have not been recommended for the better internships and hospital appointments. They have also been blocked from the more lucrative specialties, such as surgery, where men have enjoyed a virtual monopoly.[39]

38. A survey done in 1973 shows how resistant both directors and medical students are to flexible time programs in graduate medical education—see Mary C. Howell, "Patients and Family: What Does 'Responsible' Mean? The Supply and Demand of Flexible-Time Programs in Graduate Medical Education," 24, no. 11 *New Physician*, (November 1974), p. 27. Executive Order #11246, as amended by #11375, administered by the Office of Federal Contract Compliance, United States Department of Labor. Title I, Amendments to Title VII of the Public Health Service Act, Public Law 92–157, 92nd Congress, H.R. 8629, November 18, 1971.

39. *Medical Tribune*, August 14, 1974, p. 2; Dixie Sommers, "Occupational Rankings for Men and Women by Earnings," *Monthly Labor Review* (August 1974), pp. 35, 42. The mean net income (minus tax-deductible professional expenses) in 1972 was $47,945 for males and $27,558 for females according to an AMA study conducted in the fall of 1973. See Barbara H. Kehrer, "Factors Affecting the Incomes of Men and Women Physicians," Paper presented at the annual meeting of the Southern Economic Association, Atlanta, Georgia, November 15, 1974. In

As we have seen, for most of the twentieth century a woman's main concern has been to get into any internship program available. There was little chance for the women to be selective in their choices. The only published work on medical education that does include women interns is Emily Mumford's participant observation study *Interns: From Students to Physicians*. Mumford investigated two hospitals, a major institution affiliated with a medical school and a smaller suburban hospital. At the larger hospital only one of eighteen interns (5.5 percent) was a woman, while four of the ten interns (40 percent) at the smaller hospital were women. At the larger hospital ("University Hospital" in the study) emphasis was placed on careful research and training under chiefs of staff who were all full professors at the medical school. The interns planned to go into either research or prestigious specialties. The supervisors at the second institution ("Community Hospial") were engaged in local private practice; the interns there had lower objectives, either planning to go on for a residency or directly into general practice.[40]

It is more than likely that the lack of solid technical and experimental training at the smaller hospital may do much to undermine the confidence of its interns. For the women, who are entering a society that has reservations about female competence, the result may be a decision to opt for the least threatening patients—women and children, the poor, and the mentally ill. Another option is to move into public health with its captive clientele. Scholars have ignored the whole history of women's entrance into public health work in American medicine, but there are indications that many of the early pioneers became involved in the field after exclusion from other medical careers

---

addition to her income findings, Kehrer has an excellent summary of the growing literature on male-female professional income differentials.

40. Emily Mumford, *Interns: From Students to Physicians* (Cambridge, Mass., 1970); cited by Judith Lorber, "Women and Medical Sociology: Invisible Professionals and Ubiquitous Patients," in Marcia Millman and Rosabeth Moss Kanter (eds.), *Another Voice: Feminist Perspectives on Social Life and Social Science* (New York, 1975), pp. 13–15.

due to sex discrimination. It almost appears as if the American medical establishment, steadfast in its opposition to socialized medicine, had decided that women could supply a voluntary form of low-cost medical care. Around the turn of the century, the only way that many women could secure a foothold in medicine was through charity work. Even before, as the history of several hospitals owned and operated by women indicates, charity work was the means of establishing the women physicians in urban areas. In the twentieth century, females have filled a proportionately larger number of positions in public health because the salaries were too low to attract a significant number of competent male physicians. Today women physicians are still more apt to be found in the lower echelons of public health and in semicharitable institutions. As one woman physician involved in public health put it: "Only a woman can afford to work for such a small salary. . . . Most of my friends fill just such positions, low in pay and much needed. Sometimes I think we do our profession a disservice but I'm afraid we all wonder who would render some of these services if we didn't and I'm afraid the answer is no one." [41]

Finally, any discussion of women's lack of progress in medicine must take into account the decline of feminism. Dr. Alice Hamilton believed that it had been easier for a woman to become a doctor earlier in the century when feminism was still a powerful force and "a woman doctor could count on the loyalty of a group of devoted feminists who would choose a woman doctor because she was a woman." It is difficult, of course, to always distinguish between feminist forces and Vic-

41. Lopate, p. 123; Mabel Ulrich, "Men Are Queer That Way: Extracts From the Diary of an Apostate Woman Physician," *Scribner's Magazine,* June 1933, pp. 365–69; Esther Pohl Lovejoy, *Women Doctors of the World* (New York, 1957), pp. 109, 123, 381; Esther P. Lovejoy, "My Medical School, 1890–1894," *Oregon Historical Quarterly* 75 (1974), p. 8; Mary Ritter Beard, *Women's Work in Municipalities* (New York, 1915), chapter 2, "Public Health," pp. 45–96; John Kosa and Robert E. Coker, Jr., "The Female Physician in Public Health: Conflict and Reconciliation of the Sex and Professional Roles," *Sociology and Social Research* 49, no. 3 (April 1965), pp. 294–305. See also Lorber, p. 5; Glick, p. 45.

torian prudery in creating opportunities for medical women. No doubt each gave strength to the other, the result of which was the large number of insurance companies, department stores, restaurant chains, and industrial firms that regularly employed female physicians as medical examiners in the late nineteenth century and early twentieth century.[42]

By World War I the Victorian ideal of womanhood was in retreat. Although the sexual liberation of women in the 1920s has been greatly exaggerated, the forces which led some women to seek out physicians of their own sex in an effort to protect their modesty were no longer as strong as they had been in the previous era. Of even greater significance, the passage of the nineteenth amendment convinced many women that emancipation was a fait accompli and it was much more difficult to define—much less overcome—the next level of obstacles preventing women from realizing their potential in medicine. The net result of declining sexual taboos in conjunction with the waning of feminism was a shrinking of what had once been a guaranteed market for women physicians. Looking back over thirty years as a physician, Lilian Welch noted in 1927 that the demand for women doctors had become "as keen as that for a horse and buggy." [43]

Although feminism among women doctors never took on the militancy connected with the suffrage movement, it did play a vital role in their careers. For example, of the women doctors included in *Notable American Women,* 96 percent were, at one time, either affiliated with women's institutions or were leaders in the nineteenth-century woman's movement.

42. Alice Hamilton, *Exploring the Dangerous Trades: The Autobiography of Alice Hamilton* (Boston, 1943), p. 268. Elizabeth Kemper Adams, *Women Professional Workers: A Study Made for the Women's Educational and Industrial Union* (New York, 1921), pp. 66–67; Frances A. Rutherford, "The New Force in Medicine and Surgery," *Michigan Medical Society,* 1893, p. 6; Mary Ritter Beard, *Woman's Work in Municipalities* (New York, 1915), pp. 47–48; *The 50th Anniversary of the New England Hospital for Women and Children* (Boston, 1913), pp. 34–37.

43. Lilian Welch, "The Woman Doctor Struggles On," *Baltimore Sun,* magazine section, July 10, 1927.

In Boston, New England Hospital women led by Marie Zakrzewska always emphasized the fact that female physicians must prove themselves competent as doctors and in this way earn the acceptance of society and their male peers. Nevertheless, the hospital group functioned as an island of nineteenth-century feminism and was in the forefront of every organized effort to advance the cause of women in medicine. Ednah Cheney, a Boston woman's movement leader for some fifty years, considered the hospital group "nobly true to every idea that lies at the basis of the woman movement." [44]

Although not usually viewed as part of the feminist movement, the separate women's medical colleges were motivated in part by the same spirit. It is, of course, impossible to determine what would have happened had women been able to maintain a number of such institutions in addition to the Woman's Medical College of Pennsylvania. We do know that they played a vital role in women's medical education during the late nineteenth century. In 1892, for example, 63 percent of those women enrolled in regular medical schools were attending all-female ones. As late as 1926, 75 percent of the women in the American College of Surgeons had graduated from women's medical colleges, interned, or served on the staffs of female-operated hospitals for part of their career. [45]

Moreover, when women's medical colleges merged with male institutions, opportunities for women to hold faculty positions —and thus become role models for women students—were sharply curtailed. A case in point is the New York Infirmary,

44. *WJ*, January 6, 1872, p. 5. Several Boston women physicians were officers in the Massachusetts Woman Suffrage Association in its early years: Dr. Mercy B. Jackson, Dr. Lucy Sewall, Dr. Marie Zakrzewska, and Dr. Martha Ripley (an officer before she finished her M.D.). Dr. Anna Howard Shaw, as noted in chapter 6, became nationally prominent in the woman suffrage movement beginning in 1892. See also Mary Putnam Jacobi, *"Common Sense" Applied to Woman Suffrage* (New York, 1894), and also her *Address on Behalf of the Women of the City of New York* (May 31, 1894, Committee on Suffrage of the New York Constitutional Convention), pp. 199–236.

45. *MWJ* 33 (1926), p. 343; *RCE* (1892–93), pp. 1990–95.

which closed when Cornell University opened its medical department in 1899. Even Emily Blackwell, who hailed the move, regretted that "it cut short the teaching careers of a group of capable and rising young women teachers." Thirteen years later, Cornell did not have a single woman on its teaching staff or in its clinical service. The significance of a male monopoly on faculty positions was underscored by Dr. Alice Weld Tallant in an address to an alumni meeting of the Woman's Medical College of Pennsylvania in 1912: "Until I took my internship I had never seen a woman operate, and I do not think those of you who have had your training in this school can realize what it means to have never seen a woman doing that which to you seems second nature, from your student days. It must be a great incentive to the student to see what women can do; it is almost inevitable, if you never have seen a woman doing anything, to think she cannot do it quite as well as a man, no matter how strongly you feel in favor of women." [46]

The medical variety of feminism with its sense of solidarity and common purpose ebbed after the first barriers had been broken, out of the belief that the goals had been accomplished. Many physicians were misled by the victories in their state medical societies which seemed to negate the need for a women's organization as a bulwark against male institutions and as a training ground for leadership. After over thirty years of struggling to get into the Massachusetts Medical Society, it seemed foolish to move in a separate direction. But membership only let women into the society, it did not make them part of the society. In later years, the small number of women who attended the annual conventions were described in the local press as anonymous members. During the first seventy-five years of their participation in the Massachusetts Medical Society, for example, only one woman was invited to give the annual oration.[47]

46. *WMJ* 11 (1901), p. 13; *Transactions of the Woman's Medical College of Pennsylvania* (1900), p. 79; ibid. (1912), p. 78.
    47. *Boston Globe,* May 20, 1959, p. 31.

As previously demonstrated, the gradual realization by some women physicians in the early years of the twentieth century that progress was largely illusory caused a flurry of organizational activity—but with relatively little success. The American Medical Women's Association valiantly tried to recruit supporters, but the organization always remained a minority representative of a minority group. Dr. Josephine Baker spoke to this issue in the mid-1930s when women were being replaced by men in Children's Bureau appointments: "The only solution, as I see it, is a recognition by women that they must again fight if they are not to lose out in any public field. There is no one to protest to. It's up to women to fit themselves for these jobs and then to use political push. I do think that *if the [AMWA] was truly representative,* it might well be a splendid, backing force." [48]

The New England Women's Medical Society, like groups of women all over the country, remained isolated from the national group, thus limiting even its geographical representation. It was not until 1950, after several years of inactivity, that the New England group voted to become a chapter of the association and transferred its scholarship funds to Tufts Medical School for the benefit of a woman student. [49]

Merger was no solution for the declining fortunes of the parent organization. American Medical Women's Association membership also dipped 20 percent between 1963 and 1967. As older members retired or died, their places were not filled by younger women physicians, who viewed the organization as

48. Dr. Josephine Baker to Dr. Mable E. Gardner, August 6, 1936, box 11, AMWA Collection, CUA. (This box contains many references to the organizational problems of this period.)

49. Margaret Noyes Kleinert, "Medical Women in New England: History of the New England Women's Medical Society," *JAMWA* 11 (1956), pp. 63, 64, 67. This historical account is taken verbatim from the 1908 booklet of the society, with the exception of material for the period after 1910. Despite extensive search, local records for this group have not been recovered. All material pertaining to the New England Chapter in the AMWA archives was examined. In addition, local members were interviewed for memories of this period.

something of an anachronism. One intern who attended a national convention in the mid-1960s, came away with the feeling that the association provided members with an opportunity to swap stories about pre-World War I injustices to women physicians.[50]

Throughout the twentieth century a few women physicians have called for an organization that would give women a united voice, but the forces militating against such a step have so far proved insurmountable. As early as 1900, Jacobi identified one major problem, women's lack of class interest, which she believed stemmed from the traditional isolation of women from one another, "each as the center of a family and called therefore to play her hand alone." In addition to this, women have faced the dilemma that confronts every minority group: integration versus segregation. Consequently, many have viewed any step which identifies them with a woman's movement as a step away from whatever chance they have for advancement within the medical mainstream. All of this is not to argue that had women been able to maintain their organizational pressure they would have necessarily prevailed. Obviously, their ability to control events and shape their environment was limited; nevertheless, their real gains did parallel the feminist surge of the late nineteenth century.

Symbolic of the waning fortunes of twentieth-century medical feminism was the decline of New England Hospital. Where once voluntary contributions from wealthy women in combination with a dedicated staff had enabled the hospital to make steady progress, the growing costs of medical care created real difficulties. Only the large, heavily financed hospitals could afford the necessary, expensive equipment and laboratories; only the large hospital could provide the variety of cases essential to medical education. The transformation of medical education is illustrated by a comparison of the advice offered to women interns in 1899 and 1930 by the same physician, Agnes Vietor, a surgeon at New England Hospital. At the end

50. "AMWA Membership Statistics," box 9, AMWA Collection, CUA.

of the nineteenth century, Vietor felt that a good deal of surgical training did not even require a hospital: "It is possible to do at home practically all operations that do not require frequent, complicated or voluminous dressings or continued skilled nursing." But by 1930 Vietor's advice reflects the fact that the smaller institutions like New England Hospital were fast becoming inadequate; the surgical intern and resident required "a specially equipped hospital operating room, a corps of specially trained assisting doctors and nurses, and elaborate laboratories and facilities for preparing dressings, as well as specially trained nurses for the aftercare of the patient." [51]

By the end of World War II the medical center of gravity had clearly swung in the direction of what some described as the "Medical Industrial Complex." [52] New England Hospital valiantly tried to stay in the race. In 1948 it proudly announced in its annual report that it was seeking "closer connections" with Tufts Medical School, the Boston Dispensary, Boston University, and Colby Junior College. But it was too late. At this point, financial difficulties coupled with an aging physical plant had created a desperate situation. Beds were no longer filled; badly needed equipment could not be purchased; and, more tragic, it was unable to attract an adequate number of women doctors. By the mid-1950s all the interns were

51. Agnes C. Vietor, M.D., *The Making of a Woman Surgeon* (Boston, 1899); Agnes C. Vietor, "Women in Surgery," *Medical Mentor* (April 1930), p. 207. See also "Resignation of Dr. Bertha Van Hoosen," box 6, New England Hospital Collection, SSC-SC; Sam Bass Warner, Jr., has an excellent summary of the changes in hospitals in the late nineteenth and early twentieth century—see his *The Urban Wilderness: A History of the American City* (New York, 1972), p. 216, and his accompanying references; Anderson, pp. 26–36, 52–56; and, George Rosen, "The Efficiency Criterion in Medical Care, 1900–1920," *Bulletin of the History of Medicine* 50 (Spring 1976), pp. 28–44.

52. Rosemary Stevens, *American Medicine and the Public Interest* (New Haven, 1971), pp. 145 ff.; Barbara Ehrenreich and John Ehrenreich, *The American Health Empire: Power, Profits and Politics* (New York, 1970), pp. 34–39.

foreign-born, without the qualifications to obtain other appointments in better equipped hospitals.[53]

During these years a split developed between the younger members of the board of trustees at the hospital, who favored hiring male physicians, and the older group, increasingly a minority, who defended the traditional policy. The traditionalists were led by two of the oldest board members, Mrs. Oakes Ames, a former suffragist and a leader of the Planned Parenthood Movement, and Mrs. Stanley McCormick, who had been annually donating between $80,000 and $100,000 to shore up the economic base of the hospital. In 1958 the integrationists prevailed and a male physician was hired to head the gynecological and obstetrical division. McCormick resigned in protest, but by this point neither integration nor separatism could have saved the hospital. Despite McCormick's support, the hospital had only remained solvent by closing down whole wards and various services. In 1968 a professional hospital consultant was called in and as a result of his advice, the hospital was closed to bed patients the following year and transformed into an outpatient community health center.[54] Ironically, the end of this former source of medical feminism in Boston, which had emerged out of the nineteenth-century women's rights movement, came at a time when a new feminist movement was taking shape.

53. AR-NEH (1948), p. 12.
54. Mrs. Oakes Ames to Mrs. Frank A. Vanderlip, May 26, 1961, folder 49, p. 238, Kleinert Collection, SA. *New England Hospital News* 1, no. 2 (March 1954), misc. papers, Kleinert Collection, SA. See also the New England Hospital Collection, SC, and the New England Hospital Papers, SSC-SC. There are public relations and newspaper articles for the entire 1950s, collected by a newspaper clipping service in SSC-SC.

9

Will History Repeat Itself?

In October 1970 the long string of abuses in admissions to medical schools, revealed in a congressional hearing a few months earlier, led the Women's Equity Action League (WEAL) to file a class action complaint against every medical school in the country. This and other individual suits in conjunction with the federal government's requirement of affirmative action led to a sharp increase in the number of women medical students. In one year alone (1971) the number of women entering the three medical schools in Boston was double that of the previous year. In subsequent years the total number of women enrolled in medical schools has more than tripled from 3,390 in 1969–70 (9.0 percent of the total enrollment) to 11,417 in 1975–76 (20.5 percent). Moreover, the curve is clearly rising (see table 10). By the fall of 1976, the number of entering women medical students had increased more than 700 percent since 1959–60.[1]

1. On the rise of the new American feminism see Judith Hole and Ellen Levine, *Rebirth of Feminism* (New York, 1971); Jo Freeman, *The Politics of Women's Liberation: A Case Study of an Emerging Social Movement and Its Relation to the Policy Process* (New York, 1975); and Gayle Graham Yates, *What Women Want: The Ideas of the Movement* (Cambridge, Mass., 1975). For a summary of legislation on medical women see Deborah Shapely, "Medical Education: Those Sexist Putdowns May be Illegal," *Science* 184 (April 1974), pp. 449–51; *Boston Globe,* July 15, 1971, p. 33. I have had personal correspondence with Bernice Sandler, Executive Associate of the Women's Equity Action League (WEAL), October 24, 1974, to ascertain the facts involved here. Statistics of female medical school enrollment are from the Association of American Medical Colleges, Mrs. William F. Dube, personal communication, March 4, 1976, and published sources.

It takes four years for any change in enrollment at the first year of medical school to be felt at the internship level; hence, it will take a few more years before the full impact of the recent increase in the number of female medical students is felt. Moreover, it will be somewhat more difficult to measure this impact since recent changes in postdoctoral programs have meant that some doctors begin residencies immediately after

Table 10   Women Students in U.S. Medical Schools, 1961–76

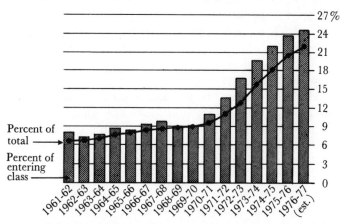

Sources: *JAMA* education issues; Association of American Medical Colleges, Central Student Records file; *J. Med. Ed.* 48 (February 1973), pp. 187–89.

completing medical school, bypassing the internship altogether. Still, between 1969 and 1973, the number of female interns had increased more than 200 percent. Also encouraging was the increased number of women in that hitherto most carefully guarded of male medical domains—surgery. For example, for the first time in their history, all three of the major teaching hospitals in Boston—Massachusetts General, Boston City, Peter Bent Brigham—simultaneously had a female surgical intern.[2]

2. Based on computations from the *Directory of Women Physicians in the U.S., 1973* (Chicago, 1974), pp. 249–53; James N. Haug, "A Review of Women in Surgery," *Bulletin of the American College of Surgeons* (September 1975), p. 22.

Quite clearly, these developments stemmed from the pressure exerted by the women's liberation movement. There were, of course, those like a Tufts Medical School spokesperson who saw the sudden upsurge as an "accident, a pure accident." Similarly, Dr. Francis Moore, Surgeon-in-Chief at Harvard's sixty-one-year-old teaching hospital, Peter Bent Brigham, denied that the appointment of the hospital's first female surgical intern was the result of any feminist pressure: "There was no agitation, whatsoever. I think we're all tired of these Women's Lib agitators." [3]

But the "agitators" seemed unwilling to go away. Significantly, in the spring of 1973, a group of feminist women physicians in Boston gained control of the regional branch of the American Medical Women's Association. As one of the newly elected officers put it: "In the past women in medicine felt a need for mutual support and communication and formed women's groups. . . . In the current atmosphere of feminist activity, many women are recognizing again the importance of providing support and obtaining information from women who have found different kinds of solutions.[4]

The net result was that for the first time in nearly seventy-five years it was again possible to be optimistic about the future of women in medicine. In the spring of 1975 a survey of American medical school deans conducted by the Association of American Medical Colleges, predicted that by the 1980s women would account for one-third of the medical students and physicians in the United States. Later in the same year, Dr. Richard Kessler, associate dean of Northwestern University Medical School was even more sanguine, forecasting that

3. *Boston Globe,* July 15, 1971, p. 33.

4. Drs. Leah Lowenstein and Carol Nadelson became the new president and vice president in the spring 1973 election. The quotation is taken from an article written by Carol Nadelson and Malkah T. Notman, "The Woman Physician," *J. Med. Ed.* 47 (1972), p. 182. I have subsequently interviewed Dr. Nadelson and Dr. Lowenstein, to verify the facts involved here.

by the end of the century at least half of the country's doctors would be women.[5]

But as we have seen, women had been there once before. They had experienced a similar upsurge and had heard similar optimistic predictions at the end of the nineteenth century. Yet their expectations were never realized, and they were soon forced to accommodate to a quota system which admitted only a small number of women to the profession each year. Today, medical women may be once more at the crossroads. Whether the current figures represent the commencement of a permanent advance or whether they merely reflect a temporary accommodation by the medical establishment remains to be seen. A few speculations will be offered here.

One can identify certain favorable factors that could guarantee continued expansion of the supply of women doctors. Medical schools, for example, no longer possess the autonomy they enjoyed at the turn of the century. The fact that more than half their annual expenditures are financed by federal funds makes them vulnerable to government influence. Although hardly a panacea, affirmative action requirements accompanied by the threat of the loss of federal funds have proven to be a useful weapon in the drive to open more medical school places to women. One result has been that medical schools and hospitals have been forced to move in the direction of making their admissions criteria more rational for students and intern appointments. Thus, just as the combined efforts of nineteenth-century women succeeded in making the barriers visible, today's struggle centers on insuring that the barriers be fair.

Equally encouraging is the evidence that some medical women are reviving the mutually supportive efforts which were used to good effect in the nineteenth century. The New England branch of the American Medical Women's Associa-

5. Joseph A. Keyes, Marjorie P. Wilson, and Jane Becker, "The Forecast of Medical Education: Forecast of the Council of Deans," *J. Med. Ed.* 50 (1975), p. 321; *Boston Globe*, November 19, 1975, p. 1.

tion is in the process of establishing task forces dealing with a variety of problems, including: increasing the admission of women into medical school, locating female role models for women medical students, discovering solutions to family and career conflicts, and coping with academic medicine—"how to advance your career in the 'male-buddy' system." [6] Similarly, faculty women have established support groups for first year women at a number of schools. One encouraging sign that a more receptive medical school climate has begun to bear dividends is the recent reduction in female medical school attrition rates. The higher dropout rate for women has long served as an excuse to limit female enrollment. But, since 1970 the female and male dropout rates have been the same.[7]

Women may be approaching a watershed in American medicine. If the present trend continues into the 1980s, the woman physician will no longer be an anomaly. The concept of the "tipping point" may be relevant to the future of women physicians. Here, the concept may be used to denote the point at which the woman doctor is no longer atypical. There is no underestimating the psychological significance if such a development were to take place.[8]

Despite these encouraging signs, one should pause before concluding that the battle has been finally won. The very fact that a previous advance faltered suggests that we could experience a similar historical cycle. One thing is clear: sexual discrimination is deeply embedded in the fabric of American medicine. From Dr. Horatio Storer to Dr. Edgar Berman, who recently argued that the menstrual cycle impaired the capacity

6. Flyer for meeting, American Medical Women's Association, New England Branch, November 18, 1975.

7. Elaine Hilberman et al., "Support Groups for Women in Medical School: A First-Year Program," *J. Med. Ed.* 50 (1975), pp. 867–75; Davis G. Johnson and William E. Sedlacek, "Retention by Sex and Race of 1968–1972 U.S. Medical School Entrants," *J. Med. Ed.* 50 (1975), p. 927.

8. Jessie Bernard, *Women, Wives, Mothers: Values and Options* (Chicago, 1975), pp. 74–89, has a discussion of "tipping points and turning points" though she does not make reference to women doctors or to specific occupations.

of women for leadership, the medical establishment has had little sympathy for feminist goals. In view of this, it would be naive to interpret the recent increase in the number of women medical students as a signal that sexual discrimination has been erased from the medical profession.[9]

The medical establishment, while retreating in the face of feminist and federal pressure, has yet to acknowledge any fundamental commitment to the medical education of women. There has never been, in fact, a willingness on the part of more than a handful of male medical leaders to recognize the fact that women as physicians can make a positive contribution to medicine. As early as 1884, when women were first allowed into the Massachusetts Medical Society, Marie Zakrzewska noted that the step had been taken out of "necessity, not the acknowledgment of the right of women to practice." Similarly, as the number of women medical students increased at the turn of the century, an editorial in the *Women's Medical Journal* attributed this rise to "expediency" and not "because it is to the best interests of medical education." And there is still no recognition that medical schools have an obligation to recruit women. Thus, a spokesman for the Wisconsin Medical School in Milwaukee, where women account for slightly over 12 percent of the student body, saw no reason to seek additional women students because the school had "plenty of women candidates."[10]

Although affirmative action programs attempt to improve women's competitive position, they have been unable to affect the problems posed by marriage and family responsibilities. Despite the success of some pioneering programs in part-time internships and residencies, a survey of 119 program directors

9. Chris Coste, "Women in Medicine: Progress and Prejudice," *New Physician* 24, no. 11 (November 1975), pp. 26–27; Dr. Edgar Berman's argument that women had "raging hormones" appeared in the *New York Post,* August 3, 1970.

10. Agnes Vietor, *A Woman's Quest: The Life of Marie E. Zakrzewska* (New York, 1924), p. 399; *WMJ* 11 (1901), p. 13; *Milwaukee Journal,* September 8, 1974.

revealed that only 15 percent were willing to implement such plans. Beyond this, the specialty choice of a woman becomes extremely constricted if she requires a part-time residency to complete her training. Two-thirds of these flexible training programs were in the areas of psychiatry and pediatrics, traditionally female fields. Across the country, only 1 percent of the female interns or residents in the nation were holding part-time appointments. The result is to leave untouched what has been suggested as the central problem for many women: combining marriage, childbearing and rearing, and a professional career in medicine.[11]

In 1920 a writer in the *Independent Woman* noted that "the modern woman labors under the handicap of not having a wife." [12] This observation is especially true in medicine where the intervening fifty-five years have continued the pattern of long and irregular hours for physicians. This is highlighted by two recent letters to two different medical journals, one from a male physician commenting on the role of the doctor's wife, and the other from a male Ph.D. who articulates the problems of the doctor's husband. The male physician declared that he could not continue without his wife's understanding and support; he pointed out that doctors need their wives at their side "ready to sacrifice part of their womanhood and their roles as wives and mothers." The husband of the woman doctor makes no statements about expecting to sacrifice part of his "manhood" in order to make his wife's career possible. If anything, he is angry at the loss of his sense of entitlement as he complains about "his wife's later hours, night duty, her incessant studying and debilitating fatigue (with its well-known and customary sexual consequences)." Such a life, he argues, "holds no benefits for the husband," and he sadly concludes, "I am not happy to be married to a woman doctor. I

11. "Medical Schools Continue Demeaning Bias, Women Say," *Medical Tribune*, August 7, 1974, p. 2; *JAMA*, Supplement on Medical Education, vol. 231 (1975), pp. 58–60.

12. Cited by William Chafe, *The American Woman* (New York, 1972), p. 280, n. 22.

would not do it again." [13] This is not to argue that it is impossible for a woman physician to enjoy a successful marriage, only that our sex-role expectations place unequal demands on the sexes, with far more obstacles for the female physician.

Equally discouraging—no less so because it originates with two women writers—is the reappearance of the hoary argument in the June 1975 issue of the *Journal of Medical Education* that the reluctance to train women physicians "has been justified by the failure of women to use their education." They estimate that women practice an average of two-fifths fewer hours over their lifetimes than do men, with the consequent loss of an educational investment of $55,000. Although the authors hope that their findings will not be used to discriminate against women in medicine, similar economic arguments have played an important role in keeping women out of medical schools in the past—despite the fact that there has always existed strong evidence to support the position that female physicians are at least as productive over their professional life as their male counterparts. One suspects that the reduced productivity argument has always found greater receptivity because it is in accord with what most medical men want to believe.[14]

There are also ominous signs that a male backlash could be taking shape which would seriously affect the chances for any further female advance. Affirmative action programs have drawn increasing fire from academicians in general. Beginning with the argument that affirmative action goals are really quotas, they have gone on to label the entire effort as one of reverse discrimination.[15] Although affirmative action has never

13. "Viewpoint: An Open Letter to the Wives of Medical Students," *New Physician* 24, no. 2 (February 1975), pp. 40–41; "Viewpoint: Spouses of Physicians-In-Training Speak Out," *New Physician* 24, no. 5 (May 1975), pp. 42–43, 51; letter to the editor from Louis T. Milic, *WP* 26, no. 4 (April 1971), pp. 217–18.

14. Judith Jussim and Charlotte Muller, "Medical Education for Women: How Good an Investment?" *J. Med. Ed.* 50 (1975), pp. 571, 577.

15. Richard A. Lester, *Antibias Regulation of Universities* (New York, 1974); Everett Carll Ladd and Seymour Martin Lipset, "Faculty Women:

measured up to its supporters' expectations, it has led to a medical school admissions policy more open than any in the past. Any diminution of its effectiveness would pose a serious threat to the future of women physicians.

Another potential problem can be located in the feminist-female physician nexus. Just as the nineteenth-century feminist movement provided the major impetus for women physicians, the women's liberation movement, more than anything else, is responsible for the recent expansion of medical opportunities for women. However, the drive to expand medical opportunities for women has not been without its own internal turmoil. As Dr. Mary Putnam Jacobi noted: "Unfortunately, it often happens with weaker parties that they intensify their own weakness by internal discords at the very moment that the closest union, the most frank and fraternal friendship, can alone save their cause and win the day." [16]

Today, a growing disagreement over methods and goals threatens women medical students and physicians with a similar loss of feminist support. On the one side, many women medical students and physicians have failed to perceive a direct connection between their improved professional possibilities and the feminist movement. This view is understandable in those women physicians who were able to squeeze through the cracks in the barriers and establish careers in the years before the recent rebirth of feminism. Nevertheless, the women's liberation movement, with its success in enabling professional women to feel better about themselves as women and its call for expanded opportunities, has created a healthier

Little Gain in Status," *Chronicle of Higher Education*, September 29, 1975, p. 2; Sidney Hook and Miro Todorovich, "The Tyranny of Reverse Discrimination," *Change: The Magazine of Higher Learning* 7, no. 10 (December–January 1975–76), pp. 42–43; Jack Magarrel, "Faculty Women's Status Deteriorated in Year," *Chronicle of Higher Education*, June 28, 1975, p. 5.

16. Mary Putnam Jacobi, "Address Before the Women's Medical Association About 1900," in *Mary Putnam Jacobi, M.D.: A Pathfinder in Medicine with Selections from Her Writings and a Complete Bibliography* (New York, 1925), p. 494.

climate for women physicians. It is the younger female students, interns, and residents who have benefitted most directly from the women's movement. No doubt there is a natural tendency on the part of many of these women to view their success as stemming solely from their own abilities. What they fail to remember is that women in previous generations were equally talented, but their talent went unrecognized because of the absence of a strong, political women's movement.[17]

Meanwhile, a number of radical feminists have begun to question the advisability of supporting the call for more women doctors. Convinced that medicine, as currently practiced in the United States, is elitist and exploitive, they have decided to concentrate on a reformation of the entire health delivery system. They see little gain in supporting women physicians who are likely to be coopted into the medical establishments and, if anything, "outman the men." There is also a feeling that attention given to the cause of women physicians comes at the expense of other female health personnel. As one writer in *HealthRight,* a national newsletter for the women's health movement, put it: "Demands for admission of more women into professions, equal pay for women doctors, and more women in high administration positions miss the point in failing to address the majority of unorganized health workers and consumers." [18]

These criticisms have stimulated some women to experiment with alternative solutions to the present health delivery system. Ironically, many of the plans to revolutionize American medicine parallel the approach taken by some nineteenth-century women. One is immediately struck by the similarities between the present women's health movement and the ladies

17. The growing disagreement over methods and goals is documented in *HealthRight,* a journal of the women's health movement. See also the review essays in the *International Journal of Health Services* 5, no. 2 (1975), "Special Issue on Women and Health"; and the various issues of *Monthly Extract.* My observations on women physicians and women medical students are based on interviews conducted from 1973–75.

18. *HealthRight* 1, no. 1 (Fall 1974), p. 4; Boston Women's Health Book Collective, *Our Bodies, Ourselves* (New York, 1973), p. 248.

physiological societies that flourished in the 1830s and 1840s. Just as nineteenth-century women frustrated with the existing medical system came together to better understand their own bodies, a number of today's women have become convinced that real liberation is impossible without control over their own reproductive system. To date, their work has led to the creation of approximately 1,200 health collectives throughout the country.[19] Whether or not these groups will be more successful than their antecedents remains to be seen. The relevant point here is that although these collectives have played a significant role in improving health care delivery, their concern with reform from the bottom up diverts attention from the need for more women physicians. Such a reduction in feminist pressure may lead to a decrease in the number of women entering medicine, and this will leave the remaining women physicians to fend for themselves.

A recent suggestion that women establish their own medical school also recalls earlier solutions. In fact, the description of the school, which is written from the view of a historian looking back from the year 1999, sounds remarkably like an account of the origins of New England Hospital or one of the women's medical colleges: "The first modern woman's health school had its origins in 1977 with the purchase of an old hospital building and the surrounding land. The money was raised by contributions from women, mostly small donations." [20] The woman physician who wrote this holds up the superior care provided by women physicians at New England Hospital as compared to the male-administered Boston Lying-In Hospital as evidence of what a female institution can do.

Both the women's health collective movement and the concept of a separate women's medical school reflect the antihierarchical concerns of one wing of the feminist movement.

19. Helen I. Marieskind and Barbara Ehrenreich, "Toward Socialist Medicine: The Women's Health Movement," *Social Policy* 6 (September/October 1975), p. 38.

20. Mary C. Howell, "A Women's Health School?" *Social Policy* 6 (September/October 1975), p. 50.

There is no question that the effort to improve the health care environment by transforming the patient from the object of care into an active participant is long overdue. But the majority of health delivery reformers continue to believe in varying degrees that modern medicine does have a body of useful scientific knowledge and technology to offer. How best to tap that source remains an unresolved question. One could, as previously suggested, undertake the creation of an independent women's medical college which would turn out primary health care practitioners trained to involve patients in the medical process. The problem with this approach is the amount of time, money, and duplication of effort involved in the creation of a viable institution. The other alternative is to somehow involve women physicians more actively in the women's health movement. Such a step would be facilitated if there were more feminist-oriented women physicians in effective leadership positions in the medical system. Unfortunately, the increasing attack on the elitist nature of medicine may serve to discourage many women from seeking positions of power.

Three-quarters of a century ago women had less ambivalence about the need to expand their power base. As an editorialist in the *Women's Medical Journal* in 1901 put it: "Women will not be content to be admitted and graduated from these so-called liberal schools. They will ask for a fair proportionment of college appointments that will rank above that of assistant [professor]." Another woman physician at an alumnae meeting of the Woman's Medical College of Pennsylvania noted that Dr. Florence Sabin was a well-known professor at Johns Hopkins in 1911 but she was not "part of the voting faculty which shapes the policy of the college." [21] Women did ask for a policy-making role but their requests went unheeded. Not only did women obtain few faculty positions but they were also denied policy-making positions in medical societies. As

21. *WMJ* 11 (1901), p. 14; *Transactions of the Woman's Medical College of Pennsylvania* (1911), p. 41.

their own hospitals, other health care facilities, and medical schools were closed, they lost the opportunity for feminist self-assertion, autonomy and role models as well.

Today, despite the spate of articles commenting on the expanding opportunities for medical women, the number of female medical leaders has largely been unaltered. There are no women deans listed in the 1975–76 American Association of Medical Colleges directory. The few women who do hold administrative positions, about one percent, are concentrated in the student affairs offices, not in key policy-making positions. And, despite affirmative action programs and the anguished cries of "reverse discrimination" by male academicians, the percentage of women on medical school faculties has remained unchanged since 1971.[22] The result is to place an impossible burden on the few women who do slip into administrative positions. As Wolman and Frank show, the individual woman in a male work group faces "a stressful situation with little leverage for changing it." [23]

The experience of Dr. Mary Howell, former associate dean at Harvard Medical School (one of the four women administrators in the nation appointed from 1971 to 1974), illustrates the truth of the solo woman theory. Howell accepted her appointment in 1972 in the hope that she could be an advocate for women physicians and medical students and a voice for change in the administration of the medical school. Moreover, as the first woman in the school's history to hold a high administrative appointment, she was regularly cited as one more example of woman's progress in the medical profession. Three years later, Howell resigned, characterizing her struggle at Harvard as an attempt to remain "sane in an insane place."

22. *Women in Health Careers: Chart Book for International Conference on Women in Health, June 16–18, 1975* (Washington, 1975), p. 48. Marlys H. Witte et al., "Women Physicians in United States Medical Schools: A Preliminary Report," *JAMWA* 31 (1976), p. 211.

23. Carol Wolman and Hal Frank, "The Solo Woman in a Professional Peer Group," *American Journal of Orthopsychiatry* 45 (January 1975), pp. 164–71.

In "An Open Letter to the Woman's Health Movement" she explained her reasons for resigning: "The problems that we are struggling against, of disadvantage and deprivation of privilege, are not the problems of individuals. They will not be solved by the mere elevation of individuals, unless those individuals are willing and able to speak and act on behalf of the disadvantaged and deprived groups they represent. We, who come from those groups—defined by our sex, skin-color, minority ethnicity, poverty, or powerlessness as patients—are not helped, and may be hurt by token appointments. Only when our representatives have a real voice in decisions will changes come about." [24]

The call for an increase in the supply of women physicians has always rested on the assumption that they can make a difference. From Harriot Hunt, who in 1856 looked forward to the time when women would become physicians and "open books that are sealed," to the feminists of today, the argument has been made that the coming-of-age of the woman physician would result in improved health care for women. In 1970, for example, Dr. Frances Norris told a congressional subcommittee that the federal government's failure to investigate sex discrimination in medicine was in large part responsible for the poor quality of medical care given women in this country.[25] Others have pointed out that not only has the paucity of women physicians in the American medical community affected the freedom of women to choose physicians of their own sex, it has also determined the priorities of medical research itself. There is a growing awareness that there is an interrelationship between discrimination against women as medical students and physicians and against women as patients —resulting in the present lack of research on breast cancer,

24. *HealthRight* 1, no. 3 (Spring 1975), p. 2.
25. *Hearings before the Special Subcommittee on Education of the Committee on Education and Labor, House of Representatives,* 91st Congress, 2nd Session on Section 805 of H.R. 16098, part 1 (Washington, 1970), p. 511.

excessive rates of hysterectomies and surgery on women, lack of concern for the hazards of birth control devices, and generally deficient health care for women. To date most research on female medical problems has been done from a male perspective. Consequently, Dr. Howard W. Jones had no apparent reservation when, in a recent paper at the National Institute of Health, he characterized menopausal women as "a caricature of their younger selves at their emotional worst." The participants invited to hear his paper were twenty-five male researchers, none of whom saw anything amiss in his analysis.[26] In a similar vein, the male author of a recent textbook on gynecology informs the gynecologists of tomorrow that the traits which comprise the core of the healthy female personality are "feminine narcissism, masochism, and passivity." [27]

The expectation that women are capable of bringing about a real transformation of medical practice, while they fuel the drive to expand the number of women physicians, is not without danger. For one, it may place an impossible demand on a group of women already weighed down by the pressures associated with seeking a career in what is defined as a male profession—a profession that produces a great deal of tension for its male practitioners.[28] If to the difficulties attached to medical school, internship, and a career, we add the job of

26. Jones's comments appear in K. J. Ryan and D. C. Gibson (eds.), *Menopause and Aging*, U.S. Dept. of Health, Education, and Welfare, Publication No. (NIH) 73-319 (Washington, 1971). See also Mary Brown Parlee, "Psychological Aspects of Menstruation, Childbirth, and Menopause: An Overview with Suggestions for Further Research" (available from the author, Department of Psychology, Barnard College, Columbia University).

27. Diana Scully and Pauline Bart, "A Funny Thing Happened on the Way to the Orifice: Women in Gynecology Textbooks," *American Journal of Sociology* 78, no. 4 (January 1973), p. 1048.

28. See, for example, Charles L. Bowden, "The Physician's Adaptation to His [Sic] Role," in Charles L. Bowden and Alvin G. Burstein, *Psychosocial Basis of Medical Practice* (Baltimore, 1974), pp. 217-23; Edith T. Shapiro et al., "The Mentally Ill Physician as Practitioner," *JAMA* 232 (1975), pp. 725-27.

reforming the medical system, we may simply be asking too much. Moreover, if women physicians are to be essentially viewed as reformers, they can expect to run into even greater resistance from the male medical establishment.

Perhaps what is necessary is for both radical feminists and women physicians to recognize the benefits each can offer the other. Women physicians must recognize the debt they owe to the feminist movement. The realization that the progress which took place in the nineteenth century was easily reversed could serve to remind them of the need for a permanent support group—a politically active women's movement. The present small number of women physicians are not going to effect a rapid reform of American medicine but it can serve as a base for future improvement. Although the professional socialization process often forces those in training to absorb the values of the dominant group, little is known about how this process affects women students specifically. This may be the result of the fact that women have historically comprised only a small portion of each medical school class or group of interns. Women physicians in large numbers could develop attitudes that do not mirror the male-dominated view of medicine; some women might be able to develop attitudes consonant with the goals of the woman's health movement.

Too often reforms of American society have been advocated as a solution to some comprehensive problems rather than as a redress of historic inequities or injustices. Women deserved the vote—not because they would cast their ballots to end corruption, but because they were entitled to it by virtue of their human talents. Similarly, women are entitled to an equal opportunity in medicine and in the other professions.

Research and Manuscript Collections Consulted

American Medical Association, Chicago, Ill.
Association of American Colleges, Washington, D.C.
Association of American Medical Colleges, Washington, D.C.
Boston City Hospital Archives, Boston, Mass.
Boston Lying-In Hospital Archives, Boston, Mass.
    Miscellaneous Papers, Uncatalogued
    Scrapbooks of Hospital History
Boston Public Library, Research Room, Boston, Mass.
    Susan Oliver Diary
Boston University Medical School Archives, Boston, Mass.
    Miscellaneous Papers, Uncatalogued
Boston University Archives, Boston, Mass.
    New England Female Medical College Records
    New England Hospital Papers, Nursing Archives
Cornell University Archives, Ithaca, N.Y.
    American Medical Women's Association Collection
    New York Women's Medical Association Collection
Francis A. Countway Library of Harvard Medical School, Boston, Mass.
    Boston Obstetrical Society Records
    Boston Medical Association Records
    Henry I. Bowditch Papers
    James Chadwick Papers
    Edward H. Clarke Papers
    Dorchester Medical Club Records
    Reginald Fitz Papers
    Samuel Gregory Scrapbook
    Harvard Medical School Papers
    Massachusetts General Hospital Records
    Massachusetts Medical Society Records

New England Hospital Records
Horatio R. Storer Papers
Harvard University, Widener Library Archives, Cambridge,
Mass.
Charles Eliot Papers
Harvard Corporation Records
Alfred Worcester Papers
Johns Hopkins Medical School Library, Baltimore, Md.
Library of Congress, Washington, D.C.
Blackwell Family Papers
Elizabeth Cady Stanton Papers
Maryland Historical Society, Baltimore, Md.
Massachusetts Historical Society, Boston, Mass.
Caroline Dall Papers
Lemuel Shattuck Papers
Massachusetts State Archives, State Capitol Building, Boston,
Mass.
Legislative Packets
National Library of Medicine, Bethesda, Md.
Horatio R. Storer Letters
Northwestern University Medical School Library, Chicago, Ill.
Enoch Pratt Free Library, Baltimore, Md.
Special Collections
Arthur and Elizabeth Schlesinger Library on the History of
Women in America, Radcliffe College, Cambridge, Mass.
Blackwell Family Papers
Dorothy Brewer Blackwell Papers
Dillon Collection
Martha Eliot Papers
Alice Hamilton Papers
Mary Putnam Jacobi Papers
Sara Murray Jordan Papers
Margaret Noyes Kleinert Papers
New England Hospital Collection
New England Women's Club Collection
Sophia Smith Collection (Women's History Archives), Smith
College, Northhampton, Mass.

Blanche Ames Collection
Connie Guion Papers
Hunt Family Papers
Margaret Long Papers
Dorothy Habel (Reed) Mendenhall Papers
New England Hospital Papers
Florence Rena Sabin Papers
Margaret (Higgins) Sanger Papers
Vida Dutton Scudder Papers
Caroline M. S. Severance Papers
Emma Frances Ward Papers
Alice Weld Tallant Papers
Emma Walker Papers
William Lloyd Garrison Papers
Tufts College Archives, Medford, Mass.
Tufts Medical College Records, 1893–1920
Tufts University Medical School Library, Boston, Mass.
University of Illinois Medical School Archives, Chicago, Ill.
Woman's Medical College of Pennsylvania Archives, Library of the Medical College of Pennsylvania, Philadelphia, Pa.
American Medical Women's Association Collection
Miscellaneous Papers
Woman's Medical College of Pennsylvania Collection

Index

Abolitionist movement, 19, 149
Abortion, 72n, 145, 145n–46n
Achievement motivation, 33n, 250 and n
Adams, Abigail, 16, 17
Adams, John, 17
Advocate of Moral Reform, 19
Affirmative action, 268–80 passim
Agassiz, Alexander, 170
Albany Medical College, 243
Alcott, William, 39
Allport, Gordon, 149, 191
American Association of Medical Colleges, 280
American College of Surgeons, 200, 262
American Institute of Homeopathy, 162
American Medical Association (AMA), xv, 110, 134, 139, 190, 229; membership of women, 154–55, 155n, 213, 217; publications, 202, 203, 224
American Medical Association Council on Medical Education, 219
American Medical Education Society, 50
American Medical Women's Association (AMWA): membership, 216–18, 264–65; and World War I, 218–19; and internships, 219, 221, 223; and World War II, 226–30
American Medical Women's Association, New England branch, 270 and n, 271–72

American Physiological Society, 40
American Sociological Association, x, 252
American Urological Association, 114n
Ames, Mrs. Oakes, 267
Amherst College, 131
Anthony, Susan B., 34n, 107
Antifeminism, 119, 190, 200–01, 203, 204n; of nineteenth-century male physicians, xii, xv, 106, 108–09. *See also* Feminism
Apprenticeship: of Hunts, xiv, 1, 20, 23–24; before *1835*, 6, 12, 13, 14
Archives of Ophthalmology and Otology, 90
Armstrong, Professor, 187–88
Army and Navy Medical Corps, 230
Associated Collegiate Alumnae, 131
Association for the Advancement of Women, 169, 179
Association of American Medical Colleges, 243, 270
Attrition. *See* Dropout rate

Baker, Josephine, 264
Baldwin, F. A. M., 43
Barbier, Emile, 140
Barringer, Emily, 229–30
Bass, Mary, 7
Batchelder, Mrs., 220n
Beecher, Catherine, 107
Bellevue Hospital, 101
Bennett, Alice, 161
Berkshire Medical College, 13n, 49
Berlin (Berlinerblau), Fanny, 91

Berman, Edgar, 272–73
Bigelow, Jacob, 119
Blacks in medicine: students, 31–32, 31n, 32n; physicians, 61, 61n–62n, 192, 194 and n, 218; medical schools, 192
Blackwell, Elizabeth, 1, 34; medical training, 27, 28, 30; unhappiness, 33, 82; and Zakrzewska, 57, 79–80, 80–81; later life, 76 and n; and New York Infirmary, 81–82, 169, 179
Blackwell, Emily, 115, 174, 179–80; unhappiness, 33, 82; later life, 76 and n; medical training, 79, 81; and New York Infirmary, 82, 169, 263
Boivin, Madame le Docteur, 28
Boston City Directory, 46–48, 47n–49n, 49, 104, 107
Boston City Hospital, 143; and women interns, 72 and n, 197–98, 220 and n, 223 and n, 269; services, 92, 96n, 113
Boston Dispensary, 266
Boston Female Medical College (later New England Female Medical College): founding, xiv, 30, 31, 35, 44; trained midwives, 47, 48n; early years, 49, 51, 51n–52n, 52; directors, 50, 51n, 53; finances, 50–55; and male prejudice against, 53 and n; merger, 53–54, 53n; graduates, 55
—students, 49; statistics on, 49. See also New England Female Medical College
Boston fire of 1872, 70
Boston Gynecological Society, 140
Boston Lying-In Hospital, 279; closed, 57 and n, 86, 92, 94; interns, 223
Boston Medical and Surgical Journal: on Blackwell, 28; on physio-

logical institute, 43; on merger of New England Female, 75; refused article by woman, 90; against women physicians, 109, 133, 135, 142, 172–73, 198; Storer's letter, 110, 117; Clarke's article, 120; Dimock's letter, 132; overcrowding, 134; editors of, 140, 162
Boston Medical Association, 46
Boston Medical Society, 53n
Boston Physiological Society, 40
Boston University Medical School, 69, 214–15, 266; coeducational, xvi, 98, 182, 195; merger with New England Female, 70–71, 75, 195; homeopathic curriculum, 71, 98, 104, 182, 195–97, 198; and women students, 187, 195–99, 242
—students, statistics on, 196, 198; women, 182, 199, 230–31, 236, 248–49, 249n
Botanism, 23n. See also Sectarian medicine
Bowditch, Henry I.: and New England Hospital, 85, 86, 93, 94n, 117, 149, 157; and Massachusetts Medical Society, 148–50, 151, 157, 161; biographical sketch, 149
Bowdoin College, 131
Bowdoin Medical College, 49
Boylston Medical Prize, 130
Boylston Medical School, 45, 52
Boys in White, x
Breed, Mary, 89
Briggs, Le Baron Russell, 209
British Medical Corps, 228
Bronson, C. P., 42
Brown, Francis, 150
Brown, Madelaine Ray, 223
Brown, Sara E., 90–91
Brown University, 49
Bryn Mawr College, 124, 175, 190
Butler, Benjamin, 176

Cabot, J. Elliott, 170
Cabot, Samuel, 100n; and New
  England Hospital, 85, 86, 93, 94n,
  117, 149, 157; and Massachusetts
  Medical Society, 117, 148–49, 156,
  157, 161
Calhoun, Arthur, 190
Call, Emma, 132, 162; and Massa-
  chusetts Medical Society, 162,
  213; and Harvard, 174, 208
Carnegie Commission, 252
Carnegie Foundation, 239
Carney Hospital (Boston), 114
Catt, Carrie Chapman, 229
Celler, Emanuel, 229
Chadwick, James: and New En-
  gland Hospital, 117, 149; and Mas-
  sachusetts Medical Society, 148–
  49, 159, 161; and Harvard, 174
Channing, Walter: and female
  midwives, 8–9, 9n; and women at
  Harvard, 27; Gregory and, 39;
  and puerperal disease, 93, 94n;
  and New England Hospital, 117
Charité Hospital (Berlin), 77, 93
Charlestown Ladies' Physiological
  Society, 42n–43n
Cheney, Ednah, 33, 88, 262
Chickering, Jesse, 126n
Children's Bureau, 264
Christian Scientists, 104. See also
  Sectarian medicine
Clairvoyants, 47, 48, 80. See also
  Sectarian medicine
Clark, Nancy Talbot, 195; and
  Massachusetts Medical Society,
  xv, 46n, 151–52, 152n, 153; med-
  ical training, 151, 202
Clarke, Edward H., 123, 151, 187,
  232; and Harvard, xv, 70n, 119,
  123, 124n, 167; and New England
  Hospital, 117, 120, 127–28; on
  women in medicine, 120–25 pas-
  sim, 133

—Sex in Education, xv, 124–27,
  124n; books responding to, 128,
  130; critics of, 128–32
Clarke, James Freeman, 64n
Clarke, Mrs. James Freeman, 33n
Cleveland Medical College, 79
Codes (of medical societies), 12,
  23n
Coeducation: opponents of, xv, 125,
  127, 171, 177, 201; effect and re-
  sistance, 187–90
Colby Junior College, 266
College of Physicians and Surgeons
  (Mass.), 182
—students, women, 203; statistics
  on, 193, 203
Collegiate Alumnae Association, 190
  and n
Columbia (College of Physicians
  and Surgeons, N.Y.), 209
Consultation, 12, 90, 150, 155, 158,
  161
Contract surgeons: in World War
  I, 218–19, 227; in World War II,
  227–28
Cooper Medical College (Calif.),
—students, women: statistics on,
  193
Cornell, William, 49, 53
Cornell University, 102, 169, 248
Cornell University Medical School,
  255, 263
Cotting, Benjamin, 85, 86
Council Bluffs Medical College
—students, women: statistics on,
  193
Councilman, William T., 177
Council on Medical Education
  (AMA), 219
Cowles, Edward, 142–43

Dall, Caroline, 107, 118, 168n, 216
Delany, Martin, 31, 32n
Denver Medical College

—students, women: statistics on, 193

Derby, Hasket, 167

Dimock, Susan, 100n, 132, 156; biographical sketch, 100; as a surgeon, 100 and n, 156; and Harvard, 100, 166–68; medical training, 100–01, 156, 166, 167; and Massachusetts Medical Society, 152n, 156–57; at New England Hospital, 156; death, 157

Doctress: and female practitioners, 4, 10n–11n, 11; and Gregory, 63, 68

Dorchester Medical Society, 135, 154

Dropout rate

—of medical students, 251–52, 255–56, 255n, 256n, 272; statistics on, 74n, 254, 254n–55n

—of physicians, 275; statistics on, 183, 252–53, 253n–54n, 254

Drury, Gardner, 64n

Duberman, Martin, 148

Duffey, E. B., 128, 129

Dykman and Stalneker, 245–46

Eclectics, xiii, 154, 241. See also Sectarian medicine

Ecole de Medicine, 99, 169

Eddes, Robert, 154

Education, 131

Electricians, 104. See also Sectarian medicine

Electropaths, 47, 48. See also Sectarian medicine

Eliot, Charles: reforms of medical school, 69, 164, 168, 171; and admission of women, 170, 172–73, 174, 175–76

Eliot, Martha, 222

Emory University Medical College, 243

Everett, Edward, 27

Ewell, Thomas, 38

Fabyan, George, 64n

Facts and Important Information for Young Men . . . , 37

Fees: for midwives, 7, 8 and n; for schoolteachers, 21 and n; for physicians, 139 and n, 183–84, 258 and n

Female Medical College of Pennsylvania (later Women's Medical College of Pennsylvania), 62, 72n, 78, 79; and Hunt, 32, 47n; merger with Boston Female, 53–54, 53n; graduates, 99, 165. See also Woman's Medical College of Pennsylvania

Female Medical Education Society, 50–56 passim. See also Boston Female Medical College

Feminism, xv, 84; and women physicians, xvi, 260–67, 270, 276–83; defined, xvii; nineteenth-century reform movement, 19–20, 44, 118; and New England Hospital, 76, 88–91, 103; and Zakrzewska, 79–80, 88–89; and antifeminism, 106, 107–08, 107n; and professionalism, 148, 214–15; and Harvard, 168 and n. See also Antifeminism

Fitz, Reginald, 117

Flexner, Abraham, 239

Flexner report, 237, 239–40

Fores, S. W., Man-Midwifery Dissected, 37–38, 38n

Fowler, Lydia Folger, 1

Free Hospital for Women (Boston), 90

Freidson, Eliot, 252–53; Profession of Medicine, x

Friendship, female, 29n, 80, 88, 89

Garrett, Mary Elizabeth, 176–77

Garrison, William Lloyd, 118

Gassett, Helen M., 50–51, 65n

Geneva Medical College, 1, 27, 28

Gibbons, Cardinal, 178
Gibbons, Dr., 155
Ginzberg, Eli (Men, Money, and Medicine), 253
Goddard, Lucy, 88
Gorgas, W. C., 226
Goulding, Anna, 49n, 59n, 67 and n
Gove, Mary S. (later Mary Gove Nichols), 41
Graham, Sylvester, 39; Lecture to Young Men on Chastity, 37n
Graham Journal, 41
Green, Charles M., 201
Gregory, George, Medical Morals, 39, 40, 41
Gregory, Samuel, 82, 85, 98, 109, 152; founded Boston Female, xiv, 31, 35, 37, 44; and role of women, xiv, 36, 50–51, 51n–52n, 57–59, 58n, 67 and n, 74–75, 76; education, 36; Facts and Important Information for Young Men . . . , 37; Licentiousness, Its Causes and Effects, 37; and male midwifery, 37, 38–39, 73, 116; Man-Midwifery Exposed . . . , 39; honorary degree, 45, 73; and certification and degrees, 47, 49, 63, 68; and finances of Boston Female, 50–55, 51n; and merger of Boston Female, 53–54; and male prejudice, 53n, 72n, 135; arguments for women's medical colleges, 55–56; and lady managers, 57–58, 58n, 64 and n, 74, 86, 96; and Zakrzewska, 58–59, 64, 74, 83, 86; and graduates, 59n, 60, 60n–62n, 63; and trustees, 64; and finances of New England Female, 66–68; and investigation, 67–68; death, 68; failure, 73–75, 117–18
Gregory Society, 196–97
Grimke, Angelina and Sarah, 29 and n
Gross Medical College (Colo.)

—students, women: statistics on, 193
Gynecological Society of Boston, 109, 116
Gynecological surgery: Storer, 110, 113–15; Sims, 115–16, 115n, 144

Hahnemann, Samuel, 195
Hahnemann Society, 196–97, 197n
Hale, Edward Everett, 69–70
Hall, Beatrice, 214
Hall, G. Stanley, 203
Hamilton, Alice, 204, 211–12, 260
Hamilton, Frederick W., 200–01
Handlin, Oscar, 144
Harvard Board of Overseers, 176; Clarke a member, xv, 119, 123; and proposed merger with New England Female, 69, 70; and women's endowments, 170–75 passim
Harvard Corporation, 175, 176; and Hunt, 27 and n, 28–29, 30–31; and Sewell and Tyng, 165; and admission of women 1944, 232–33
Harvard Medical School, 15, 44, 45, 85, 270; professors at, 8, 109, 112–13, 119, 149, 201, 211–12; licensing, 13; Ware's speech to, 32n, 74 and n; Clarke's speech to, 120–22; competition about menstruation, 130; against new medical schools, 134n; curriculum reforms, 164
—admission of women, xiv, xv, 105, 106, 123, 127, 147, 148, 160, 181, 187, 207–08; Hunt's applications, xiv, xv, 20, 26–32, 27n, 35, 108, 151, 153, 164–65, 166; effect of World War II, xiv, 231–33, 242; proposed merger with New England Female, 69–70, 168; Dimock and Jex-Blake's applications, 100–01, 166–68; arguments for admission, 164; Sewell and Tyng's ap-

Harvard Medical School (*continued*)
plication, 165–66; efforts to buy
admission, 168–76; *1905* petition,
208; effect of World War I, 209–
11; and Hamilton, 211–12; policies in *1930s*, 231; first woman
dean, 280–81
—students: internships, 219; women,
statistics on, 233
Harvard University, 131, 208
Hawkins, Jane, 5
HealthRight, 277
Heinzen, Karl, 122n
Hewkin, Elizabeth H., 235
Higginson, Thomas Wentworth, 128
Holmes, Oliver Wendell: and Hunt,
28, 30, 31; on puerperal disease,
92–93; and Massachusetts Gen-
eral Hospital, 101; and Dimock
and Jex-Blake, 166
Home economics movement, 189–90
Homeopathic Medical College for
Women (Cleveland), 180
Homeopathy, xiii, 47, 48; and Bos-
ton University, 71, 104; and Za-
krzewska, 83–84, 104; *New En-
gland Medical Gazette,* 118; and
Massachusetts Medical Society,
154, 162; decline, 195–96, 241. *See
also* Sectarian medicine
Horner, Matina, 250
Hovey, Marion, 169
Hovey fund, 169–72, 176
Howard University, 98
Howe, Julia Ward, 129
Howell, Mary, 280–81
Hunt, Harriot K., 46, 79, 89, 281;
applications to Harvard, xiv, xv,
20, 26–32, 27n, 34, 35, 108, 151,
153, 164, 165, 166; apprenticeship, xiv, 1, 20, 23–24; first woman
physician, xiv, 5, 20, 181; began
practice, 1, 2, 24–25; and sectarian
medicine, 1, 25, 26 and n; early

years, 20; schoolteacher, 20–22;
decision to enter medicine, 22–
23; and regular medicine, 25; and
woman's rights movement, 25n,
29–30; and Grimke sisters, 29 and
n; honorary degree, 32, 47n; silver wedding anniversary, 33–34;
and New York Infirmary, 33n,
82; last years, 34; and physiological societies, 42n–43n; and Zakrzewska, 82–83
Hunt, Sarah: began practice, 1, 2,
24–25; apprenticeship, 1, 23–24;
birth, 20; illness, 22, 23; left
medicine, 26
Hurd-Mead, Kate, 103, 217
Hutchings, Martha E., 167n
Hutchinson, Anne, 16
Hydropaths, xiii. *See also* Sectarian
medicine
Hysteria, 19n, 203

Illinois State Medical Society, 155
Income. *See* Fees
Independent Woman, 274
Indian doctresses, 47, 48. *See also*
Sectarian medicine
Ingegno, Alfred, 252
International   Ladies   Garment
Workers Union, 229
*Interns: From Students to Physi-
cians,* 259
Internships, xviii, 207; at New
England Hospital, xiv, 60, 97–99,
102–03, 104, 123; at New York In-
firmary, 83; at Massachusetts
General Hospital, 147; in nine-
teenth century, 219–21; and
World War I, 221–22, 223n; and
World War II, 233–35; and
women's aspirations, 259; and af-
firmative action, 271
—statistics on: 83n, 219–22, 224 and
n, 233–34, 269

Irregular medicine, 22; and women, xiii, 83–84, 182; and Hunt, 1; in nineteenth century, 15; and medical societies, 207; decline, 241. *See also* Sectarian medicine

Jackson, Mercy Bisbee, 59n, 63
Jackson College, 201
Jacobi, Mary Putnam: opinions on issues, 59–60, 112, 116 and n, 178, 200, 249, 251, 265, 276; medical training, 60, 99 and n; biographical sketch, 99 and n; "Mental Action and Physical Health," 130; study refuting Clarke, 130–31; and Dimock, 156; and women's endowment, 169, 173, 174; in woman's movement, 215n
Janeway, Margaret, 227
Jarvis, Edward, 117
Jensen, Richard, xii
Jews in medicine, 192, 194, 221–22
Jex-Blake, Sophia: and women's medical education in Britain, 100, 101–02; medical training, 100–01, 166, 167; applications to Harvard, 100–01, 166–68; biographical sketch, 100–02
Johns Hopkins Medical School: and admission of women, 176–77, 178, 179, 206, 207; effects of admitting women, 181, 187, 279
—students, 177n, 222, 251–52; statistics on, 193, 205; internships, 219
Jones, Howard W., 282
Jones, Jane Gaudette, 255–56, 256n
Jones, Margaret, 5
Journal of Medical Education, 236, 275
Journal of the American Medical Association, 134, 143 and n

Journal of the American Medical Women's Association, 234, 257
Journal of the Gynecological Society of Boston, 110n, 114n
Joy, Nabby, 87

Kansas Medical College
—students, women: statistics on, 182, 193
Kansas medical society, 155–56
Kaplan, H. S., 257
Kenyon, Dorothy, 229
Kessler, Richard, 270–71
Kimball, Helen F., 88
King, Dexter Stillman, 51n

La Chapelle, Madame, 77
Ladies Catholic Charities of New York, 229
Ladies Medical Academy, 59n, 61n
Ladies' Medical Oracle, 22
Ladies Physiological Institute of Boston, 42–43
Laing, Daniel, 31
Laura Memorial Woman's Medical College (Cincinnati), 180
Lawyers, women, 108 and n
Lecture to Young Men on Chastity, 37n
Lee, Rebecca, 61, 61n–62n
Lewis, Dio, 45
Lewis, Winslow, 52 and n, 54
Licensing: effect on women physicians, xvii, 3, 15, 237–39; before *1835,* 10, 11–12, 11n–12n; at Harvard, 13; in later nineteenth century, 45, 150–54 passim; and internships, 219–22; statistics on exams, 238–39
Licentiousness, Its Causes and Effects, 37
London School of Medicine for Women, 102
Longshore, Hannah, 53

Lowell, A. Lawrence, 211, 212
Lowell, Josephine, 178
Lowenstein, Leah, 270n
Loyola Medical School, 243
Lyman, George, 163

Mackensie, Colin, 6
McCormick, Mrs. Stanley, 267
Magnetists, 104. See also Sectarian
    medicine
Mandigo, Pauline, 229
Manliness, cult of: books on, 144
Man-Midwifery Dissected, 38
Man-Midwifery Exposed, 39
Marlowe, Leigh, xvii
Marsh, Bela, 50
Marvel, L. H., 131
Massachusetts Bureau of Labor Sta-
    tistics, 131
Massachusetts General Hospital,
    149; services, 92, 96n, 113
—internships: for Harvard, 147,
    164; women's efforts for, 100-01,
    153, 167, 168, 220, 221-22, 234;
    statistics on women in, 222, 234
    and n; in surgery for women,
    234, 269
Massachusetts Institute of Technol-
    ogy, 189, 191n
Massachusetts legislature: and Mas-
    sachusetts Medical Society, 11;
    and Female Education Society,
    50; scholarships for women, 55;
    and New England Female, 56,
    67-68, 72n; and New England
    Hospital, 86
Massachusetts Licensing Act of 1895,
    237-38
Massachusetts Medical Society, 23n,
    42, 141-42; and licensing, 11, 13,
    154; and Storer, 114n; exams,
    152 and n; and Massachusetts
    General Hospital, 153, 168; and
    Harvard, 170, 171-72; and ho-

meopaths, 195; and Woman's
    State Medical Society, 215-16
—admission of women, xiv, xv, 15,
    104, 105, 106, 133, 147, 148, 164;
    Clark's application, xv, 46 and
    n, 151-52, 152n; Zakrzewska's ap-
    plication, 86, 152 and n; advan-
    tages of membership, 150, 151;
    Dimock's application, 152n, 156-
    57; arguments for admission, 153-
    54; Middlesex resolution, 157-58;
    1882 meeting, 159-60; 1883 meet-
    ing, 161; first woman member,
    161-62, 213, 273; opinions on
    admission, 162-63
—members, 13n, 49, 117, 149, 208,
    263; honorary memberships, 152n;
    statistics on women, 213
M.D. degree, 45, 46-48, 47n-49n,
    74n, 102
Medical College of Chicago. See
    Woman's Hospital Medical Col-
    lege
Medical Department, University of
    Colorado
—students, women: statistics on,
    193
Medical Economics, 252
Medical Morals, 39, 40, 41
Medical Register of Boston, 91
Medical Reserve Corps, 226-27
Medical School Admission Require-
    ments, 243
Medical schools, 15; curriculum,
    xv, 44, 66, 164; development of,
    3, 12-14, 23n, 44; statistics on,
    14, 192, 240; numbers of, 44-45,
    69, 182, 225; effect of World War
    II, 228, 230-33; effect of affirma-
    tive action, 280
—black: statistics on, 192
—coeducational: in Boston, xvi,
    98, 182, 187, 195-202 passim;
    started as, 54, 177; increase and

decline, 191, 192, 193, 199, 205–06, 207; effect of World War II, 228, 230–31; statistics on, 240, 244
—homeopathic, 206; Boston University, 182, 195–97, 198, 242; statistics on, 198
—irregular, 1, 71, 98, 104
—regular: benefits of, 1–2, 207; statistics on, 182, 183, 193, 241
—women's medical colleges: first, xiv, 35; male physicians against, 59n, 71–72, 72n; statistics on, 179, 180, 182, 240, 262; decline and disappearance, 191, 192, 206, 262–63; and licensing exams, 238; recent proposal for, 278–79
Medical societies, 15; and women, xv, 104, 151, 155–56, 207, 213–14, 215, 229, 263–65; development, 3, 10, 12; statistics on, 14, 159; and classification of physicians, 45–46; special interest, 213–14. See also Licensing; Massachusetts Medical Society
Medical Students: statistics on 14; social class, 62n; dropout rate, 74n, 254, 254n–55n, 255–56, 256n, 272
—black, 31–42, 31n, 32n, 194n
—Jewish, 192, 194
—women: numbers, ix, x, xvi; quota system, xviii, 224–25, 228, 242–44, 245, 252, 271; and male prejudice, 97, 98, 120; effect of affirmative action, 268, 271, 273, 275–76; effect of feminism, 276–77
—women, statistics on: percent of total, xvi, 183, 230, 236, 245, 268, 269, 270; percent of increase, xviii, 268, 269; numbers, 181, 240; percent at various schools, 182, 193, 244; percent at types of schools, 191, 241, 262; applicants, 225, 242, 248

Medical Woman's Journal, 233
Medicine before 1835, women in, 2–15
Meigs, Charles, 111
Men, Money, and Medicine, 253
Mendenhall, Dorothy, 177n, 191n
Menstruation as argument against women physicians: Storer's, xv, 110–11, 118, 155; Clarke's, xv, 125–26, 127 and n, 128–32; Hall's, 203; Berman's, 272–73
"Mental Action and Physical Health," 130
Michigan medical society, 155–56
Middlesex resolution, 157–58
Midwifery: female, 2–10 passim; as a field, 5–9, 9n; male, 6–8, 37–39; classification, 47, 48; at Boston and New England Female, 47, 49, 61n
Mills, C. Wright, xviii
Minor, William Thomas, 64n
Minot, Francis, 117
Moore, Francis, 270
Mosher, Elizabeth, 102, 122
Mott, Elizabeth: Ladies' Medical Oracle, 22, 24; and Hunts, 22–24, 25
Mott, Lucretia, 19
Mott, Richard D.: and Hunts, 22, 23–24
Mt. Holyoke Female Seminary, 55, 60, 131
Mumford, Emily: Interns: From Students to Physicians, 259

Nadelson, Carol, 270n
National Institute of Health, 282
National Normal University (Ohio)
—students, women: statistics on, 193
National University (D.C.)
—students, women: statistics on, 193

National Woman Suffrage Association, 215

National Women's Medical Association, 216

National Women's Party, 229

New England Female Medical College (formerly Boston Female Medical College), 85, 86, 180; chartered, $47n$–$49n$, 56, $72n$; first use of name, 52; and Zakrzewska, 64–66, $65n$, 82–83, 98; finances, 66–69; investigation, 67–68; proposed merger with Harvard, 69–70, 168; merger with Boston University, 70–71; 75, 195; male physicians against, 71–72, $72n$, 109; failure, 71–75, 76. *See also* Boston Female Medical College

—graduates, 59–61, $59n$–$62n$, 165, 220; statistics on, $60n$

—hospital: plans for, 52; lady managers' role, 56; opened, 57 and n; and Gregory, 64, 73; closed, 66 and n

—lady managers, $36n$–$37n$, 88; formation, 56–57; and Gregory, 57–58, $58n$, 64 and n, 66, 74, 86; and New England Hospital, 84, 96

—students, 62–63, $62n$, 68, 72 and n; statistics on, $62n$, $74n$

—trustees: formation, 56; and lady managers, 57, 58; and Gregory, 63–64, $64n$; and Zakrzewska, 64–66; and investigation, 66–68; fundraising, 68; and mergers, 69, 70, 71

New England Hospital for Women and Children, $66n$, $122n$, $146n$; founding, xiv, 65, 66, 76, 84; and feminism, xiv, 85, 88–91, 103, 104–05, 262; students, 60, $98n$, 99–102, $99n$, 122, 123, 166; support from men, 84–86, 149, 157; finances, 86–88; success, 87 and n, 96–97, 117; services, 91–97; male opposition, 109, 127; and Storer, 109–17 passim; staff, 132, 156, 162, 163, 165, 208; decline and close, 265–67; current model, 278

—internships: objectives, 97, 220, 221; statistics on, 98 and n, 223; program, 98–99, 102–03; and irregulars, 104; at Massachusetts General Hospital, 153; effects of World War I, 222

New England Hospital Medical Society, 104, 105, 174, 216. *See also* New England Women's Medical Society

New England Journal of Medicine, 256

New England Medical Gazette, 118

New England Woman Suffrage Association, 88

New England Women's Club, 88, 89, 123

New England Women's Medical Society, 216, 264. *See also* New England Hospital Medical Society

New York College of Pharmacy, 99

New York Female Moral Reform Society, 19, 20

New York Free Medical College for Women, 180

New York Hospital for Women, 115–16

New York Infirmary for Women and Children, 130; fundraising for, $33n$, 82, 85, 169; founding, 82; internships, 83, 221; graduates, statistics on, 179; closed, 179, 262–63

New York Woman's Medical College, 180, 206

Nichols, Mary Gove. *See,* Gove, Mary S.

Norris, Frances, 242, 281
Northwestern University Medical School, 61, 204, 205, 270
Northwestern University Woman's Medical College (formerly Woman's Hospital Medical College), 180, 204–05
Notable American Women, 261
Nursing: women predominate, x; male physicians' attitude toward, 142–43, 143n; at New England Hospital, 156; effect on women physicians, 246; statistics on, 246

O'Hara, Dwight, 252
"Old boy" network, xviii, 213, 258
Oliver, Edward, 140–41
Oliver, Susan, 140–41
Ordway, Mabel, 223n
Osler, William, 177
Overcrowding (in medical profession), 134 and n, 194

Parrish, John, 248
Part-time training, 257–58, 258n, 273–74
Pendleton, Ellen, 211
Penn Medical College, 45, 54
Pennsylvania Hospital, 97, 120
Pennsylvania Medical Society, 72, 161
Peter Bent Brigham Hospital: women interns, 222, 269, 270
Phelps, Charles, 236
Philadelphia County Medical Society, 72, 120
Phrenologists, 104, *See also* Sectarian medicine
Physicians: statistics on, 14, 134n; nineteenth-century social stratification, 81n; dropout rate, 254
—black, 61, 61n–62n, 192, 194 and n, 218
—Jewish, 194

—women: ignored by scholars, x–xii; male opposition to, xii, 90–91, 116, 132–46, 133n–34n, 139n; and medical societies, xiv, 148, 150, 153–54, 207, 213–14, 215–18, 263–65; numbers, xvii, xviii, 219, 241; and institutional power, xvii, xviii, 279–81; effect of professionalization, xvii, 3, 10–15, 237–39; and sectarian medicine, 26n; problems of classification, 46–48, 47n–49n, 91, 104; and abortion, 72n, 145, 145n–46n; and feminism, 89–91, 276–83; novels about, 180–81; in Boston *1890's*, 182–83; dropout rate, statistics on, 183, 252–53, 253n–54n, 254, 275; income, 183–84, 258 and n; and marriage, 184, 251–58, 251n, 274–75; and suffrage movement, 214–15, 215n, 262n; and World War I, 218–19, 226, 227; and World War II, 225–30; explanations of twentieth-century decline, 244–67
—women, statistics on: in United States, ix, xvi, 181, 185, 186, 194, 270–71; in Boston, xvi, 5, 107–08, 181–82, 185, 186, 191, 216, 238; marriage, 184, 251
Physiological movement, 39–44
Physiological societies, 40; female, 42–44, 42n–43n, 80, 277–78
Physiomedicals, 241. *See also* Sectarian medicine
Pope, C. Augusta, 132, 208
Pope, Emily, 132, 208
Population problems, 126 and n
Preceptorships, 23n, 73, 74n
Presbyterian Hospital and Woman's Medical College (Cincinnati), 180
Preston, Ann, 62
Professionalization in medicine: effect on women physicians, xvii,

Professionalization (*continued*)
3, 10–15, 237–39. *See also* Licensing; Medical schools; Medical societies
Profession of Medicine, x
Public health, 259–60
Puerperal disease, 57n, 92–95
Pusey, Nathan, 212
Putnam, C. P., 93, 94n

Quota system: on women, xviii, 194, 211, 224–25, 228, 242–44, 245, 252, 271; on Jews, 192, 194

Radcliffe College, 208, 209, 210
Ramey, Estelle, 249
Regular medicine, 15; and women, xiii, 182, 241; irregulars' views on, 22, 25, 195; and Zakrzewska, 83–84, 104; and Massachusetts Medical Society, 150, 154
Residency. *See* Part-time training
Restelle, Madame, 63
Rhode Island medical society, 155–56
Richards, Ellen, 189
Ripley, Martha, 197–98
Rogers, Edith Norse, 229
Rolfe, Enoch C., 47, 49, 50; disagreements, 49, 51n, 53, 72n; on Gregory, 64n; and investigation, 67 and n
Roosevelt, Eleanor, 229
Roosevelt, Franklin D., 226, 230
Rothstein, William G., 81
Rudolph, Frederick, 189
Russell, LeBaron, 170, 171–72

Sabin, Florence, 279
St. Elizabeth's Hospital (Boston), 114
St. Louis Woman's Medical College, 180
Salisbury, Sarah W., 220

Sanford, Amanda, 123
Sanger, George Partridge, 64n
Schmidt, Joseph, 77–78
Sears, Willard, 51n
Sectarian medicine: in nineteenth century xiii; and Hunt, 25, 26 and n; sects, 47, 48; and Massachusetts Medical Society, 104, 150. *See also* Irregular medicine
Seneca Falls convention, 19–20, 44
Severance, Caroline, 79–80, 82
Sewell, Lucy: letters from Zakrzewska, 85, 132; at New England Hospital, 87, 95, 100, 102, 112, 165; medical training, 89, 165; application to Harvard, 165–66
Sewell, Samuel: and Boston Female, 51n, 64–66, 65n, 68; and New England Female, 70n, 71
Sex in Education: Clarke's book, xv, 124–27; books responding to, 128, 130; critics of, 128–32
Sexual hygiene, 37n
Shattuck, George Brune, 162, 163
Shattuck, George Cheyne, 160, 165, 166
Shaw, Anna Howard, 214–15
Shaw, Mrs. Robert G., 87
Shipley, Simon G., 51n
Shippen, William, 6, 7
Simmons College, 210
Sims, J. Marion, 115–16, 115n, 144
Sinclair, Andrew, 240–41
Smellie, William, 7
Smith College, 191, 192
Snowden, Isaac, 31
Sparkman, John, 229
Sparkman-Johnson Bill, 230
Special Subcommittee on Education, Discrimination Against Women, 244
Spiritualist, 80. *See also* Sectarian medicine
Stanton, Elizabeth Cady, 19, 34n

State Normal School (Mass.), 60
Statistics. *See* Internships; Medical
   schools; Medical students; Phy-
   sicians, women
Status of women before *1835*, 10,
   10*n*–11*n*, 15–16, 17–20
Stedman, Charles Ellery, 135–36,
   137, 138
Stephenson, John H., 94*n*
Stevenson, Sarah Hackett, 155 and *n*
Stillé, Alfred, 154–55
Stimson, Barbara, 228
Stone, Lucy, 89
Storer, David Humphreys, 109
Storer, Horatio, 120, 272; attack on
   women physicians, xv, 109–11,
   117, 118, 121, 133, 155; at New
   England Hospital, 84–85, 94*n*,
   109–16 passim, 165; at Harvard,
   109, 112–13; and Gynecological
   Society of Boston, 109, 116; and
   American Medical Association,
   110; and gynecological surgery,
   110, 113–15, 114*n*; infection and
   retirement, 119 and *n*; on nymphomania, 144–45; on abortion,
   145 and *n*
Storer, Malcolm, 113
Sturtevant, Georgia, 101
Suffolk District Medical Society, 46
Suffrage movement, 214–15, 215*n*,
   262*n*. *See also* Woman's rights
   movement
Syracuse University
—students, women: statistics on,
   193

Talbot, Israel, 195, 196
Tallant, Alice Weld, 263
Taylor, William R., 141
Thaxter, Adam Wallace, Jr., 64*n*
Thomas, M. Carey, 124, 126, 175,
   178, 190, 201
Thompson, Mary Harris, 61

Thomsonianism, 22, 24
Toledo Medical College
—students, women: statistics on,
   193
Towsley, Matilda, 167*n*
*Transactions of the Woman's Med-
   ical College of Pennsylvania*, 238
Tremont Medical School, 45
"True womanhood," cult of, 9, 18,
   32, 38, 56
Tufts Medical School, 264, 266;
   major coeducational school, xvi,
   182; opened, 134*n*; and admission of women, 187, 199–202, 242,
   252, 270
—students, women: statistics on,
   182, 193, 199, 200–01, 200*n*, 202,
   203*n*, 230–31, 244
Tufts University, 200–01, 202
Twentieth-Century Club, 215
Tyng, Anita, 110, 165–66

University of Arkansas Medical
   School, 228
University of Buffalo Medical
   School
—students, women: statistics on,
   193
University of California Medical
   School
—students, women: statistics on,
   193
University of Michigan Hospital,
   223
University of Michigan Medical
   School
—students, women, 98, 102, 122,
   123; statistics on, 182, 193, 205–
   06, 244
University of Oregon Medical
   School
—students, women: statistics on,
   182, 193

University of Pennsylvania Medical School, 6, 123
University of Southern California Medical School
—students, women: statistics on, 193
University of Zurich Medical School, 100, 156

V-12 program, 230
Van Hoosen, Bertha, 204–05, 213, 218
Vesey, Lawrence, 188
Vietor, Agnes, 265–66

Wakefield, Dr., 159–60
Walker, Minerva, 102
Ward, Mrs. Montgomery, 205
War Department, 227, 228, 229
Ware, John, 32n, 74 and n, 135
Weiskotten, Herman, 225
Welch, Lilian, 261
Wellesley College, 191, 192, 210, 211, 212
Wellington, W. W., 156–57
Western Reserve Medical School, 151, 201–02
West Philadelphia Hospital for Women, 221
Wisconsin Medical School, 273
Woman Citizen, 215n
Woman Physician, 248
Woman's Hospital and Foundling Home (Detroit), 221
Woman's Hospital Medical College (later Northwestern University Woman's Medical College), 61, 180, 204
—students: statistics on, 204
Woman's Hospital of Philadelphia, 221
Woman's Journal, 89–91, 127, 143, 215

Woman's Medical College (Baltimore), 180
Woman's Medical College (Cincinnati), 180
Woman's Medical College (Kansas City), 180
Woman's Medical College (St. Louis), 180
Woman's Medical College (St. Louis, homeopathic), 180
Woman's Medical College of Georgia and Training School for Nurses, 180
Woman's Medical College of Pennsylvania (formerly Female Medical College of Pennsylvania), 72n, 174, 180; last women's medical college, 73, 179 and n, 206, 262; students, 98, 102, 123; in twentieth century, 219, 226, 263, 279. See also Female Medical College of Pennsylvania
Woman's Medical College of the New York Infirmary for Women and Children, 180. See also New York Infirmary
Woman's rights movement, 140; and women physicians, xvi, 261; and Hunt, 1, 25n, 29–30; Seneca Falls convention, 19–20; and physiological movement, 42, 43; and suffrage, 44; Zakrzewska and, 79; and feminism, 88. See also Feminism
Woman's State Medical Society of Massachusetts, 215–16
Women in medicine before 1835, 2–15
Women's and Children's Home (San Francisco), 221
Women's and Children's Hospital (Chicago), 221
Women's Army Auxiliary Corps (WAACS), 227–28, 229

Women's Bureau, 242
Women's Equity Action League (WEAL), 268
Women's liberation movement, 270, 276–79. *See also* Feminism
Women's Medical Journal, 216, 273, 279
Woody, Thomas, 188, 189
Woolf, Virginia, xviii–xix
World War I, 207; and women medical students, 209–11; and women physicians, 218–19, 226, 227; and internships for women, 221–22, 223n
World War II, 207; and women physicians, 225–30; and medical schools, 228, 230–33; and internships for women, 233–35
Wright, Mary, 222
Wyman, Morrill, 160
Wyman, Morris, 170

Yale Medical School, 209, 243
Yale University, 36, 131

Zakrzewska, Marie, 97, 109; founded New England Hospital, xiv, 65, 76, 84; and New England Female, 36n, 57, and n, 61n, 62, 64–66, 65n, 75, 82–83, 98; and Blackwell, 57, 79–81, 82; and puerperal disease, 57n, 93; and Gregory, 58–59, 64, 74, 83, 86, 152; students, 60, 100; and Samuel Sewell, 64–66, 65n, 68; and merger of Harvard and New England Female, 70 and n, 168; on irregular medicine, 71, 83–84, 98, 104; early life, 76–77; medical training, 77–78, 79–80, 84, 93, 202; emigration, 78–79; and woman's rights movement, 79; feminist support, 79, 80, 88–89; and New York Infirmary, 81–82, 85; ideas about Boston's liberality, 82, 108–09, 152; and male physicians, 85–86, 117, 132; and Massachusetts Medical Society, 86, 149, 152 and n, 163, 273; medical practice, 87–88, 99; and New England Women's Club, 89; and *Woman's Journal*, 89; goals for New England Hospital, 91–92, 97, 103; and hospital's services, 95, 96; tactics for women physicians, 105, 118, 168n, 262; and Storer, 110, 117–18, 120; and Clarke, 120, 127–28; and medical science, 122n; and women's endowment, 173, 174